4TH EDITION

Neeb's Fundamentals *of* Mental Health Nursing

Linda M. Gorman, RN, MN, PMHCNS-BC, FPCN
Clinical Nurse Specialist/Nursing Consultant
Private Practice
Studio City, California

Robynn F. Anwar, MST, MSN, Ed
Nursing Faculty/CNA and Multi-Skilled Coordinator
Camden County College, Camden Campus
Camden, New Jersey

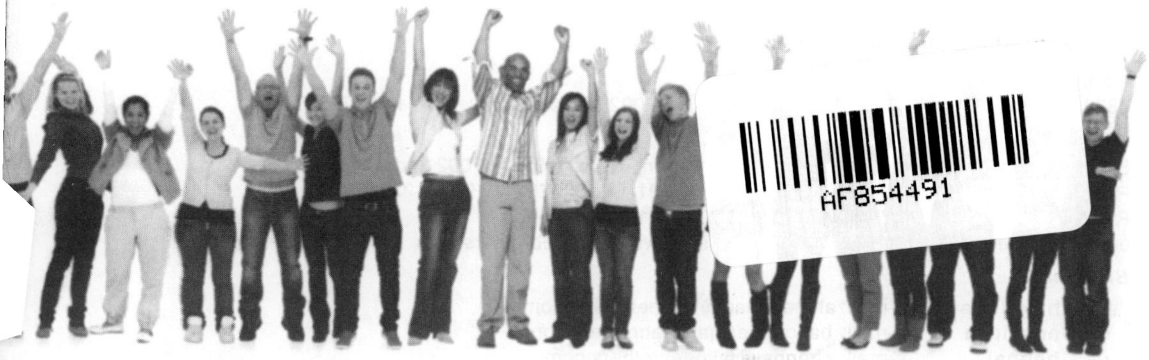

F.A. Davis Company • Philadelphia

JAYPEE The Health Sciences Publisher

FIRST INDIAN EDITION 2015

As new scientific information becomes available through basic and clinical research, recommended treatments and drug therapies undergo changes. The authors and publisher have done everything possible to make this book accurate, up to date, and in accord with accepted standards at the time of publication. The authors, editors, and publisher are not responsible for errors or omissions or for consequences from application of the book, and make no warranty, expressed or implied, in regard to the contents of the book. Any practice described in this book should be applied by the reader in accordance with professional standards of care used in regard to the unique circumstances that may apply in each situation. The reader is advised always to check product information (package inserts) for changes and new information regarding dose and contraindications before administering any drug. Caution is especially urged when using new or infrequently ordered drugs.

Printed in India

Published by

Jaypee Brothers Medical Publishers (P) Ltd

Corporate Office
4838/24, Ansari Road, Daryaganj, **New Delhi** 110 002, India, Phone: +91-11-43574357

Registered Office
B-3, EMCA House, 23/23B Ansari Road, Daryaganj, **New Delhi** 110 002, India
Phones: +91-11-23272143, +91-11-23272703, +91-11-23282021, +91-11-23245672
Rel: +91-11-32558559 Fax: +91-11-23276490, +91-11-23245683
e-mail: jaypee@jaypeebrothers.com Website: www.jaypeebrothers.com

Branches

- **Ahmedabad** e-mail: ahmedabad@jaypeebrother.com
- **Bengaluru** e-mail: bangalore@jaypeebrothers.com
- **Chennai** e-mail: chennai@jaypeebrothers.com
- **Lucknow** e-mail: lucknow@jaypeebrothers.com
- **Hyderabad** e-mail: hyderabad@jaypeebrother.com
- **Kochi** e-mail: kochi@jaypeebrothers.com
- **Kolkata** e-mail: kolkata@jaypeebrothers.com
- **Mumbai** e-mail: mumbai@jaypeebrothers.com
- **Nagpur** e-mail: nagpur@jaypeebrothers.com

ISBN 978-93-5152-796-1

To Corie, who saw me as an author many years ago.
(LG)

To Mayme, I realize how much easier this journey would have been if you were here. Wasim and Andrea, I appreciate your belief in my abilities. "Mom Bessie," who renewed her practical nurse license at age 94. Linda, thank you for being my mentor through this process. Shirley, Toni, and Ted—Thank you.
(RA)

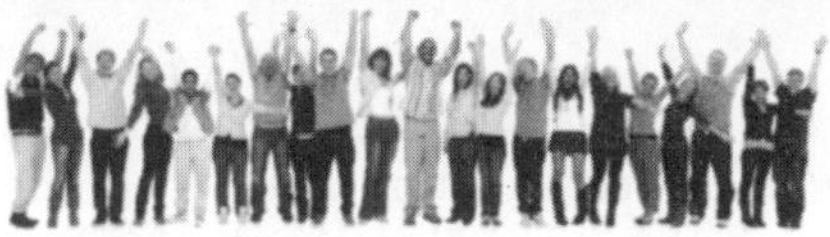

Neeb's Fundamentals of Mental Health Nursing is a psychiatric nursing text tailored specifically to the needs of the LVN/LPN student. We understand that many students at this level of preparation do not have the opportunity for clinical experience in a psychiatric setting, but they will encounter patients with mental health issues in their rotations. Students will encounter patients and their families with psychiatric diagnoses as well as a variety of psychosocial issues and behaviors that challenge them. This text will provide the basic knowledge and skills to address many of these challenges, with an emphasis on communication. This new edition also brings enhancements via the Internet through Davis*Plus*.

Our goal with this text is to provide basic information about mental health theories, personality development, coping and communication styles, psychiatric diagnoses, and nursing actions, all as they pertain to the practice of the LVN/LPN.

The impact of psychiatric disorders continues to be a concern in the United States. Depression, anxiety, eating disorders, and substance abuse continue to be major health problems. How society responds to debilitating mental illness has been the subject of much debate. Clearly the need for nurses to have education in caring for people with mental health issues is essential.

The Fourth Edition of *Neeb's Fundamentals of Mental Health Nursing* brings new authors who have expanded on the foundations that Kathy Neeb created so successfully in the first three editions. The new authors bring broad experience in psychiatric nursing, education, and clinical practice. New chapters in this Fourth Edition include postpartum issues as well as separate chapters on depressive and bipolar disorders. We have added more features to enhance the concepts and make them more meaningful and current.

Chapters 1 to 9 provide the basics of mental health nursing concepts, with an emphasis on communication. Chapters 10 to 22 are "clinical" chapters in that they cover specific diagnoses and/or populations. Many of the chapters include the following new or enhanced key features:

- *Neeb's Tip* will give a "clinical pearl" that succinctly describes a key take-away from the chapter.
- *Critical Thinking Questions* are expanded and interspersed in the chapters to emphasize a concept and challenge the student to apply the concept just covered. Many of these include case-based scenarios.
- *Toolbox* provides additional resources for students who want more information. These can be further explored on the book's Web site.
- *Pharmacology Corner* in Chapters 10 to 20 and 22 covers important current information about medications used for the specific population that will pertain to the LVN/LPN scope of practice.
- *Clinical Activities* are suggestions for the student to utilize when caring for patients with a particular disorder.
- *Classroom Activities* include suggestions for projects or actions that students and faculty can use in the classroom to enhance learning.
- *Case Studies* are in-depth, with questions to help the student apply knowledge learned in the chapter.
- *Multiple Choice Questions*—At least 10 questions are provided at the end of the chapters, with the answers/rationales in Appendix A. Additional NCLEX questions are on the book's Web site.
- Sample Care Plans are provided in the clinical chapters.
- Appendix E, which is new, matches common behaviors with nursing diagnoses.

Internet-based enhancements include podcasts, updated references, and other resources such as drug monographs and Neeb's blog. Neeb's blog will provide an opportunity for the student to reflect on learning and experiences that can be shared with others. For the instructor, this Fourth Edition provides access to PowerPoint presentations, test bank questions, and other expanded features.

This edition coincides with the publication of the *DSM-5, Diagnostic and Statistical Manual for Mental Disorders* by the American Psychiatric Association that was published in 2013. The terminology used throughout this edition reflect the changes in this major psychiatric reference. Although the LVN/LPN student will not be using the *Manual* routinely, a familiarity with the terminology that is used by other health-care professionals is essential. The chapter titles reflect the new terminology where changes have been made.

We, as practitioners and educators in the field of mental health, have seen the impact of mental health issues on our patients and society. We hope that the students who utilize this book will gain a new perspective that includes up-to-date knowledge as well as empathy for the suffering these disorders can cause. We hope this book will contribute to knowledgeable and compassionate LVNs/LPNs.

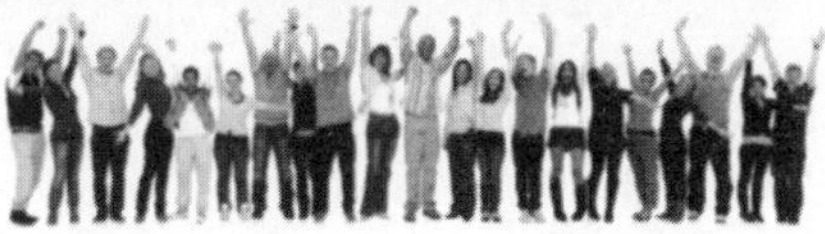

Reviewers

Patti Alford, RN, BSBM
Instructor
Kilgore College
Longview, Texas

Ruth Fee Blackmore, MSN, RN, CNOR
Faculty of Nursing
Isabella Graham Hart School of Practical Nursing
Rochester, New York

Reneé T. Burwell, AASN, BSN, MSEd, EdD
Coordinator of Health Science Programs
Charlotte Technical Center
Port Charlotte, Florida

Joyce Canavan, BS Ed, MSN, RN
Mental Health, Lead Instructor
Anamarc College
El Paso, Texas

Tammie Cohen, RN, BSN
Nursing Instructor, Faculty Advisor Chairperson
Western Suffolk BOCES
Northport, New York

Wendy C. Farr, RN, BSN, MSN Ed, Ins
Practical Nursing Instructor
Southern Crescent Technical College
Thomaston, Georgia

Brian Fonnesbeck, RN, MN, BSN, ADN
Associate Professor of Nursing and Health Sciences
Lewis-Clark State College
Lewiston, Idaho

Cheryl Gilbert, RN, BHA
Assistant Director, Vocational Nursing Program
Chaffey College, Chino Campus
Chino, California

Peggy Grady, RN, ASN
Assistant Director, PN Program
Clinical Instructor
Southern Crescent Technical College
Griffin, Georgia

Deborah B. Harris, BSN, MSN, RN
Director, Practical Nursing Program
Valley Vocational Technical Center
Fishersville, Virginia

Eula Jackson, ADN, BS, MSN, CNE, PhD
Nursing Facilitator/Clinical Instructor
Reid State College and University of Phoenix
Evergreen, Alabama

Linda Johnson, RN, PHN, MSN, DHA
Assistant Director Vocational Nursing Program
Los Medanos College
Pittsburg, California

Ethel Jones, EdS, DSN, RN, CNE
Nursing Instructor
H. Councill Trenholm State Technical College
Montgomery, Alabama

Tammy Krell, MSN, RN
Coordinator of PN Program
Western Wyoming Community College
Evanston, Wyoming

Susan R. Leferson, RN, BSN, MSBA, COHC
Nurse Educator
Medical Careers Institute, School of Health Sciences of ECPI University
Manassas, Virginia

Rimina Lewis, MSN/Ed, RN
Instructor, Practical Nurse Program
Savannah Technical College
Savannah, Georgia

Gayla Love, MSN, BSN, RN, CCM
Program Coordinator, Practical Nursing
Southern Crescent Technical College
Griffin, Georgia

Kimberly K. McClure, MSN, RN
Vocational Nursing Instructor
Victoria College
Victoria, Texas

Carol A. Miller, BSN
Nursing Instructor
Southeastern Technical Institute
Easton, Massachusetts

John H. Nagelschmidt, MSN, RN
Nursing Instructor
Assabet Valley Regional Technical High School
Marlborough, Massachusetts

Diana Nobleza, MSN, RN
Instructor and CFO
Pinelands School of Practical Nursing & Allied Health, Inc.
Toms River, New Jersey

Sallie Noto, RN, MS, MSN
Director, CTC School of Practical Nursing
Career Technology Center
Scranton, Pennsylvania

Mary A. Olson, MA, RN
PN Program Director
St. Paul College
Saint Paul, Minnesota

Kristi Pfeil, MSN, RN
VN Nursing Faculty
Victoria College
Victoria, Texas

Maryellen Picchiello, MS, RN
LPN Instructor
Ocean County Vocational Technical School
Toms River, New Jersey

Jennifer Ponto, RN, BSN
Instructor, Vocational Nursing
South Plains College
Levelland, Texas

Cindy Price, MSN, RN
Practical Nurse Instructor
Mid-East Career and Technology Center
Zanesville, Ohio

Cynthia Roberts, MS, RN
Program Director
Isabella Graham Hart School of Practical Nursing
Rochester General Health System
Rochester, New York

Phyllis Rowe, DNP, RN, ANP
Professor, Nursing
Riverside City College
Riverside, California

Ellen Santos, MSN, RN, CNE
Instructor of Practical Nursing
Assabet Valley Regional Technical School
Marlborough, Massachusetts

Judith M. Shaffer, RN, BSN, MSN Ed student
Practical Nursing Educator
ECPI University
Raleigh, North Carolina

Claudia Stoffel, MSN, RN, CNE
Professor of Nursing, Practical Nursing Program Coordinator
West Kentucky Community and Technical College
Paducah, Kentucky

Kendra Strenth, RN, MSN, DNP, BC
Instructor
Bishop State Community College
Mobile, Alabama

Barbara Taylor, RN, MSN
LPN Instructor
Walton Career Development Center
DeFuniak Springs, Florida

Sandra D. Thompson, RN
Coordinator
Mercer County Technical Education Center
Princeton, West Virginia

Peggy Valentine, RN, BSN, MSNc
Director of Nursing
Skyline College
Roanoke, Virginia

Faye Warner, RN, MSN
LPN Instructor
Kaynor Regional High School
Waterbury, Connecticut

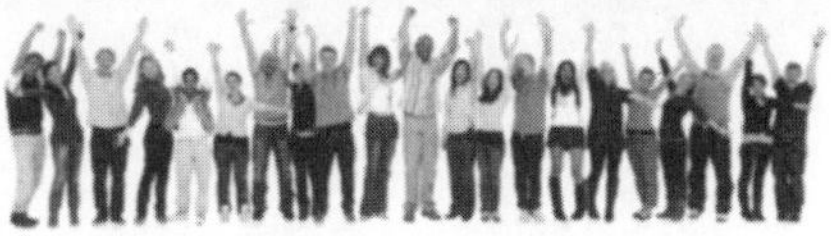

Consultants to Previous Editions

Brenda Agee, RN, MSN
Nursing Instructor
Delaware Technical and Community College
Georgetown, Delaware

Ethel Avery, RN, MSN, EdS
Instructor
H. Councill Trenholm State Technical College
Montgomery, Alabama

Sharon M. Erbe, RN, BSN, MSN(c)
Nursing Coordinator
WSWHE BOCES
Hudson Falls, New York

Gloria Ferritto, RN, BSN, PHN
Assistant Director, Vocational Nursing Program
Maric College
Vista, California

Frances Francis, RN, BS
Practical Nursing Instructor
Hazard Regional Technology Center
Hazard, Kentucky

Sue Garland, RN, MSN, ARNP
Division Chair, Allied Health and Related Technologies
Practical Nursing Program Coordinator
Big Sandy Community and Technical College
Paintsville, Kentucky

Nancy T. Hatfield, RN, BSN, MA
Instructor, Practical Nursing Program
Career Enrichment Center
Albuquerque Public Schools
Albuquerque, New Mexico

Christine D. Herdlick, RN, BA
Nursing Instructor
Marshalltown Community College
Marshalltown, Iowa

Debra Hodge
Licensed Practical Nursing
West Virginia Academy of Careers and Technology
Beckley, West Virginia

Phyllis Lilly, RN, BSN
Instructor
Isabella Graham Hart School of Practical Nursing
Rochester General Hospital
Rochester, New York

Maureen L. McGary, RN, MSN, NP-C
Former Program Head, Practical Nursing
Virginia Western Community College
Wirtz, Virginia

Betty Richardson, RN, PhD, LPC, LMFT, CS, CNAA
Instructor, Practical Nursing Program
Austin Community College
Austin, Texas

Robin A. Spidle, RN, PhD
Payson, Arizona

Judy Stauder, RN, MSN
Coordinator
Practical Nursing Program of Canton City Schools
Canton, Ohio

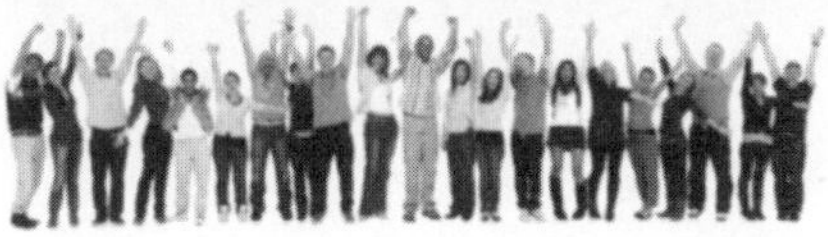

ACKNOWLEDGMENTS

We want to acknowledge our Development Editor, Julie P. Scardiglia. Julie guided us through the writing process. Her enthusiasm, encouragement and, of course, her attention to detail kept us on track throughout the revision process. Her suggestions, responsiveness, availability for many conference calls, and organization skills helped us produce a revision that taps into today's student's needs. She worked closely with us every step of the writing process. We are thankful for all her help.

Jacalyn Clay, our Project Editor from F.A. Davis, provided us with the support and resources to develop a project that expands on Kathy Neeb's original ideas. We appreciate all the guidance she provided to us.

—LINDA GORMAN
ROBYNN ANWAR

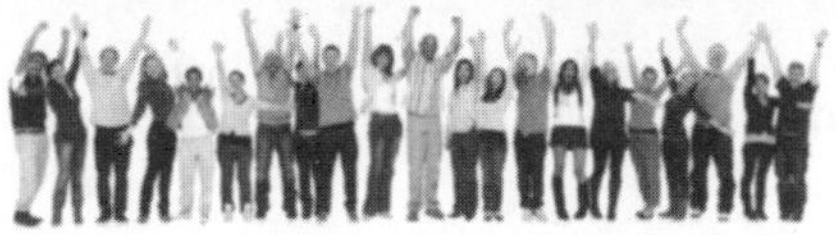

TABLE OF CONTENTS

Appendices

UNIT 1

Foundations *for* Mental Health Nursing

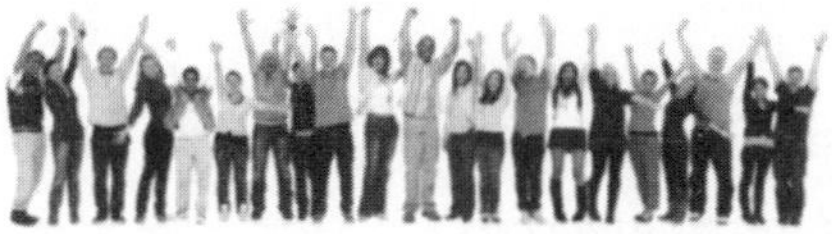

CHAPTER 1

History of Mental Health Nursing

Learning Objectives

1. Identify the major trailblazers to mental health nursing.
2. Know the basic tenets or theories of the contributors to mental health nursing.
3. Define three types of treatment facilities.
4. Identify three breakthroughs that advanced mental health nursing.
5. Identify the major laws and provisions of each that influenced mental health nursing.

Key Terms

- American Nurses Association (ANA)
- Asylum
- Deinstitutionalization
- Free-standing treatment centers
- National Association for Practical Nurse Education and Service (NAPNES)
- National Federation of Licensed Practical Nurses (NFLPN)
- National League for Nursing (NLN)
- Nurse Practice Act
- Psychotropic
- Standards of care

The Trailblazers

For centuries, nurses have been many things to many people. People have nurses to thank for cooking, cleaning, and ministering to those who fought battles.

Long before people knew what aerobic or anaerobic microorganisms were, nurses knew when to open or close the windows. Nurses helped women give birth to their young and nursed the babies when mothers were unable to or when mothers died during or shortly after giving birth. The first flight attendants were nurses. For centuries, nurses have gone about the business of caring for people, but they have not always done that quietly. Who were the nurses who took the risks? Who were the ones who spoke out on behalf of the patient and the profession? In times when nursing was considered only "women's work," and when women were not politically active, the major trailblazers were female.

Florence Nightingale

Florence Nightingale (1820–1910) (Fig. 1-1). has been called the founder of nursing. Her story and her contributions are numerous enough to fill many volumes. She was born of wealth and was highly educated. When she was very young, she realized she wanted to be a nurse, which did not please her parents. Conditions in hospitals were poor, and her

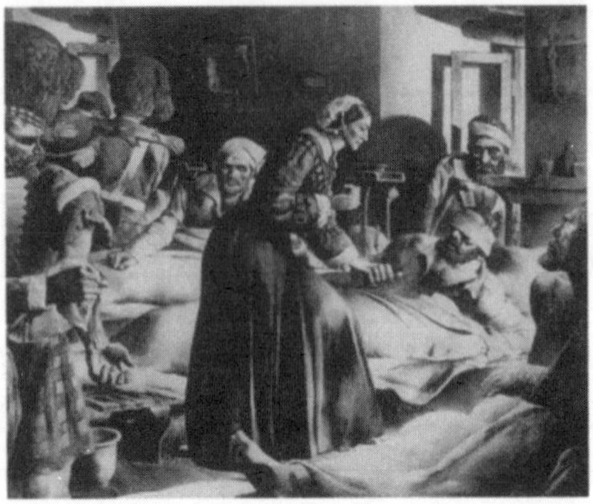

Figure 1-1 Florence Nightingale at work during the Crimean War.

parents wanted her to pursue a life as wife, mother, and society woman.

Florence worked hard to educate herself in the art and science of nursing. Her mission to help the British soldiers in the Crimean War earned her respect around the world as a nurse and administrator. This was no easy task because many of the soldiers at the Barrack Hospital at Scutari resented her intelligence and did what they could to undermine her work.

The relationship between sanitary conditions and healing became known and accepted due to her observations and diligence. Within 6 months of her arrival in Scutari, the mortality rate dropped from 42.7% to 2.2% (Donahue, 1985, p. 244). She insisted on proper lighting, diet, cleanliness, and recreation. She understood that the mind and body work together and that cleanliness, the predecessor to today's sterile techniques, is a major barrier to infection and promotes healing. She carefully observed and documented changes in the conditions of the soldiers, which led to her adulation as "The Lady with the Lamp" (from the poem "Santa Filomena" by H. W. Longfellow).

Santa Filomena

by Henry Wadsworth Longfellow

Whene'er a noble deed is wrought,
Whene'er is spoken a noble thought,
Our hearts, in glad surprise,
To higher levels rise.
The tidal wave of deeper souls
Into our inmost being rolls,
And lifts us unawares
Out of all meaner cares.
Honour to those whose words or deeds
Thus help us in our daily needs,
And by their overflow
Raise us from what is low!
Thus thought I, as by night I read
Of the great army of the dead,
The trenches cold and damp,
The starved and frozen camp,
The wounded from the battle-plain,
In dreary hospitals of pain,
The cheerless corridors,
The cold and stony floors.
Lo! in that house of misery
A lady with a lamp I see
Pass through the glimmering gloom,
And flit from room to room.
And slow, as in a dream of bliss,
The speechless sufferer turns to kiss
Her shadow, as it falls
Upon the darkening walls.
As if a door in heaven should be
Opened and then closed suddenly,
The vision came and went,
The light shone and was spent.
On England's annals, through the long
Hereafter of her speech and song,
That light its rays shall cast
From portals of the past.
A Lady with a Lamp shall stand
In the great history of the land,
A noble type of good,
Heroic womanhood.
Nor even shall be wanting here
The palm, the lily, and the spear,
The symbols that of yore
Saint Filomena bore.

She was a crusader for the improvement of care and conditions in the military and civilian hospitals in Britain. Among her books are *Notes on Hospitals* (1859), which deals with the relationship of sanitary techniques to medical facilities; *Notes on Nursing* (1859), which was the most respected nursing textbook of the day; and *Notes on Matters Affecting the Health, Efficiency and Hospital Administration of the British Army* (1857) (Donahue, 1985, p. 248).

The first formal nurses' training program, the Nightingale School for Nurses, opened in 1860. The goals of the school were to train nurses to work in hospitals, to work with the poor, and to teach. This meant that students cared for people in their homes, an idea that is still gaining in popularity and professional opportunity for nurses. Florence Nightingale died at the age of 90.

Dorothea Dix

Dorothea Dix (1802–1887) (Fig. 1-2) was a schoolteacher, not a nurse. She believed that people did not need to live in suffering and that society at large had a responsibility to aid those less fortunate. Her primary focus was the care of prisoners and the mentally ill. She lobbied in the United States and Canada for the improvement of **standards of care** for the mentally ill and even suggested that the governments take an active role in providing help with finances, food, shelter, and other areas of need. She learned that many criminals were also mentally ill, a theory that is borne out in studies today. Because of the efforts of Dorothea Dix, 32 states developed **asylums** or "psychiatric hospitals" to care for the mentally ill. There is a monument to her that symbolized her efforts on the Women's Heritage Trail in Boston.

Linda Richards

While Dorothea Dix was working for political help in mental health, a nurse named Linda Richards (1841–1930) (Fig. 1-3) was pushing to upgrade nursing education. She was the first American-trained nurse, and in 1882 she opened the Boston City Hospital Training School for Nurses to teach the specialty of caring for the mentally ill. By 1890, more than 30 asylums in the United States had developed schools for nurses. Linda Richards was among the first nurses to teach and work seriously with planning and developing nursing care for patients. In cooperation with the **American Nurses Association** (ANA) and the **National League for Nursing** (NLN), she was instrumental in developing textbooks specifically for nurses that had stated objectives for outcomes of nursing education and patient care.

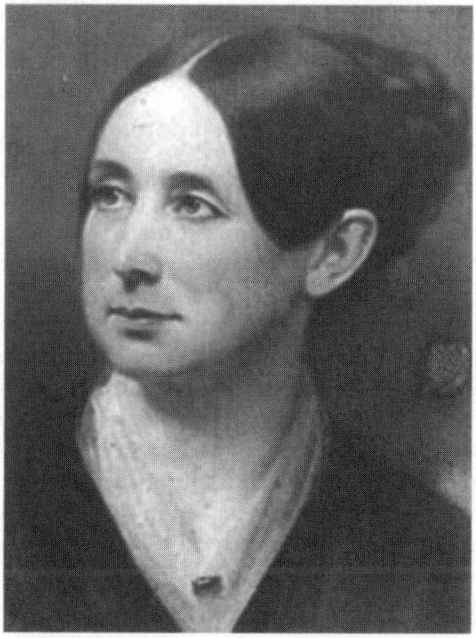

Figure 1-2 Dorothea Dix.

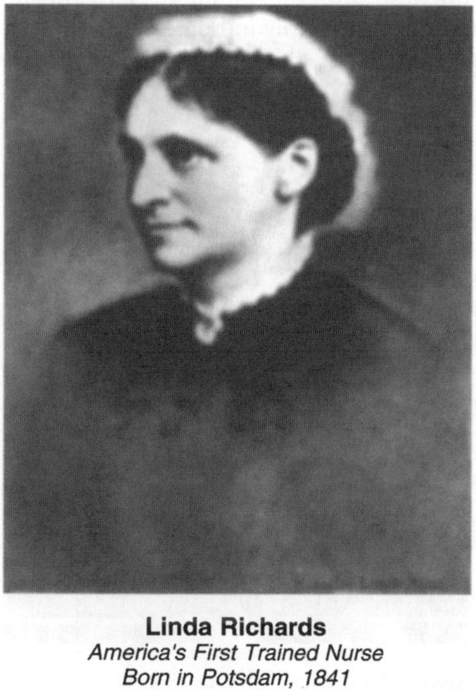

Figure 1-3 Linda Richards.

Harriet Bailey

The first textbook focusing on psychiatric nursing was written in 1920 by Harriet Bailey. It included guidelines for nurses who provided care for those with a mental illness. Bailey understood that nurses caring for these patients needed proper training. After she published her book, the NLN began requiring all student nurses have a clinical rotation in a psychiatric setting (Videback, 2013).

Effie Jane Taylor

Effie Jane Taylor (Fig. 1-4) initiated the first psychiatric program of study for nurses, in 1913. She is also well known for her development and implementation of patient-centered care, putting emphasis on the emotional and intellectual life of the patient. Effie Taylor received a diploma in nursing from Johns Hopkins School of Nursing, later to become a nursing professor in psychiatry (American Association for the History of Nursing, Inc., 2007).

Mary Mahoney

Mary Mahoney (1845–1926) (Fig. 1-5) is considered to be America's first African-American professional nurse. Her contributions were primarily in home care and in the promotion of the acceptance of African Americans in the field of nursing. An award in her name is presented at the annual ANA convention to a person who has worked to promote equal opportunity for minorities in nursing. During her career, it was necessary to open separate schools of nursing for African American students because they were banned from the schools for white students. Two of these separate schools were Spelman Seminary (currently known as Spelman College) in Georgia and Tuskegee Institute in Alabama.

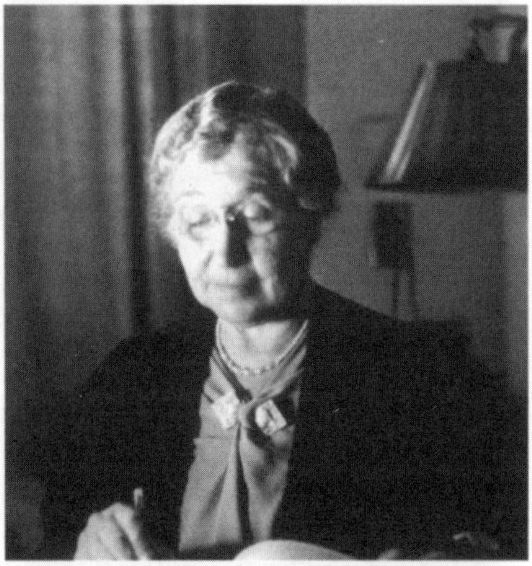

Figure 1-4 Effie Jane Taylor. *(From Yale University, Harvey Cushing/John Hay Whitney Medical Library.)*

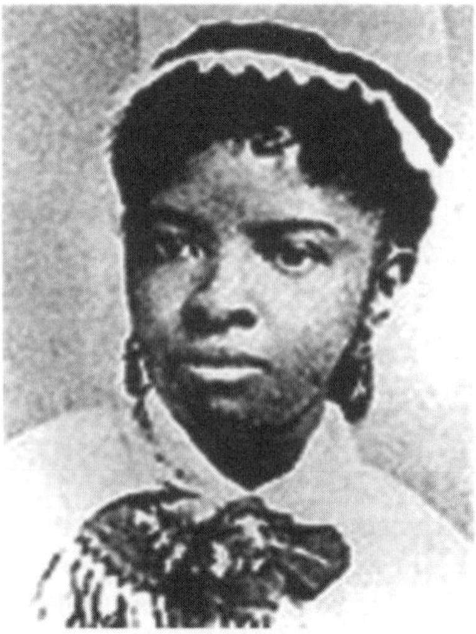

Figure 1-5 Mary Mahoney.

Hildegard Peplau

Dr. Hildegard Peplau (1909–1999) (Fig. 1-6) was a nurse ahead of her time. She believed that nursing is multifaceted and that the nurse must educate and promote wellness as well as deliver care to the ill. In her book, *Interpersonal Relations in Nursing* (1952), Dr. Peplau brought together some interpersonal theories from psychiatry and melded them with theories of nursing and communication. She believed that nurses work in society—not merely in a hospital or clinic—and that they need to use every opportunity to educate the public and follow role models in physical and mental health. Peplau saw the nurse as:

1. *Resource person.* Provides information.
2. *Counselor.* Helps patients to explore their thoughts and feelings.

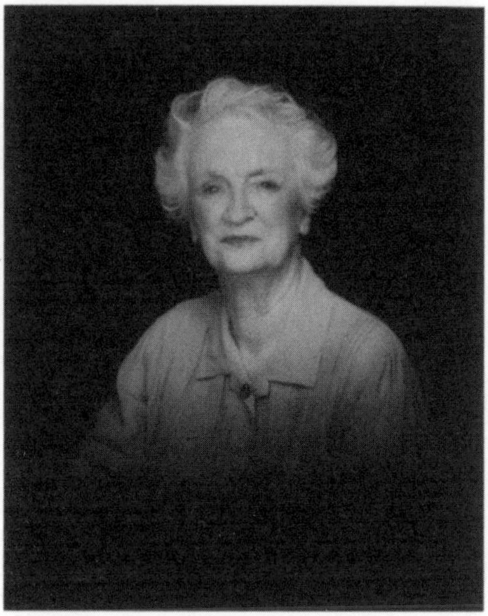

Figure 1-6 Hildegard Peplau.

3. *Surrogate.* By role-playing or other means helps the patient to explore and identify feelings from the past.
4. *Technical support.* Coordinates professional services (Peplau, 1952).

In addition to this, she believed in building a collaborative therapeutic relationship between the nurse and the patient. In her book she cites four stages of this relationship (Peplau, 1952):

1. *Orientation.* Patient feels a need and a will to seek out help.
2. *Identification.* Expectations and perceptions about the nurse-patient relationship are identified.
3. *Exploration.* Patient will begin to show motivation in the problem-solving process, but some testing behaviors may be seen; patient may have a need to "test" the nurse's commitment to his/her individual situation.
4. *Resolution.* Focus is on the patient's developing self-responsibility and showing personal growth.

In 1954, the first graduate-level nursing program was developed by Dr. Peplau at Rutgers University to provide training for clinical nurse specialists for psychiatric nursing.

Hattie Bessent

In the early 1980s, the National Institute of Mental Health granted money to be used for the education and research of minority nurses who were choosing to upgrade to master's and doctorate levels of practice. Hattie Bessent (Fig. 1-7) is credited with the development and directorship of that program. In 2008 the ANA presented Dr. Bessent with its Hall of Fame Award.

Critical Thinking Question

The "trailblazers" were risk takers. One of the professional responsibilities of nursing is to try to give something back to our profession. How will you, as an individual, become a trailblazer? What direction should nursing as a whole take to strengthen the profession? What criteria should be important when deciding what level of preparation in nursing should allow the nurse to be a specialist in mental health?

Classroom Activity

- Have students (and colleagues) research trailblazers in nursing and, on an assigned day, come to class with a prop and a brief explanation of the trailblazers and their contributions to nursing.

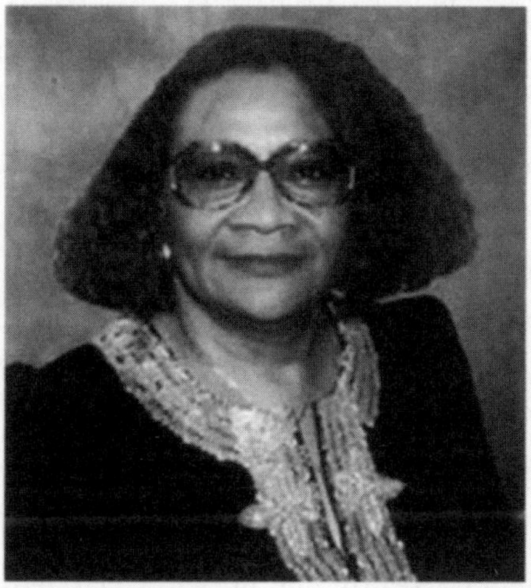

Figure 1-7 Hattie Bessent.

The Facilities

People who have mental illnesses are everywhere; popular statistics say that about one in every three Americans will experience some form of mental illness at some point in life. The trailblazers in nursing realized that mental illness is different from medical-surgical disorders. They understood that each person's mind is truly unique and therefore nurses need information and training specific to those illnesses. To help meet those needs, they took action to improve the quality of care for those patients. This was not enough, however, and it became evident that persons with moderate to severe mental disorders were often better served through care in special facilities.

Asylums

These special facilities were called asylums, which Webster Online, in part, defines as "1: a place of refuge; 2: protection given to criminals and debtors; 3: an institution for the care of the needy or sick and especially of the insane." Patients in asylums were frequently treated less than humanely. Custodial care was provided, but patients were often heavily medicated. Nutritional and physical care was minimal, and often these patients were volunteered for various forms of experimentation and research.

One of the largest asylums in the United States was known as ByBerry, later to be renamed Philadelphia State Hospital (Fig. 1-8). This facility reportedly provided inhumane treatment to its patients. With the onset of deinstitutionalization and due to the poor conditions, this facility saw its last patient in 1990.

Hospitals

As treatment facilities evolved, the term asylum and the connotations associated with it became unpopular. In 1753, Pennsylvania Hospital established a facility to treat those with mental disorders. The hospital was established by Dr. Thomas Bond and Benjamin Franklin. Until the Community Mental Health Act of 1963 was passed, housing of this clientele was primarily handled by individual state hospital systems.

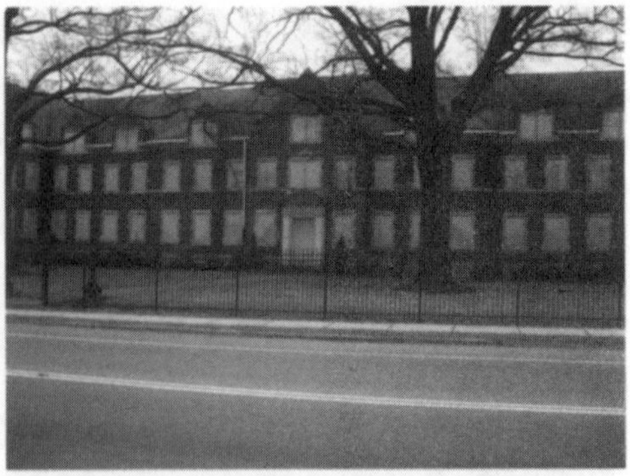

Figure 1-8 ByBerry, later to be renamed Philadelphia State Hospital.

Today, hospitals handle patients with psychological needs according to the size of the hospital and its resources. To comply with regulations surrounding mental health issues, in smaller communities these patients may be seen in a hospital emergency room and then referred to other clinics or hospitals. Communities large enough to support such programs may provide in-house mental health treatment as well as outpatient treatment and aftercare. Metropolitan areas commonly provide treatment via several options, including hospitals and free-standing treatment centers.

Free-Standing Facilities

Free-standing treatment centers may be called detoxification (detox) centers, crisis centers, or similar names. Most people are familiar with the Betty Ford Center. Many free-standing treatment centers provide care ranging from crisis-only to more traditional 21-day stays. As with the Betty Ford Center, a stay can last up to 120 days. This, too, depends largely on the size and needs of the individual community. More discussion on the types of treatment facilities occurs in the section on The Laws.

The Breakthroughs

It was not until 1937 that formal clinical rotations in mental health began for nurses. Today, these rotations are required for students in nursing programs, but students in practical or vocational nursing are usually exposed to mental health theory and very short observational experiences. In 1955, theory relating to mental health nursing became a requirement for licensure for all nurses.

Throughout the 1800s and early 1900s, progress was made in developing humane, effective treatment of mental illnesses. With the best knowledge available to them as a profession, nurses were forward thinkers in providing specialized care to people unfortunate enough to have illnesses that were somehow different from the tuberculosis, smallpox, and influenza that filled hospitals. There was one major difference, however: Medicines existed to help in treating those diseases. At that time, no one had been able to find pharmacologic help for people with emotional, behavioral, or physical brain disorders. That would change in the 1950s.

Psychotropic Medications

In the early 1950s, chemists were experimenting with combinations of chemicals and their effects on people. In 1955, a group of **psychotropic** medications called phenothiazines was discovered to have the effect of calming and tranquilizing people. One well known phenothiazine is Thorazine. What a world of possibility this opened for people living with and caring for those with mental disorders! Suddenly it was possible to control behavior to a degree, and patients were able to function more independently. Other forms of therapy became more effective because patients were able to focus differently. Some patients improved so dramatically that it was no longer necessary for them to remain hospitalized and dependent on others. Between the mid-1950s and the mid-1970s, the number of patients hospitalized with mental illnesses in the United States was cut approximately in half, mainly because of the use of psychotropic drugs.

Deinstitutionalization

The use of phenothiazines (see Chapter 8) became so effective that state hospitals and other facilities dedicated to the care and treatment of people with mental illness saw a large decline in population. It became costly to run these large buildings and continue to employ staff. The combination of these effects, as well as new laws pertaining to the care of the mentally ill, resulted in a movement called **deinstitutionalization.** People who had formerly required long hospital stays were now able to leave the institutions and return to their communities. Once discharged, some went to group homes and others to their own homes. Deinstitutionalization was and still is a controversial issue, but it was a huge step in returning a sense of worth, ability, and independence to those who had been dependent on others for their care for so long.

Critical Thinking Question

The laws have said that people who have mental illnesses should be treated using the least restrictive alternative. Deinstitutionalization allows these people to live among us in the community. Consider the following scenario: Your city has just purchased the house next door to you, and the plan is to develop this into a halfway house for women who have been child abusers. You are the parent of a 3-year-old and you are also a mental health nurse. What would you do? What are your thoughts and feelings about this situation?

Nursing Organizations and Recommendations

A natural progression from the breakthroughs that were happening in nursing was the development of organizations for nurses. The American Nurses Association (ANA) is recognized as an organization for registered nurses (RNs). One of its goals is to promote standardization of nursing practice in the United States. It also promotes the certification of nurses who meet specific criteria. The concept of psychiatric nurse specialists, clinicians, or advanced practice nurses is a result of the work of the ANA. The American Psychiatric Nurses Association provides leadership in recommending standards of care for nurses who care for people with mental illness. This organization invites nurses who are RN-prepared. Further information can be obtained at its Web site, www.apna.org.

Classroom Activity

- List the standards of psychiatric/mental health clinical nursing practice and give an example of a nursing behavior or action that correlates with each standard. (www.nursingworld.org/scopeandstandardsofpractice)

The National League for Nursing evolved from the National League for Nursing Education and became known as the NLN in 1952. NLN is the accrediting agency for many schools of nursing across the United States with its specific focus on nursing education.

Every state has adopted its own code or set of rules by which all nurses are expected to perform. This is called the **Nurse Practice Act** and is based on federal guidelines that have been adapted to the needs of the individual state. The Nurse Practice Act is discussed in more detail in Chapter 3.

Sigma Theta Tau is an honor society for nurses who have shown special talents in research or leadership. It is open to baccalaureate-degree nursing students, graduate students in nursing, and leaders in the nursing community.

Specific to the licensed practical/vocational nurse are two organizations: **National Federation of Licensed Practical Nurses** (NFLPN) and **National Association for Practical Nurse Education and Service** (NAPNES). NFLPN welcomes licensed practical nurses (LPNs), licensed vocational nurses (LVNs), and practical/vocational nursing (PN) students in the United States. In September 1991, a new category of affiliate membership was established to allow those who have an interest in the work of NFLPN but who are neither LPNs nor PN students to join. The NFLPN has a published set of Nursing Practice Standards for the LPN (Appendix D). The standards can be found online at www.nflpn.org/practice-standards4web.pdf.

NAPNES was founded by practical nurse educators in 1941 and identifies itself as the world's oldest nursing organization dedicated exclusively to the promotion of quality nursing service through the practice of LPNs and LVNs. NAPNES is a multidisciplinary organization of individuals, facilities, and schools that advocate for professional practice of practical and vocational nursing. Visit the NAPNES Web site at www.napnes.org to read the NAPNES position paper, dated July 18, 2004, "Supply, Demand and Use of Licensed Practical Nurses."

Tool Box | Organizations for Practical and Vocational Nurses

National Federation of Licensed Practical Nurses, Inc. (NFLPN)
www.nflpn.org
National Association for Practical Nurse Education and Service, Inc. (NAPNES)
www.napnes.org

The National Coalition of Ethnic Minority Nurse Associations (NCEMNA) is made up of five national ethnic nurse associations: Asian American/Pacific Islander Nurses Association, Inc. (AAPINA), National Alaska Native American Indian Nurses Association, Inc. (NANAINA), National Association of Hispanic Nurses, Inc. (NAHN), National Black Nurses Association, Inc. (NBNA), and Philippine Nurses Association of America, Inc. (PNAA). Goals include advocating for equity and justice in nursing and health care for ethnic minority populations and endorsement of best practice models for nursing practice, education, and research for minority populations. More information can be located at its Web site, www.ncemna.org.

The American Assembly for Men in Nursing (AAMN) provides a framework for male nurses, as a group, to meet to discuss and influence factors that affect men as nurses. Among its objectives is to encourage men of all ages to become nurses and join together with all nurses in strengthening and humanizing health care. The organization also supports men who are nurses to grow professionally and demonstrate the increasing contributions being made by men in the nursing profession. As do the other professional organizations, AAMN advocates for continued research, education, and dissemination of information about men's health issues, men in nursing, and nursing knowledge at the local and national levels.

Tool Box |▶ Nursing Organizations
ANA: American Nurses Association:
www.nursingworld.org/
APNA: American Psychiatric Nurses Association:
www.apna.org/
NLN: National League for Nursing:
www.nln.org/
NFLPN: National Federation of Licensed Practical Nurses:
www.nflpn.org/
NAPNES: National Association for Practical Nurse Education and Services:
www.napnes.org/
NCEMNA: National Coalition of Ethnic Minority Nurse Associations:
www.ncemna.org/
AAPINA: Asian American / Pacific Islander Nurses Association, Inc.:
www.aapina.org/
NANAINA: National Alaska Native American Indian Nurses Association:
www.geronurseonline.org/ (see partner organizations)
NAHN: National Association of Hispanic Nurses:
www.nahnnet.org/
NBNA: National Black Nurses Association:
www.nbna.org/
PNAA: Philippine Nurses Association of America:
www.mypnaa.org/
AAMN: American Assembly for Men in Nursing:
http://aamn.org/

Appendix C of this text provides more contact information for these and other agencies designed to promote and assist nurses, particularly at the LPN and LVN level of preparation.

■ THE LAWS

Over the years many changes and advancements have been made in medicine and nursing in general. But mental health has remained a challenge. There were ethical considerations that had not surfaced in earlier years. Psychotropic and (also known as psychoactive) medications were benefiting many patients but had their own problems as well; side effects were not always pleasant. More drugs were being developed, and more questions arose: How much is too much to give people? Do we keep them completely sedated? People were asking which was worse: the illness or the medication? People are still asking that question. Other concerns have arisen, for example, how some psychotropic drugs are associated with diabetic mellitus.

Nonetheless, it was necessary to begin regulating the health-care industry a bit more. A series of laws governing various aspects of care for persons with mental illnesses were passed. The laws have changed somewhat and have been renamed in some cases, but the collective intention is to provide funding, treatment, and ethical care for this segment of society.

■ ■ ■ Critical Thinking Question
Your employer has announced that your company is changing its medical insurance policy. The company will be providing you with a set amount of money to spend on insurance benefits. The three insurance services you have to choose from offer either family coverage or mental health services. You are a single parent with two preschoolers. You also have a diagnosis of bipolar disorder for which you need medications, therapy, and periodic hospitalization. What will you choose?

Hill-Burton Act

In 1946, Senators Lister Hill and Harold Burton collaborated and created the Hill-Burton Act, a federal law. It was the first major law to address mental illness. It provided money to build psychiatric units in hospitals. Today, the many soldiers returning from the Afghanistan war who suffer from post-traumatic stress disorder know they will not be turned away because of financial difficulties, as the Hill-Burton Act protects those who have no insurance coverage.

National Mental Health Act of 1946

The National Mental Health Act of 1946 was a result of the first Congress held after World War II. It provided money for nursing and several other disciplines for training and research in areas pertaining to improving treatment for the mentally ill. The National Institute of Mental Health (NIMH) was established as part of the National Mental Health Act of 1946. The NIMH continuously updates the public on mental health issues. Since 1999, NIMH has been researching autism. The agency also started the Army Study to Assess Risk and Resilience in Service Members (Army Starrs). The Army Starrs will look at the many factors that will be facing those who had to encounter battle.

Community Mental Health Centers Act of 1963

The Community Mental Health Centers Act resulted from President John F. Kennedy's concern for the treatment of the mentally ill. Its main purpose was to provide a full set of services to the people living in a particular community. These services were to include inpatient care, outpatient care, emergency care, and education. This was to be a national effort, funded federally at first. The goal was for the centers to generate enough services so that, eventually, the community could support it financially.

In 1981, the bill was amended in Congress. Called the Omnibus Budget Reconciliation Act (OBRA), it allows money to be allocated differently. There is currently less money available in the federal budget, and that money can be withheld at any time. Unfortunately, with the turmoil in the insurance and health-care delivery systems today, mental health benefits are often among the first services to be cut back or eliminated.

Patient Bill of Rights

In 1980, the image of the patient was changing. The Civil Rights Movement of the 1960s was giving way to the provision of rights for all groups of people. Patients were beginning to be identified as "clients" who purchase services from health-care providers. Persons of very young or very old age or persons with certain physical, intellectual, or communication difficulties became politically recognized as "vulnerable." The outcome was the development of the Patient Bill of Rights, which is discussed in more detail in Chapter 3.

Tool Box | Community Mental Health Act 1963
www.mass.gov/eohhs/gov/departments/dmh/about-the-department-of-mental-health.html
Omnibus Budget Reconciliation Act
www.gpo.gov/fdsys/pkg/BILLS-103hr2264enr/pdf/BILLS-103hr2264enr.pdf

Clinical Activity

Discussion Questions: In clinical post-conference, discuss your answers to these questions.

1. Identify ways that (a) the delivery of psychiatric/mental health nursing and (b) roles, functions, activities, and settings have changed.
2. What issues or trends do you perceive in psychiatric/mental health in the future.

Key Concepts

1. Mental health nursing has a long and rich history. It has evolved from very rudimentary skills before the time of Florence Nightingale to the specialty area of nursing today.
2. Patients with mental illness are treated in many different types of facilities, depending on the diagnosis and the availability of care in the particular community.
3. The 1950s were important years in the mental health field. The first psychotropic medications were developed, making it possible for people to return to their homes and communities (deinstitutionalization). These medications also allowed other treatment forms to be used more effectively.

4. Nurses at all levels of preparation are integral parts of the mental health treatment team. Our observations, documentation, and interpersonal skills make nurses effective tools in patient care.
5. Since 1955, all nursing curriculums are required to provide mental health theory.
6. A series of laws over the past 50 years have provided for money, education, research, and improvements in the care of the mentally ill. Financial difficulties in the insurance and health-care industries contribute to cutbacks in money and services for care and treatment of the mentally ill.

REFERENCES

American Association for the History of Nursing, Inc, (2007). *Euphemia (effie) jane taylor.* Retrieved from www.aahn.org/gravesites/taylor.html.

Donahue, M.P. (1985). *Nursing, the Finest Art.* St. Louis: CV Mosby.

Henry, G.W. (1921). Nursing mental disease, by Harriet Bailey, R.N. Bangor, Maine, 175 pages. (New York: The Macmillan Company, 1920). *The American journal of psychiatry, 77*(3), 473–474. Retrieved from www.focus.psychiatryonline.org/data/Journals

Peplau, H.E. (1952). *Interpersonal Relations in Nursing.* New York: GP Putnam's Sons.

Longfellow, H.W. (1857) *Santa Filomena. The Atlantic Monthly, 1*(1) 22–23.

Verghese, M. (2010). *Essentials of Psychiatric and Mental Health Nursing.* 3rd ed., pp. 254–255. Kalk, New Delhi: Elsevier.

Videbeck, S. L. (2013). *Psychiatric-Mental Health Nursing.* 6th ed. Philadelphia: Lippincott Williams & Wilkins.

Webster Online (2004). www.merriam-webster.com

Test Questions

Multiple Choice Questions

1. The main goal of deinstitutionalization was to:
a. Let all mentally ill people care for themselves.
b. Return as many people as possible to a "normal" life.
c. Keep all mentally ill people in locked wards.
d. Close all community hospitals.

2. A major breakthrough of the 1950s that assisted in the deinstitutionalization movement was:
a. The Community Mental Health Centers Act
b. The Nurse Practice Act
c. The development of psychotropic medications
d. Electroshock therapy

3. The set of regulations that dictates the scope of nursing practice is called:
a. National League for Nursing
b. American Nurses Association
c. Patient Bill of Rights
d. Nurse Practice Act

4. As a result of deinstitutionalization and changes in the health-care delivery system, nurses can expect to care for people with mental health issues in which of the following settings?
a. Psychiatric hospitals only
b. Outpatient settings only
c. Medical-surgical hospital settings
d. All of the above

5. Which of the following trailblazers in nursing was not a nurse?
a. Hildegard Peplau
b. Linda Richards
c. Harriet Bailey
d. Dorothea Dix

6. The following nursing organizations specifically represent minority nurses. *(select all that apply)*
a. NACE
b. AAPINA
c. NAPNES
d. PNAA
e. NANAINA

7. In the past facilities that housed patients who were needy, sick, or insane were known as:
a. Detox centers
b. Asylums
c. Outpatient clinics
d. Hospitals

8. What institute was established as result of the National Mental Health Act of 1946?
a. NLN
b. NFLPN
c. Hill-Burton Act
d. NIMH

9. Florence Nightingale's focus in the Crimean War was:
a. Mental health
b. Upgrading education
c. Clean environment
d. Writing care plans

10. The first psychotropic medications were introduced in the:
a. 1950s
b. 1930s
c. 1980s
d. 1920s

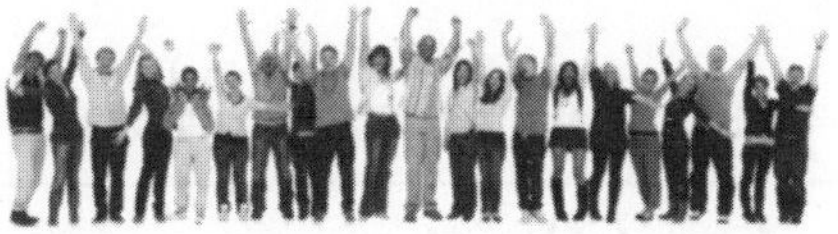

CHAPTER 2

Basics of Communication

Learning Objectives

1. Identify three components needed to communicate.
2. Differentiate between effective and ineffective communication.
3. Identify six types of communication.
4. Identify five challenges to communication.
5. Identify common blocks to therapeutic communication.
6. Identify common techniques of therapeutic communication.
7. Identify five adaptive communication techniques.
8. Define key terms.

Key Terms

- Aggressive communication
- Aphasia
- Assertive communication
- Communication
- Communication block
- Dysphasia
- Hearing-impaired
- Ineffective communication
- Laryngectomy
- Message
- Neurolinguistic programming (NLP)
- Nonverbal communication
- Receiver
- Sender
- Social communication
- Therapeutic communication
- Verbal communication
- Visually impaired

Human beings communicate. Everything people do or say has a message and a meaning. Sometimes, the words and the actions send different meanings to different people. For example: Sally and Jim meet for shift report in the morning. Sally's eyes are red and swollen, and she is unusually quiet. Jim asks her if something is wrong, and she responds, "No, everything is just fine." Jim has observed some changes in Sally's behavior and appearance. Sally has verbally communicated that nothing is wrong. What is really being communicated here?

People of different cultures communicate differently. Men and women communicate differently. **Hearing-impaired** people communicate differently from people who are not hearing impaired. A hearing-impaired person may use a hearing aid, technology, and amplifiers. People in the medical professions communicate differently from people in business professions by using terminology which relates to the medical profession rather than to the business world. People communicate all the time in everything they do. **Communication** is an ongoing process of sending and receiving messages.

Communication Theory

Sender, Receiver, and Interpretation of Message

One of the challenging parts of communicating with others is that the process requires three parts: a **sender,** a **message,** and a **receiver** (Fig. 2-1). That means the sender is only partially responsible for the communication. Sally cannot totally control Jim's interpretation of her message.

Sally is the sender, sending a message to Jim, the receiver, in the above scenario. As it turns out, Sally is a victim of severe allergies. She was visiting her friend who has cats. Sally is very allergic to them, and the redness and swelling were symptoms of her allergic response. She simply did not wish to burden Jim with her problem during shift report, so she opted to respond by telling him everything was "just fine."

> **Classroom Activity**
> - What was your initial interpretation of what Sally was communicating? On what did you base your interpretation? What "spoke" louder to you: Sally's words or her actions and appearance? What is the danger in making this assumption about Sally's message?

It is very important for the sender and receiver to double-check the message. In nursing, this is crucial because nurses use their own professional "language"; when dealing with the health and safety of patients, nurses need to be very sure that there are not "mixed" or "missed" messages.

Figure 2-1 A basic flow of communication.

Types of Communication

Verbal and Written Communication

Verbal communication is the process of exchanging information by the spoken or written word. It is, therefore, the subjective part of the process. In the example given earlier, Sally's reply that "everything is just fine" is an example of verbal communication. The expertise a nurse develops in the areas of written and verbal communication is largely responsible for the credibility of that nurse. Critical thinking is essential to understanding Sally's reply.

> **Neeb's Tip**
> In a discussion class on the topic of words and gestures and what they mean, one African American female student spoke up. She shared with the class that "gals" in her world was a demeaning term relating to the degrading role of the African American woman in history. It is important to know that the meaning of a word can change from one generation to the next. In the 1950s and 1960s, being part of the "guys" or the "gals" was a good thing. It demonstrated acceptance and belonging to one's social group.

Nonverbal Communication

Nonverbal communication is more subtle, but it is the greatest influence on communication. It consists of people's actions, tone of voice, the way they use their body, and their facial expressions. It is more subjective since nonverbal communication can be interpreted many different ways by the receiver (Fig. 2-2). In the example above, Sally's body language communicated that she was not "fine."

This points out the need to be careful with hand gestures that can be misinterpreted. Many people use hand gestures when speaking. People do it often without thinking.

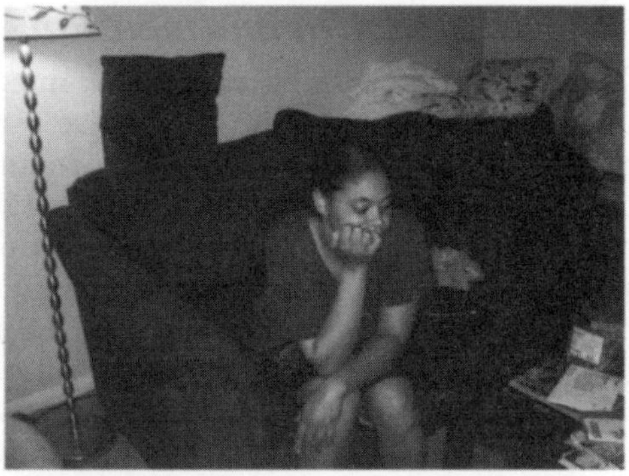

Figure 2-2 Nonverbal communication is estimated to be 70% of the message we send. The old saying is true: A picture is worth a thousand words!

However, making the "OK" sign with one's fingers, which is normally a sign of encouragement, agreement, or congratulations, is a vulgarity in some cultures.

> **Cultural Considerations**
>
> Identify the diverse cultures and generations in your community and define a gesture that you use that means something different to others.

People must be ready to learn from each other every day. Nurses need to be prepared to make known those terms or gestures that are uncomfortable for them and their patients. They must make a conscious effort not to use those words when in the company of those they may offend (Box 2-1.)

Aggressive and Assertive Communication

The terms *aggressive* and *assertive* are sometimes used interchangeably in American culture, but they have very different meanings.

Aggressive Communication

Aggressive communication is communication that is not self-responsible. Aggressive statements most often begin with the word "you." Aggressive communication, like aggressive behavior, is meant to harm another person. It is a form of the defense mechanism projection, or blaming, and it attempts to put the responsibility for the interaction on the other person. Aggressive communication is also highly subjective as demonstrated in nonverbal communication.

EXAMPLE

"You make me so angry when you don't help with the housework!"

Box 2-1 Examples of Communication With Cultural Implications

Words that are seemingly harmless to some people can be very hurtful to others. People do not usually know that until they take the time to ask! These are the examples of communication that may have different cultural implications. How many more can your class identify?

- Eye contact with strangers or those in perceived positions of power or respect is not considered appropriate among some populations.
- Hand gestures may communicate different meanings to different groups of people.
- Slang terms may be inappropriate or offensive, or may exclude people who do not understand the meaning of the word.
- Gender-reference terms such as "you guys" when the group is mixed or not male.
- Terms such as "master" and "slave" frequently used in computer-related issues may offend African American people and others.
- African American women displayed in subservient roles.
- Distortion or omission of important developments in the lives of African Americans.
- Pictures or photographs that do not portray accurate skin tones, hair texture, and physical features of certain ethnic groups.

Assertive Communication

Assertive communication, on the other hand, is self-responsible. Assertive statements begin with the word "I." They deal with thoughts and feelings, and they deal with honesty.

EXAMPLE

"I feel angry when you don't help with the housework!"

Assertive behavior and communication are also techniques of personal empowerment. People *choose* to think or feel a certain way; others do not have the power to make people think or feel anything they do not choose to think or feel. To be able to say "I think" or "I feel" keeps people in control of their emotions, yet it allows honest, open expression of the feelings they have as a result of someone else's behavior. Still, the feelings and thoughts belong to the person choosing them, not to anyone else.

> **Critical Thinking Question**
>
> Write one feeling statement and one thinking statement for the following situation: A co-worker who is a BSN-prepared nurse is routinely coming late to work and overstaying breaks, causing patients to have unsafe care and you to have extra work. You speak to your nurse manager, who appears to ignore your concerns, so you approach the co-worker.

Social Communication

People usually alter their style of communicating according to who is receiving the message. **Social communication** is the day-to-day interaction people have with personal acquaintances. For example, teenagers usually communicate with their peer group in a different manner than they do with their parents. So, too, do nurses communicate differently with their patients than they do with their friends or family.

Nurses may use slang or "street language," and they may be less literal and purposeful in their social interactions. Quite simply, social interaction has a different purpose than a nurse's professional communication.

Therapeutic Communication

In **therapeutic communication,** the nurse understands that in order to acquire certain desired information from the patient, unique techniques of communication will have to be instituted. They will be individualized to the patient as well as to the mental health disorder. Therapeutic communication is a language of its own. It requires testing new methods of communicating and new ways of listening. Therapeutic communication is purposeful: Nurses are trying to determine the patient's needs. Sometimes, for various reasons, the patient is not comfortable sharing his or her needs and concerns. At those times, it is up to the nurse to try to uncover the problem by using two tools: techniques of therapeutic communication and "active" or "purposeful" listening (or "listening between the lines"). The techniques and blocks to them will be discussed at the end of this chapter. In addition it is essential to identify the components of any mental health disorder to provide effective therapeutic communication.

Neurolinguistic Programming

Neurolinguistic programming (NLP) is a form of communication developed primarily by Milton Erickson, a hypnotherapist; John Grinder, a psychologist and linguistics professor; and Richard Bandler, a mathematician and editor (Grinder & Bandler, 1981). It is a way of framing statements and questions while attempting effective communication. One of the theory's tenets, not unlike other communication theories, is that humans cannot fail to communicate. The theory builds on the idea that humans tend to communicate in basically three ways: hearing, seeing, and touching. Choice of wording can make a difference in how the words a nurse says to a patient are actually "heard" by that patient, as communication must have a sender and a receiver. NLP is one method being taught to health-care providers to assist in the successful completion of the communication loop.

NLP is not hypnosis; it is a form of communication. NLP can be used in conjunction with hypnosis and other treatment modalities. In most states, hypnosis can only be performed legally by professionals specially trained and licensed to do so.

Further explanation and some simple examples of NLP phrasing are provided in Chapter 9.

> **Critical Thinking Question**
> Turn the following aggressive statements into assertive statements.
> - "You make me so angry when you stop at the bar before you come home."
> - "You always take the 'easy' assignment, and that's not fair."
> - "Mark always gets the days off he asks for; why can't I?"

Challenges to Communication

Communicating is something that humans often take for granted—until they no longer can do it: for example, answering the telephone while having laryngitis; signing a check while your arm is in a cast; or reading traffic signs after your eyes were dilated. These are uncomfortable situations, but for the most part, they are temporary. What about patients and coworkers for whom disabilities are permanent?

> **Clinical Activity**
> Community Resources Worksheet
>
> Contact a community agency in your community. Explain that you are a student nurse and that you are trying to determine the resources available in your community.
> 1. Your name:_________
> 2. Name of agency:
> 3. Who are the target groups for this agency?
>   a. Gender
>   b. Age
>   c. Specific disabilities, such as speech, hearing, and visual or other impairments.
> 4. How do people access this agency?
> 5. What are the agency's fees for services?
> 6. What types of insurance does the agency accept?
> 7. What hours is the agency open?
> 8. Do people need appointments to come to this agency?
> 9. Where does the agency keep patient records?
> 10. What is your impression of this agency?
> 11. Would you feel comfortable coming to this agency or referring a patient here? Why or why not?

People Who Are Hearing-Impaired

The nurse must be very patient when communicating with people who are hearing-impaired. A nurse needs to be aware that the hearing-impaired person's frustration is even greater than that of the nurse in trying to communicate. Try to establish a trusting, team-approach relationship with hearing-impaired patients. Let them know you will try whatever it takes for you to be able to understand each other. Find out what has worked for that person in the past.

Not all hearing-impaired people use sign language; some use lipreading. However, lipreading may be inaccurate and could lead to incorrect communication. Sometimes writing a note or providing the patient with a journal is an effective way to communicate with a person who is deaf or hard of hearing. Keep in mind the key factor is communication and not the patient's grammatical or spelling abilities.

People Who Are Visually Impaired

When a person is **visually impaired,** the nonverbal part of communication can be a challenge. Nursing is a highly affective art, so certain nonverbal cues, such as tone of voice, body position, and facial expressions, "speak" most strongly to patients. How does a sightless person or someone who is severely impaired visually interpret these nonverbal cues?

Nurses must learn to become detail-oriented storytellers. It is important to learn to describe to a visually impaired patient the location of the call signal, what the call signal sounds like, what the people in the hall are laughing at, why the voices suddenly switch to a whisper when another person enters the room, and who has just entered. Imagine walking into a crowded lunchroom, and everybody stops speaking. How does that feel? Similarly, sightless people cannot see a wave of the hand or see when someone leaves or enters a room; these events must be verbalized.

Patient teaching takes on a new dimension because it involves physically moving, touching, or verbally explaining in much more detail than usual. Learning to eat can be difficult for a newly sightless person. Usually, the teaching involves relating the food position to the numbers on a clock face. Sightless patients need to rely on their other senses to compensate for the eyes they cannot use.

Sometimes individuals have more than one need to be considered when the nurse communicates with them. For example, some people are both hearing impaired and visually impaired. When communicating with these individuals, a nurse needs to be creative. Investigate methods that have worked for this person in the past and explore methods such as a conversation board or printing the message on the person's palm.

As emphasized in any nursing fundamentals class, when beginning and exiting the patient's room, the nurse needs: to identify him-/herself, explain what procedure is being performed, make sure the patient is safe, and identify when leaving.

People Who Have Laryngectomies

Some people live with partial or total **laryngectomy**—the removal of their larynx ("voice box"). Imagine what it would be like to be able to speak one day and have no voice at all the next. The larynx is a body part that is very much taken for granted. How do such people answer the phone? How does a person order a pizza? How would such people express their emotions? Call for help?

People With Language Differences

Today's society is global. Even though English is the predominant language in the United States, it may not be the primary language for many of the people nurses work with and care for. As a nurse, you may find yourself in an area where you are the one who does not speak the primary language. How will you communicate? How will you ensure safe care of your patients? If the physician with a thick accent gives a verbal order, how will you know you have heard it correctly? What about those people who say they are speaking English, but you are not able to understand them? It can be very embarrassing and potentially insulting for all parties involved. Techniques for ensuring understanding are discussed at the end of this chapter.

People Who Have Aphasic/Dysphasic Disorders

A person with **aphasia/dysphasia** has either no speech or great difficulty with speech. The amount of speech a patient possesses is related to many things, such as age, cause of difficulty, and severity of involvement. There are different types of aphasia (Table 2-1).

Table 2-1 Types of Aphasia

Types of Aphasia	Description
Expressive	Difficulty expressing himself or herself in written or verbal forms of communication
Receptive	Difficulty interpreting or understanding written or verbal forms of communication.
Global	Combination of receptive and expressive forms of aphasia

It is up to the physician and the speech therapist to determine the cause and extent of involvement, but the nurse will be part of the plan of care. This will be a very individualized type of communication skill. Patients may know that the nurse has asked them for the comb; they may think they are handing the nurse the comb, but they actually hand the nurse the coffee cup. A patient may try to read aloud a passage from a book, but what comes out of the patient's mouth may be a long line of obscenities. The patient would be very embarrassed if he or she knew what was said. The nurse must be very understanding and willing to try repeatedly to have correct communication with persons with various forms of aphasia. Nurses also must remember that any "nasty words" are not to be taken personally; chances are very good that those words are really a sincere attempt by the patient to say, "Thank you, nurse." See the section headed "Adaptive Communication Techniques."

> **Classroom Activity**
> - Contact a representative from Americans with Disabilities, your state's Services for the Blind, or any of your local agencies that serve populations with special communication needs. Invite someone from one of these agencies to be a guest speaker.

> **Clinical Activity**
> In a clinical rotation, assign students (simulate if in the classroom) to care for a person with a communication challenge. Have the students describe how they altered their usual communication patterns to work with this individual.

Therapeutic Communication

It is possible to have a helping, therapeutic conversation with most people, but it takes some practice. These "techniques" need to be practiced in much the same way that one learns any other language: by hearing them, practicing them, and making them part of one's professional (and social) vocabulary.

Before reviewing therapeutic communication techniques, ineffective ones will be reviewed. There is an old saying that "the road to defeat is paved with good intentions." Sometimes, nurses' good intentions get them in trouble with their communication skills. Nurses can sometimes unintentionally set themselves up for **ineffective communication.** The following is a list of ways nurses "block," or impede, helpful interactions with patients:

1. *False reassurance/social clichés.* These are phrases nurses use in an effort to sound supportive. In social communication they sound friendly, but in a therapeutic relationship they invalidate the patient's concerns.

EXAMPLE	*EFFECT ON PATIENT*
"Don't worry! Everything will be just fine."	• Tells patient his or her concerns are not valid • May jeopardize patient's trust in nurse

2. *Minimizing/belittling.* These, too, are used socially to try to relieve the tensions of others. There is security in numbers, and sharing that many people are experiencing the same thing as the individual is somehow supposed to make the problem seem lighter. In therapeutic use, the implications are different.

EXAMPLE	*EFFECT ON PATIENT*
"We have all felt that way sometimes."	• Implies that the patient's feelings are not special.

3. "*Why?*" This simple word needs to be eliminated in therapeutic interactions. "Why" connotes disapproval or displeasure. "Why ask why?" is a good question for the health-care provider to remember. The patient often does not know "why" and can end up feeling responsible for providing an answer anyway. The nurse often needs to know "why," but there are other ways to ask that are less stress-producing for the patient.

EXAMPLE	***EFFECT ON PATIENT***
"Why did you refuse your breakfast?"	• Patient feels obligated to answer something he or she may not wish to answer or may not be able to answer • Probes in an abrasive way

4. *Advising.* Alcoholics Anonymous sometimes uses the statement, "Don't 'should' on yourself." Nurses also must not "should" on their patients. This sets the stage for expectations that the patient may not be able to meet. It also sets up, in the patient's mind, some sort of value system that puts the nurse's value as the "right" one. It can sound very judgmental.

EXAMPLE	***EFFECT ON PATIENT***
"You should eat more." "If I were you, I would take those pills so I would feel better."	• Places a value on the action • Gives the idea that the nurse's values are the "right" ones • Sounds parental

5. *Agreeing or disagreeing.* Socially, people agree or disagree for several reasons. Sometimes people are just expressing their opinion. Sometimes they are trying to make a favorable impression. Therapeutically, it is wise for nurses to avoid statements that express their own opinions or values. Even though some situations appear similar, there may be factors, which make them different.

EXAMPLE	***EFFECT ON PATIENT***
"You were wrong about that." "I think you're right."	• Places a "right" or "wrong" on the action

6. *Closed-ended questions.* These are forms of questions that make it possible for a one-word "yes" or "no" answer. They discourage the patient from giving full answers to the questions. Closed-ended questions are those that start with such phrases as "Can you," "Will you," "Are they," and "May I." It does not help to add *please*, as in "Please, may I ask you a question?" or "Will you please take out the trash?" This courtesy still leaves the possibility for the receiver to say "yes" or "no." The *please* makes it sound more polite in social venues, but the same questions can be made assertive and therapeutic by stating or asking for what one wants ("I need to ask you a question" or "Please take out the trash").

The general rule for making an open-ended question from a closed-ended question is to simply drop off the first one or two words.

This can also be accomplished by adding words like *how* and *what* to the beginning of the question.

Closed: "Can I help you?"

Open: "How can I help you?" or "What can I do to help you?"

EXAMPLE	***EFFECT ON PATIENT***
"Can you tell me how you feel?" "Do you smoke?" "Can I ask you a few questions?"	• Allows a "yes" or "no" answer • Discourages further exploitation of the topic • Discourages patient from giving information

7. *Providing the answer with the question.* This is a technique that television interviewers use frequently. The interviewee may say, "The interviewer put words into my mouth." For instance, a question that answers itself is, "Didn't you know that the committee would reject the proposal?" Occasionally, the body language of the interviewer or the sender may influence the answer. A better way to ask this question is, "What were your thoughts about how the committee might react?"

EXAMPLE	***EFFECT ON PATIENT***
"Are you afraid?" "Didn't the food taste good?" "Do you miss your mom today?"	• Combines a closed-ended question with a solution • Discourages patient from providing his or her own answers

8. *Changing the Subject.* Nurses sometimes do this inadvertently. When schedules are busy and several patients need a nurse's attention at the same time, the nurse's agenda takes over, and the nurse starts to see to personal needs. It is very easy for a nurse to give a quick answer to a patient's question and then proceed with one's own agenda. Unfortunately, that may send the message to the patient that the nurse does not care or that this problem is not worthy of a nurse's time. This patient may be reluctant to offer more information to that nurse in the future.

Changing the subject may also reflect the nurse's comfort (or discomfort) level with the subject. If the nurse just experienced the death of a loved one from a heart attack, for example, it may be very uncomfortable to answer a patient's questions about recovery and prognosis following his or her bypass surgery. The nurse may answer quickly and move on to a more comfortable topic, such as, "Well, your physician has advanced your diet; that's good news!"

EXAMPLE	*EFFECT ON PATIENT*
The patient is asking a question about his/her prognosis and the nurse responds with, "Did the doctor say anything about discharging you today?"	• Discounts the importance of the patient's need to explore personal thoughts and feelings • May be a reflection of the nurse's own discomfort level with this topic

9. *Approving or Disapproving.* This is similar to minimizing or agreeing. The patient perceives a value system that puts the nurse in the position of the expert, and, in many ways, the nurse is. That puts a big responsibility on a nurse's shoulders, however, and that responsibility includes being supportive without being judgmental or portraying a personal idea of what is right or wrong, good or bad.

The nurse is in a partnership of sorts with the patient. The nurse collaborates with the patient to determine the best way to help the patient help himself or herself. If the nurse can look at the relationship with that attitude, there is no "right" or "wrong," because each person is different. No two patients are the same, so what is helpful to each one is "right" for that patient.

EXAMPLE	*EFFECT ON PATIENT*
"That's the way to think about it! Good for you!" "That's not a good idea."	• Can sound judgmental • Can set the patient up for failure if the approval or disapproval does not help; can lower the nurse's credibility

Techniques of Therapeutic/ Helping Communication

Hildegard Peplau envisioned the nurse as a "tool" for ensuring positive interpersonal relationships with patients. Nurses are with the patient for approximately 8–12 hours daily. Compare that with the amount of time a physician is able to spend with the patient, and it is easy to see how the nurse becomes the therapeutic tool that helps the patient help himself or herself. This observation was noted by Florence Nightingale in her book, *Notes on Nursing* (Nightingale, originally published in 1859).

Patients develop a different kind of rapport with nurses because they learn to trust them. Although nurses' technical skills are very important and must never be allowed to get rusty, it is the appropriate use of their verbal and nonverbal communication skills that cements the relationship with patients and that ultimately promotes their healing.

The previous section pointed out some of the bad habits of conversation. It is now time to learn new effective methods of communication. These will feel awkward at first, but with practice and trust, they will help improve the quality of interactions not only with patients, but in most interpersonal communication as well. They are "tricks of the trade" that may be as small as a one-word change in the way a sentence or request is presented, but they get a lot of mileage in the way people respond.

Neeb's Tip The listed communication methods will not all work for all people in all circumstances, but if you use them faithfully you will see improvements in the way you relate to your patients and in the way they respond to you.

1. *Reflecting, repeating, parroting.* This technique seems to be the easiest to learn and therefore is used the most often. Parrots are often trained to repeat words or phrases, such as "Polly want a cracker?"

Reflecting, repeating, and parroting refer to this technique because that is what the nurse does: He or she picks a word or phrase that seems to be a key word or idea in what the patient is trying to communicate. It sometimes involves a degree of guessing on the part of the nurse to check out the perceived message. For instance, if the patient says, "I want to get out of here; everyone is against me," the nurse has several options for checking the main concern of the patient. The nurse will repeat a word or phrase from the patient's statement to reflect, or parrot, whatever is perceived to be the main concern. The nurse could say "Everyone?" or "Against you?" to try to encourage the patient to expand on these ideas. *Caution:* Because this technique might seem obvious to the patient, use parroting sparingly. It will not take the patient too many times of hearing his or her words repeated before perhaps suggesting that the nurse look into having a good audiometric examination!

EXAMPLE	***EFFECT ON PATIENT***
Patient: "I'm so tired of all of this." Nurse: "Tired?"	• Encourages exploring the meaning of the statement • *Caution: Use sparingly, can be irritating if overused.*

2. *Clarifying terms.* People live and work in a global society. Nurses interact with many different people as patients and coworkers. Nurses sometimes use words in different ways. The American vocabulary pronounces many words the same but spells them differently.

English is a very complex language to learn. Some people use terms very literally. Nursing is a profession that is filled with inference and nuance; it is highly affective. Because of that, it is very important to clarify terms with patients and other workers. Nurses must be sure that the terms they choose are correct and mean the same thing to all parties involved in the interaction. The technique is easy to learn: Simply asking "When you say 'I can't do that,' what do you mean?" is one way of clarifying a statement. The patient may mean "I am not physically able" or "I am not morally able" or "I do not know how to do that" or any number of things that the word *can't* may mean. If the nurse does not try to clarify that simple word, she could incorrectly infer the patient's level of ability or cooperation.

EXAMPLE	***EFFECT ON PATIENT***
"When you say 'tired,' do you mean it in a physical way or an emotional way?"	• Encourages patient to restate the comment • Improves chances that the message sent is the message received

3. *Open-ended questions.* These are the essence of successful nurse-patient communication. They are also among the hardest techniques to learn, because people are constantly bombarded with incorrect usage in social interaction and in the world of talk shows and news reporters.

One of the goals of helping communication is to get the patient to participate, so it is important that the nurse present questions in a way that will encourage the patient to provide information without the nurse's sounding persistent or intrusive. Such a perception by the patient will be a major interference in future attempts at communication. The nurse needs to be able to detect cues provided by the patient when they would like to discontinue communication.

In some instances, "yes" or "no" may be all the nurse needs to know or all that the patient is capable of responding at the time. In those instances, closed-ended questions may be used until the patient is able to provide more information. Otherwise, open-ended questions will get more productive results.

EXAMPLE	***EFFECT ON PATIENT***
"How are you feeling today?" "What can I do to help, Mr. Jones?"	• Discourages "yes" or "no" answers • Encourages patient to express self in his or her own terms

Using open-ended questions can be helpful in understanding the patient's pain level. Asking the patient "Are you in Pain?" (closed-ended question) may not bring an accurate picture. Depending on the patient's culture or religious preference, or both, "pain" may or may not be acceptable. The patient may answer "yes" or "no" on the basis of those beliefs. If Ms. Green has a chemical dependency that has not been shared with you, she may say "yes" to get the benefit of the pain medication. Pain is a very individual experience and is subjective. What one person considers to be extreme pain, another might brush off as a minor irritation. The closed-ended nature of this question does not require the patient to provide useful, measurable information that allows the nurse to be helpful or therapeutic. A more helpful form of this question would be in an open-ended format, such as, "Ms. Green, on a scale of 0 to 10, how do you rate your pain?" or "Ms. Green, please tell me about your pain."

4. *Asking for what you need or want.* This relates to the discussion on assertive versus aggressive communication. Nurses can ask for what is needed and wanted from patients and coworkers and still maintain a pleasant, professional tone of voice. This technique requires the user to start the sentence with the words "I want" or "I need." Taking the direct approach with people is usually the safest way to be sure that the receiver gets the message the sender intended to send.

These two examples show ways to be assertive, direct, and self-responsible while still maintaining politeness and allowing the patient to have some control over his or her care.

EXAMPLE	***EFFECT ON PATIENT***
"Mrs. Smith, I need to ask you a few questions, please." "I want to switch shifts with Mary next Tuesday, please."	• States purpose for the interaction • Keeps speaker assertive and self-responsible

5. *Identifying thoughts and feelings.* This is another difficult technique to master. Because words, which convey thoughts and feelings, are used incorrectly more frequently than not, it is hard to reinforce proper usage. The rule is simple: A feeling is an emotion. A "feeling statement" must identify an emotion that one is experiencing or is trying to explore with a patient. For example, "I feel proud that I earned this promotion" or "I feel frightened to walk alone at night."

A thought is an opinion, idea, or fact that one wishes to express. "I think I deserve this promotion" and "I think security needs to be improved in the parking area" are examples of "thinking statements."

"I feel security needs to be improved in the parking area" and "I feel the patient needs a different pain medication" are incorrect uses of the word "feel." There is no emotion identified in these statements. "Feeling" is certainly implied, but implied thoughts and feelings need to be clarified to avoid mistaken conclusions. In both of these statements "feel" should be replaced with "think" for correct usage.

Using words pertaining to thought and feeling correctly will minimize the amount of time the nurse must spend clarifying and will maximize the quality of the interaction. In the mental health specialty, it becomes even more important for the nurse to use such terms appropriately to help the patient identify and label his or her emotions and thoughts to facilitate therapy.

EXAMPLE	*EFFECT ON PATIENT*
"I feel angry when you are not honest with me." "I think honesty is important in all relationships."	• Helps the patient to identify and label thoughts and emotions • May give insight to underlying concerns or complications of healing

6. *Using empathy.* Empathy is also tied into feelings. There is a big difference between sympathy and empathy. Sympathy is used socially when people wish to share emotional experiences. It is not a therapeutic technique because it involves experiencing the emotion. Empathy involves identifying emotions without experiencing the emotion. Nurses need to use empathy with patients. They need to be able to identify the emotion and relate to it while keeping the focus on the patient's needs. Nurses must help patients deal with their feelings and still maintain professional control of the situation; the nurse needs to remain the helper.

Sympathy often allows both persons to become emotionally invested in the moment. The focus is shared by both people. In therapeutic relationships, the focus must remain on the patient.

Consider the following situation: A nurse notices a patient crying in the lounge. The nurse wants to help, so he approaches the patient, sits down, and offers his assistance. The patient tells the nurse of the news that that she just found out that her pet died. The pet had been her "family" since her divorce. The pet had always "been there for her," and the pet has died while she has been in the hospital and could not be there. The nurse's response options are:

Sympathy: Remembering his own favorite pet who died, the nurse says, "I understand your feelings; my pet died suddenly, too."

OR

Empathy: Remembering his own pet who died, the nurse allows himself to feel that pain and then says, "I am so sorry. It must be very painful to lose something you feel so close to. I'd like to hear about your pet when you think you'd like to talk about it."

Socially, chances are that the nurse might take the "sympathy" option, which would be appropriate with people who are not patients. Patients need the nurse to be sensitive but still be the helper. The "empathy" option is more appropriate in most therapeutic situations.

EXAMPLE	*EFFECT ON PATIENT*
"It must feel very demeaning when others are dishonest." "I can only imagine how difficult this has been."	• Acknowledges patient's feelings • Keeps nurse in position of control and helpfulness

7. *Silence.* Silence serves many functions in communication, yet many people are very uncomfortable with it. American society seems to value conversation. People use vocabulary and the ability to talk about a variety of topics as a measure of intelligence and social grace. Watch what happens at a social gathering or in the break room when a short silence occurs. Often, people fidget nervously or make "small talk" just to break the silence.

Silence, as a therapeutic technique of communication, serves two main purposes: First, it allows the nurse and the patient a short time to collect their thoughts and, second, it shows patience and acceptance on the part of the nurse. Sitting quietly for a period of time, usually 2 to 3 minutes, and maintaining an open body posture sends the message that the nurse is willing to wait if the patient has more to say or that the nurse accepts the fact that the interaction may be over for the present. Silence can be just as powerful and effective as any verbal interaction.

Caution: Do not allow the silence to go on too long. If nothing has been said by either party within 2 to 3 minutes, it is wise to suggest to the patient that it might be time for a rest. Then the nurse should take cues from the patient's response. Perhaps the conversation will begin again, or maybe the patient will be grateful for the suggestion to rest. Either way, the nurse can let the patient know that he or she is there if the patient wants to talk again at another time.

EXAMPLE	*EFFECT ON PATIENT*
Sit quietly near the patient	• Shows the nurse is comfortable with whatever the patient says and willing to hear more • Allows both to collect their thoughts

Neeb's Tip Silence demonstrates that the nurse is willing to hear more.

8. *Giving information.* This is very different from the **communication block** of giving advice. Giving information relates to the helping relationship because it involves a form of teaching.

As mentioned earlier, physicians are usually with their patients for very short periods of time, whereas nurses are usually with the same patients for an 8–12 hour shift. It is very natural for nurses and patients to have more quality time for talking. This is one reason patient teaching is becoming a bigger part of a nurse's responsibility in all levels of nursing.

Nurses provide information in all phases of hospitalization, from preoperative teaching to discharge planning. It involves using pamphlets, videos, resource manuals, or other resource persons.

Neeb's Tip Most state nurse practice acts still place the stipulation that the nurse may not legally give information to the patient before the physician has given the *initial* information. This means that nurses may not give lab reports, read diagnostic information, talk about possible treatments, and so forth until these have first been discussed between physician and patient. How do nurses know this has occurred? Nurses use therapeutic techniques that allow them to ask questions that get results.

Using this combination of offering assistance and asking an open-ended question serves several purposes: The nurse has maintained rapport and has gotten Mrs. Brown to divulge her level of prior knowledge, and the nurse has let Mrs. Brown know that the nurse presumes she has had a conversation with the physician. What if Mrs. Brown hesitates or tells the nurse outright that the physician has not been in yet? The nurse should use the techniques of stating his or her needs and using empathy, and tell the patient very honestly, "Mrs. Brown, I can sense your frustration, but I cannot legally (or ethically) give you that information until you and your physician have discussed it first. I'll be happy to call your physician to let her know that you wish to see her as soon as possible. After you have talked, I'll be happy to answer any questions you may have."

EXAMPLE	*EFFECT ON PATIENT*
"Mrs. Brown, I would be glad to explain this diagnosis to you. Tell me what the doctor has said, and I'll clarify it for you any way I can."	• Increases rapport • Eases patient's anxiety • Honestly confirms that the physician has given prior information • Suggests collaboration

9. *Using general leads.* This is a method of encouraging the person to continue speaking. It lets the speaker know that one is listening and interested in hearing more. The technique is fairly simple: It involves verbal and usually nonverbal communication. Examples of general leads are saying "Yes?" while maybe raising the eyes, "Go on" while maintaining eye contact and possibly nodding the head in an affirmative motion, or just saying "and then?" if the person pauses in the middle of a statement or concern.

EXAMPLE	*EFFECT ON PATIENT*
"Go on" while nodding head and maintaining eye contact	• Feels valued and listened to

10. *Stating implied thoughts and feelings.* This takes a combination of skills. It requires using some guessing (as in reflecting), using empathy, and making an observation about a behavior or condition the nurse sees in the patient.

This technique is helpful in initiating conversation that might be difficult to start with other techniques. It is hard to deny that something is not right when someone identifies a specific behavior or action that supports the suggestion that something is different about the patient. Nurses are assessing their patient's physical and emotional states all the time.

When a patient is reluctant to share this situation, the nurse can preface the question with an observation and then follow with an educated guess at the emotion that is being experienced.

EXAMPLE	*EFFECT ON PATIENT*
"Ms. Johnson, you're not smiling today like you usually do. I sense something is bothering you. How can I help?"	• Lets the patient know you are paying attention to him or her • Identifies a specific behavior or change in behavior, which lowers the chance of denying it • Patient hears that the nurse cares and wishes to help

Adaptive Communication Techniques

Some populations of people, such as those mentioned in the previous section, require special considerations when nurses are communicating with them. These are some ways of facilitating communication with people who live with certain disabilities or who have varied amounts of ability.

People Who Are Hearing-Impaired

When communicating with a patient who is hearing-impaired, it is important to know the extent of the impairment. Does the person speech-read (also called lip-read)? Is he or she reliant on a hearing aid? What is the emotional attitude of the patient?

Communicating can be very frustrating for hearing-impaired patients as well as for the nurse. Hearing-impaired patients often use sign language, but most "hearing" people do not know sign language. Sometimes writing with pencil and paper is effective, but it is slow. Speech reading is helpful to some hearing-impaired people, but it is not always accurate. Because many words that look the same are in fact very different in meaning, and because not all speaking people say words the same way (because of dialect or different primary language from that of the hearing-impaired person), speech reading can be misleading at best.

Tool Box ▶ This Web site can be used to access American Sign Language vocabulary: http://commtechlab.msu.edu/sites/aslweb/browser.htm

People Who Are Visually Impaired

Adaptive devices such as audio books, Braille-prepared computers, and seeing-eye dogs can be extremely helpful. The type of adaptive device depends on the type and severity of the impairment. Technology has provided some methods, such as the ability to change the font size on a computer up to 500%. Visually impaired people often have heightened senses of hearing, touch.

Neeb's Tip Do not assume that visually impaired people may be hearing impaired, too. It usually is not necessary to talk slower or louder to a person with a visual impairment.

People Who Have Laryngectomies

Technology has developed several different aids that amplify the vibrations of speech. For some patients with laryngectomies, placing an amplifier over the area of the larynx and talking will produce a buzzing sound that replicates their former voice. It is a monotone sound, but it greatly improves the ability of these patients to communicate in a more natural manner. Not everyone can use these devices, however. Some people need to rely on communication boards and pictures to communicate. Some people make use of new computer-assisted devices. The patient will be in close contact with a speech therapist. Nurses need to be involved with the therapist as well, so that the patient has continuity of therapy and good evaluation of the ability to use the devices. The patient's plan of care needs to identify how the speech therapist treatment plan can continue when the patient is discharged from therapy. The goal is to restore the person to his or her surgical maximal ability of speech. It can be a frightening and frustrating time for the patient and the health-care team, but the rewards are great when speech, at whatever level, begins to return.

People With Language Differences

Honesty is the best policy here. This discussion comes up in several sections of this text, but it is much better to apologize and admit when one is not receiving the sender's message. Serious mistakes can be made when one assumes the meaning of the message. It is also important to remember that communicating is often a highly cultural activity; people are not always comfortable asking for correction or clarification from someone of a different gender, age, or social or professional status. Using assertive, honest communication skills will usually get positive results.

Neeb's Tip As a caregiver, the nurse needs to practice active listening. When not positive about the meaning of a message, ask!

People Who Have Aphasic/ Dysphasic Disorders

This is another area that offers many options for adaptive techniques. Nurses must be aware of the type and degree of aphasia/dysphasia for each patient. The physician and speech pathologist or therapist are excellent resource people to help in deciding what type of adaptive technique will be the most effective. The nurse's documentation of the responses of a patient to the various techniques will also help in these decisions.

Techniques range from changing the rate or pitch of speech to using objects, pictures, spelling boards, or computerized equipment if the patient has access to them (Fig. 2-3). However, nurses should not answer for the patient. Finishing sentences or trying to play guessing games with people who have these types of disorders is usually not in the best interest of the patient. It may take a longer time for these patients to process the information

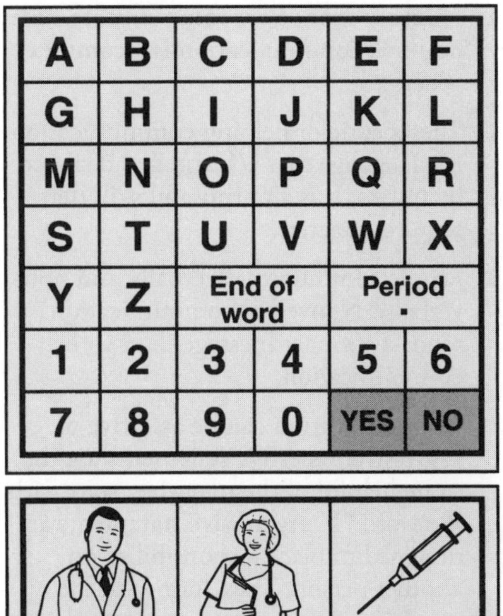

Figure 2-3 Picture board for patients with aphasia.

and get the answer out. Be patient. When the patient is getting frustrated or is truly unable to respond properly, it may be because the words the nurse used were unfamiliar or maybe too much time has passed and the patient has forgotten the question. Gentle hints or rephrasing the question may be enough to help the patient. It may be just one word that makes the difference between the patient's being successful or not.

Communication in all forms is essential to the work of a nurse. Taking the time to learn and use these techniques can make relationships with patients and coworkers very pleasant and rewarding.

■■■ Key Concepts

1. Humans cannot *not* communicate. Interpersonal communication is a complex process.
2. Therapeutic or helping communication is a language that is learned and shared by nurses. It is a purposeful skill that requires practice.
3. People communicate verbally and nonverbally. Nonverbal communication sends a stronger message than verbal communication.
4. Communication can be assertive or aggressive. Assertive statements are the more helpful of the two; they start with the word "I." Aggressive statements are designed to place responsibility on another person. They start with the word "you."
5. Nurses need to be aware of what blocks therapeutic communication.
6. Nurses need to be aware what techniques to use to encourage effective, helping communication with patients.
7. Special techniques are used when communicating with populations who have special communication needs.

REFERENCES

Grinder, J., and Bandler, R. *Trance Formations—Neuro-Linguistic Programming and the Structure of Hypnosis*, Moab, Utah: Real People Press, 1981.

Nightingale, F. (1969). *Notes on Nursing: What It Is, and What It Is Not.* New York: Dover Publications.

Townsend, M.C. (2012) Psychiatric Mental Health Nursing. 7th ed. Philadelphia: F.A. Davis.

Test Questions

Multiple Choice Questions

1. Which of the following is an example of a therapeutic, open-ended question?
a. "Why did you do that, Mrs. Jones?"
b. "How can I help you, Mr. Thompson?"
c. "Can I help you, Ms. Greene?"
d. "Please, can I ask you a question, Mark?"

2. The purpose of "therapeutic communication" is to:
a. Develop a friendly, social relationship with the patient.
b. Develop a parental, authoritarian relationship with the patient.
c. Develop a helping, purposeful relationship with the patient.
d. Develop a cool, businesslike relationship with the patient.

3. You observe a patient in the family lounge. She appears to be talking to herself. You want to find out what is wrong. Your best approach to her might be:
a. "Who are you talking to?"
b. "Please stop talking. You are disturbing the other people."
c. "I saw your lips moving. Can you tell me what you are talking about?"
d. "Why are you talking to yourself?"

4. Your patient asks you the results of his blood tests. You respond:
a. "They are all negative."
b. "Why do you want to know?"
c. "I think you should wait until your physician comes in."
d. "I am not able to tell you right now, but I will call your physician and have her stop in to explain them to you."

5. Your patient is a single parent who has just been diagnosed with terminal cancer. She is concerned about returning to work and asks many questions. Finally, the patient says, "What do you think I should do?" You say:
a. "I think you should just stay busy."
b. "I wouldn't worry about it."
c. "What are your thoughts about returning to work?"
d. "Oh, you'll be just fine. There are lots of people worse off than you."

6. Your patient has refused all of your attempts to care for him. You say:
a. "I'd like to help you; what can I
b. "Why don't you like me?"
c. "What is the matter with you?"
d. "You must do this; physician's o

7. Your patient is Jewish and refuses t non-kosher food. You say:
a. "I will ask the dietitian to come talk with you."
b. "The dietitian will come to see y
c. "It's the best we can do. You nee to eat."
d. "You're right. The hospital food leave much to be desired!"

8. Your patient is commenting that t physician has not been in to visit f two days. You say:
a. "I hate it when that happens!"
b. "What do you need to know?"
c. "Well, he is very busy!"
d. "You feel ignored by your physic

9. Your patient, who is usually very talkative, does not respond to you when you enter the room. You say
a. "Ms. Smith, you are so quiet thi afternoon. Is something botheri you?"
b. "Ms. Smith, is something bothe you?"
c. "Can I help you?"
d. "Why are you so quiet this afternoon?"

10. Ms. Smith responds to your questi (see #9), "I feel like nobody cares." respond:
a. "Why do you say that?"
b. "Like nobody cares? Please try t describe the emotion you are tr 'feeling.'"
c. "Ms. Smith, you're wrong about Of course we care."
d. "Ms. Smith, maybe the doctor c change the dosage of your medi tion. You'll feel better."

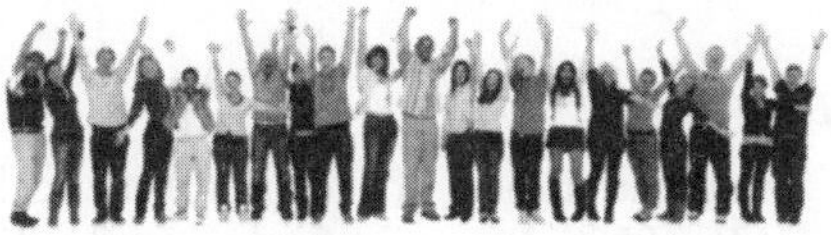

CHAPTER 3

Ethics and Law

Learning Objectives

1. Define professionalism.
2. Demonstrate understanding of the Nurse Practice Act.
3. State the importance of honesty and accuracy in verbal reporting and written documentation.
4. State the importance of confidentiality.
5. Define HIPAA and its role in health-care delivery.
6. Define the Joint Commission and its role in health-care delivery.
7. Explain the Good Samaritan Act.
8. Explain involuntary commitment.
9. Define patient advocacy.

Key Terms

- Accountability
- Advocacy
- Civil law
- Commitment
- Confidentiality
- Culture
- Culture of nurses
- Doctrine of privileged information
- Ethics
- Health Insurance Portability and Accountability Act (HIPAA)
- Intentional
- Patient Bill of Rights
- Professional
- Proxemics
- Responsibility
- Tort
- Unintentional

Professionalism

Professional is a word with many different meanings. Merriam-Webster Online defines *professional* as an adjective meaning "characterized by or conforming to the technical or ethical standards of a profession." It may be a term that requires a nurse to rely on the therapeutic communication skill of clarifying.

Nursing is a profession. Nurses care for patients and perform designated services for a salary. As a profession, however, the different levels of nursing disagree as to who is a "professional nurse." All nurses receive pay for their work, yet it is commonly accepted that only registered nurses (RNs) are considered professional nurses; the licensed practical nurse (LPN) or licensed vocational nurse (LVN) is considered a nonprofessional. In areas with union representation in nursing, the two levels usually belong to separate organizations. Some nursing groups believe that only RNs who are baccalaureate-prepared and beyond are considered professional.

Nevertheless, all nurses are expected to behave in a professional manner; they are to perform at the highest level of preparation they have achieved. Nurses are to abide by federal, state, and local guidelines. Another aspect of professionalism is the duty to stay informed in the nursing field. Participating in professional organizations and continuing education programs is important.

Professional behavior is maintained despite any personal problems a nurse is experiencing. A nurse's personal problems are to be handled outside of the work environment. Nurses are expected to be respectful of the beliefs of their patients and coworkers and not to force their personal beliefs on others at work. Nurses are expected to perform honestly. They are expected to report any infractions they notice in other nurses. In short, nurses are expected to behave and perform in a manner that promotes the pride and reputation of the nursing profession, and not as a detriment to that profession.

Critical Thinking Question

You are an LPN or an LVN on the surgical unit of the county hospital. In shift report, you are told that you will be getting a new postoperative patient within the hour. When the patient arrives, a police officer is in attendance. The officer tells you that this patient is a suspect in a homicide. The officer instructs you to report anything the patient says to you. When you begin your postoperative vital signs, the patient says, "Nurse, I shot the guy and he deserved it. I'll do it again if I have to. I can tell you, because you can't tell anyone!" How will you handle this situation?

Ethics

Part of being a professional is to conduct oneself in an appropriate and ethical manner. Nurses deal with ethical issues on a daily basis, so it is important to consider one's own values and professional **ethics.** The Codes of Ethics of the American Nurses Association and the National Federation of Licensed Practical Nurses (Appendix D) have established guidelines for the nursing profession. These guidelines provide a framework for action rather than give answers to questions.

Tool Box ▶ The Code of Ethics from the American Nurses Association can be reviewed at: www.nursingworld.org/codeofethics

Standards of Care

The National Federation of Licensed Practical Nurses (NFLPN) has adopted Standards of Nursing Practice for LPNs/LVNs (see Appendix D). These standards include a code of conduct. The American Nurses Association (ANA) has written a variety of standards of care covering topics important to the nursing profession. Some of these are relevant to LVNs/LPNs. The purpose of the ANA is fostering high standards of nursing practice, promoting the rights of nurses in the workplace, projecting a positive and realistic view of nursing, and lobbying Congress and regulatory agencies on health-care issues affecting nurses and the public. A set of Standards of Psychiatric–Mental Health Clinical Nursing Practice, written by the American Psychiatric Nurses Association (APNA), is available at the APNA Web site as well as ANA Web site. The revised standards are to be published in 2014.

Tool Box ▶ ANA materials can be accessed at: www.nursingworld.org
Standards of Psychiatric–Mental Health Clinical Nursing Practice draft Web site: www.apna.org/files/public/12-11-20-PMH_Nursing_Scope_and_Standards_for_Public_Comment.pdf

Nurse Practice Act

Nurses must be aware of their state's Nurse Practice Act and perform within its parameters. The Nurse Practice Act dictates the acceptable scope of nursing practice for the different levels of nursing. When a nurse is questioning whether or not to perform a certain skill or perhaps is accused of wrongdoing, the Nurse Practice Act typically is consulted to find out if that nurse is performing at the accepted level of preparation. For example, if a state does not allow the LPN/LVN to supervise patient care yet an LPN or LVN is the only licensed staff on duty on the night shift, the Nurse Practice Act for that state may have been ignored, and that nurse could be held liable for damages in a court of law.

This can be an ethical dilemma as well. It may be the facility's interpretation that it is permissible to allow that LPN/LVN to function as supervisor if an RN is on call. This may or may not be the interpretation of the particular state. The Board of Nursing in a particular state can give the answer. Any nurse has the right and responsibility to make that phone call.

> **Classroom Activity**
> - In Appendix E, review NFLPN Nursing Practice Standards Legal/Ethical Status. Write a paragraph on how each of these standards relates to a practical/vocational nurse.

Accuracy

The ultimate goal of the helping person in health care is to "do no harm." Safety for their patients and themselves must be in nurses' thoughts at all times.

Harm can be described as **intentional** or **unintentional** and falls under the category of a **tort,** which relates to civil law. **Civil laws** protect patients/persons and their property.

A nurse's best defense is the quality of verbal and written communication. In her book, *Legal, Ethical, and Political Issues in Nursing,* Tonia Aiken indicates that spelling errors are crucial in liability cases, as they reflect on a nurse's general ability to care for patients. Legally, the general assumption is "if it is not charted, it has not been done." Some situations can impede nurses' efforts at accuracy in charting. First of all, nurses are busy. Patient care is the primary focus of a nurse's workday. Many times, it seems that the shift is over before it starts. Charting may be scaled down to a minimum, especially if the employer does not pay for overtime. As accurate charting is part of nursing care, this became the rationale for developing different types of charting.

Some facilities use a form of charting that may be called "charting by exception." This type of documentation is based on flow-sheet charting. Normal values, the guidelines for which are established at the facility, are written on the chart form, and the nurse uses a series of check marks and arrows to indicate assessments of all systems have been made. The nurse then initials the check marks and arrows and uses a full signature at the bottom of the page. Only situations outside of the established normal parameters are mentioned in some sort of nurse's note. Although this type of charting saves time, it is sometimes challenged legally because it is not always enough documentation. Yet flow sheet charting is gaining popularity in documenting health care.

Many facilities use flow-sheet charting, and an increasing number are using electronic programs designed for patient charting that are specific for a facility. "Epic" is one of the electronic programs used by many facilities.

> **Neeb's Tip**
> The nurse needs to be proficient in reading, writing, and spelling skills. Nursing programs use a system including testing to determine if nursing candidates are proficient in reading, writing, and math prior to being admitted into a program (e.g., HESI's, TEAS V). Not only might gaps in reading, writing, and spelling be a source of extreme embarrassment to the nurse, but they are also unacceptable as professional, safe nursing practice. It is important to note as well that this is a much more common problem in the United States than one might think and that it is not just people from other countries who experience this difficulty. Basic computer skills are also increasingly required.

It is imperative that the nurse take (subjunctive) as much time as necessary to carry out complete, accurate documentation on each patient. A nurse's competency to practice nursing can be questioned if for some reason the documentation is subpoenaed in a court case and spelling and grammar are of poor quality according to American standards.

All agencies have an established method for verbal reporting. It may be a taped shift report, a grand rounds type of report, or a one-on-one report with the patient's care plan. Again, it is important for the nurse to spend as much time as needed to get the message from his or her day's work to the receiver for the oncoming shift. Be thorough but as concise as possible. It is usually standard procedure to discuss vital signs, physical assessments, any visits from physicians or visitors, new orders, responses to medications and treatments, and any change in condition. An area that is sometimes forgotten is the mental, emotional, and behavioral status of the patient, especially on a medical surgical unit. Usually, the patient's mental, emotional, and behavioral status is mentioned only if something seems inappropriate. Physical healing is to a large extent a result of attitude and emotional condition; therefore, nurses should include the patient's psychological status in their verbal report. A nurse should always check with the incoming nurse to be sure that there are no further questions and inform that nurse of anything he may not have completed.

Critical Thinking Question

You are the nurse who is supervising care on the shift 2100 to 0700. Another nurse who works this shift routinely has poor-quality charting. Nothing is hidden or omitted from the chart, but it contains many misspelled words and many grammatical errors. You decide to "keep the peace" and say nothing because you get along well with this nurse and the patients like the individual. Patient X falls out of bed on your shift, and the family sues for negligence. The other nurse is found incompetent by virtue of written documentation that the lawyers cannot decipher. To your dismay, you are also implicated as the supervising nurse on that shift because you did nothing to improve the quality of this nurse's writing skills. What are your feelings? What might this mean for you? What will your defense be to the court? How will you handle this differently in the future?

Honesty

It may seem insulting to discuss honesty and integrity with nursing students. After all, honesty, or "veracity" as it is also called, is one of the qualities of professionalism. The discussion is necessary, though, because honesty means different things to different people. It may mean "surviving" or "helping someone less able than myself" or "telling the physician what he or she wants to hear." Honesty is a concept that can be highly cultural.

The professional choice is always to tell the truth. It may be painful, frightening, or embarrassing to admit personal conflicts or errors or omissions in patient care, but nurses will avoid further potential harm to their patient as well as to their professional reputation by admitting to mistakes and taking the appropriate corrective measures. Nurses are human. Despite their best efforts and multiple medication checks, nurses make mistakes. Recognizing them, admitting them, and taking corrective measures to ensure the patient's safety are the signs of sound judgment and professional nursing behavior. Honesty can also mean the difference between keeping and losing your nursing license.

Impaired Nurses

Inappropriate use and misuse of mind-altering chemicals such as alcohol or prescription and nonprescription drugs can render a nurse legally unsafe. Continuing to practice nursing while using these chemicals displays unprofessional behavior and poor judgment. A nurse in this situation who is fearful of losing his or her license or unable to seek help may consider inaccurate charting, omission of certain charting, or blatant lying about a situation as a way to remain employed. The patient's safety is not the nurse's primary concern when this happens. Most states have developed programs to assist impaired nurses as a way to protect the public. According to the Recovery and Monitoring Program (RAMP) in New Jersey, if a health professional is impaired and working with patients, an occupational hazard eventually will occur, possibly causing an injury or even a death.

Critical Thinking Question

You are working on an Oncology unit, and a nurse who has been considered reliable and accountable by all of his/her coworkers in the past is now suspected of some type of impairment due to recent changes in behavior. This nurse frequently offers to give your patients pain medicines if you are busy. The nurse's coworkers have noted that immediately before or after giving a narcotic, the nurse usually has to use the bathroom. How would you approach this situation?

Culture of Nurses

A commonly accepted definition of **culture** includes nonphysical traits, rituals, values, and traditions that are handed down from generation to generation. Nursing is an occupation that passes its professional values, rituals, and traditions from generation to generation (Fig. 3-1). The affective, or attitudinal, components of nursing are behaviors that nurses typically learn from role modeling other nurses. This concept spawned the term **culture of nurses** (Neeb, 1994).

As mentioned earlier, nurses live and work in a global community. Nurses were born and raised in many different places. They have different ideas about politics and social issues. However, when nurses come together as a profession, they meld these ideas into consistent behaviors to provide their patients with the best possible care. Nurses may need to give up some personal ideas while working to make the whole of nursing greater than the sum of its parts. This means that skills such as spelling and grammar that may be "correct" or actually considered unimportant in personal situations are not acceptable for practicing nursing in the United States (Aiken, 2004). This is not an issue of labeling a nurse's personal or cultural belief system as right, wrong, good, or bad. Rather, it means that nurses must remember the components of professionalism and basic tenets of communication.

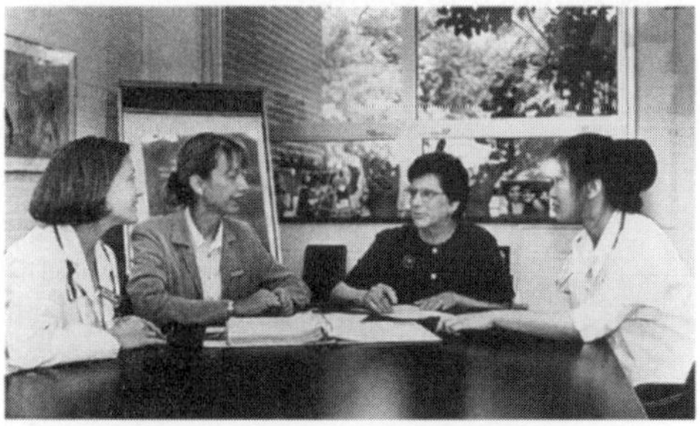

Figure 3-1 The culture of nursing. Through role modeling, professional values, rituals, and traditions are passed from one generation of nurses to the next. *(From Sorrell and Redmond (2007):* Community-Based Nursing Practice: Learning Through Students' Stories. *Philadelphia: F.A. Davis Company, with permission.)*

The field of study called **proxemics** is also cultural. Proxemics concerns space, time, and waiting, which are all influenced by one's culture. If you have ever traveled between the northern and southern tier of the United States, you may have noticed a cultural difference in time and waiting. People in the northern states tend to be much more rushed. They may watch the clock in restaurants, in classrooms, and while on hold on the telephone. In the southern states, life is a bit slower-paced. That hamburger does not have to be served in 2 minutes; people just wait and relax. This is not an issue of right or wrong, good or bad. It is an issue of differences in the way people are acculturated.

For nurses from countries in which timeliness is not an issue, punching a time clock or serving a medication within the allotted time may not be a priority. As nurses know, however, this sort of timeliness is a very important part of nursing culture. A patient who is in pain and asks for a pain medication expects the nurse to be prompt with it. If the nurse replies, "I'll be there in a minute," the patient might hear the word "minute" and take it quite literally. After all, the patient is the one in need. It may actually have taken the nurse 15 minutes to return with the medication, and in that time he or she may have answered two more call signals, helped someone to the bathroom, and taken a physician's order. However, that patient who is waiting for the medication knows only that the nurse did not return in a minute. Depending on that patient's culture, he may have used the call signal immediately after 1 minute passed or may feel it is grossly disrespectful to ask again and thus suffer silently.

Space and distance also constitute a big part of nursing culture. Nurses must touch patients in order to do their jobs. Nurses make full body assessments, catheterize, give suppositories, and perform prenatal and postnatal checks. Male and female nurses work on male and female patients. In a way, nurses become desensitized to these functions, as they become a routine part of their jobs.

Some patients are very timid and modest. In some cultures, strangers may not touch strangers in certain ways, and these individuals may prefer to have family members perform those tasks. Some nurses feel uncomfortable waking postoperative patients for their routine vital signs check because in their culture it is not proper to awaken sick people; it is proper to let them sleep and not disturb them. Nurses need to be aware of four types of spaces: public, social, personal, and intimate. Nurses are often in intimate space in their practice, especially when giving direct care.

Proxemics is a very complex field of study; this discussion has touched only on some basics. It is important for nurses to understand, however, that the concepts of space, time, and waiting are highly cultural in their interpretation.

Tool Box |▶ 2011 A guide to cross-cultural etiquette and understanding can be found at www.culturecrossing.net/

Nurses must work together for the betterment of patient care. When in doubt, ask. Learn from each other. There is no better way for personal and professional enrichment.

■ Confidentiality

Confidentiality is so important that it is singled out as one of the federal and state patient rights. Confidential means (1): marked by intimacy or willingness to confide; (2): private, secret (*confidential* information); (3): entrusted with confidences, and (4): containing information whose unauthorized disclosure could be prejudicial to the national interest (Merriam-Webster online).

Trusting a friend with a secret only to hear that secret had been repeated to someone else is a break in confidentiality. In a manner of speaking, a patient's diagnosis and plan of care are a secret to everyone but the patient and the health-care team; this information is very private and must be kept that way. But what happens when the patient shares something that must be passed on?

The **doctrine of privileged information** is a bond between patient and physician. Under this doctrine, the physician has the right to refuse to answer certain questions (e.g., in a court of law) and can cite "privileged physician-patient information." Nurses are usually not included in this relationship. If information is requested of nurses in a legal situation, they must answer as truthfully as they can. How does one maintain honesty and confidentiality at the same time? First and foremost, a nurse should communicate honestly to the patient that he or she cannot make promises. When the nurse senses that the patient is revealing information that is potentially legally sensitive, it is a good idea to tell the patient right away that nurses are not protected by the doctrine of privileged information. The nurse should tell the patient that he or she can call the physician, but if the patient still chooses to share such information, a good technique is to tell the patient the information will have to be shared with a supervisor or others involved in the patient's treatment. The 1976 case of *Tarasoff vs. Regents of the University of California* is the standard for the doctrine of privileged information. The doctrine also protects intended victims of patients who may be hospitalized or incarcerated. A nurse should inform the patient that only those parts of the conversation that are directly related to his or her care will be shared, but that if information is requested by a legal representative, the nurse will be required to answer.

Neeb's Tip When you sense that the patient is telling you information that is potentially legally sensitive, it is a good idea to tell the patient right away that you as a nurse are not protected by the Doctrine of Privileged Information.

Temptations are common, especially for the student nurse. It is fun and exciting to learn new information and to see your skills making a difference in someone's recovery. It is easy to start chatting about your experiences to another student or to a staff nurse, but be careful. The person nearby (e.g., in the elevator with you) may be a friend or family member. Unless specifically indicated by the patient, these people do not ordinarily have rights to information about the patient. There are many horror stories about innocent conversations that were overheard by the "wrong" people, which resulted in negative consequences to the patient and/or the nurse involved.

Whoever said hospitals were quiet places probably never worked in one. Nurses and physicians talk often, and usually not quietly. "Dr. X is on the phone about Mrs. D's bowel surgery," calls the unit coordinator to the nurse across the hall. "Is Mr. B's insulin up yet?" asks the nursing assistant from the kitchenette. "Nurse Y needs to know." This happens not only in the hospital, but also in physicians' offices. Consider a situation in a physician's office where a nurse shouts from the front desk that she just received Mrs. A's urine specimen results. "My goodness! Mrs. A has enough *E. coli* in her urine to kill a horse." Unfortunately for Mrs. A, she was the last person to enter the office with the last name starting with an "A". The physician's office was not equipped with a glass partition between the waiting room and the front desk.

How many other patients or people passing through the area might have heard those interchanges? How would the patient feel if he or she knew that personal information had been handled so thoughtlessly? Remember that patients can interpret messages differently than a nurse. These breaches of confidentiality happen all the time, but that does not make them acceptable. Nurses must take the extra steps required to give or receive information quietly to the appropriate people (Fig. 3-2).

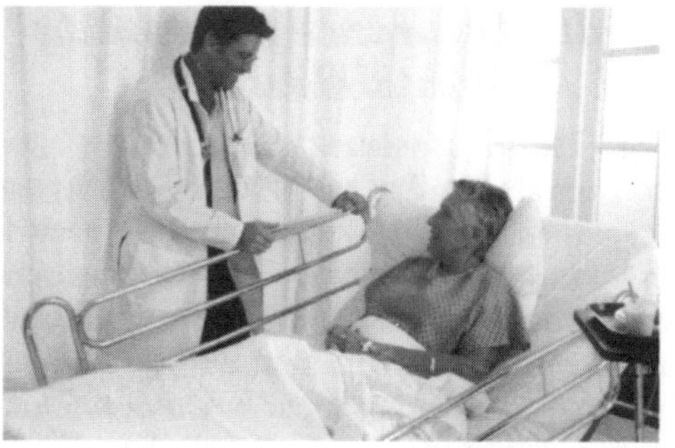

Figure 3-2 Maintaining privacy is a patient right and conveys caring to the patient. *(Photograph by Wendy Hope.)*

Charts, too, can put confidentiality at risk. How many eyes may have seen a chart accidentally left open when the nurse went to answer a call signal? What about the report sheet? Some nurses call these sheets their "brain's cheat sheet." Nurses should be sure to keep their reports with them at all times. Here is an example how a simple act of dropping a piece of paper led to a major event. The nurse's "cheat sheet" was found on the floor. The report sheet had fallen from a nurse's pocket and had been picked up by a patient's family member. This person could have brought the paper to the desk immediately and the story would have ended there, but that was not the case. At the end of the shift, the family member brought the piece of paper to the nurse in charge. None of the items on the list had been carried out, according to the family member who had been there the greater part of the day. Unfortunately for the nurse, the tasks had been charted as being completed. This display of unprofessional and irresponsible behavior was one thing; the family member maintained, however, that anyone could have picked up that piece of paper and learned many personal things about the patient. It contained information not only about that patient but perhaps information about other patients assigned to that nurse. The family member sued for breach of confidentiality and won the suit. Granted, this is a drastic example of what can happen, and laws regarding these situations vary from state to state. The story emphasizes that nurses must be careful with patient information of any kind and always maintain honesty in documentation. In these days of computerized, paperless documentation, nurses are vulnerable to breeches of confidentiality. The **Health Insurance Portability and Accountability Act of 1996 (HIPAA)** and the **Joint Commission** (JC) are intimately involved in documentation and privacy issues.

Health Insurance Portability and Accountability Act

The Health Insurance Portability and Accountability Act of 1996 (HIPAA) was developed by the Department of Health and Human Services to provide national standards pertaining to the electronic transmission and communication of medical information between patients, providers, employers, and insurers. HIPAA allows more control on the part of the patient as to what part of his or her information is disclosed. It addresses the security and privacy involved with medical records and how that information is identified and passed between care providers. For example, Social Security numbers, which were routinely used as a patient identifier in the recent past, now are either not used or are used in some manner that is difficult to track, such as a partial number or a backward number. HIPAA was implemented in April of 2003. Some areas of health care, such as workers' compensation, are either exempt from HIPAA rules or are slightly less stringent in the passing of information.

> **Clinical Activity**
> During your clinical rotation, observe the facility's Health Insurance Portability and Accountability Act (HIPAA) policy. Where is the policy located? Note during your clinical experience if the HIPAA policy is violated by whom and how many times.

In June of 2004, the U.S. Department of Health and Human Services Substance Abuse and Mental Health Services Administration Center for Substance Abuse Treatment published a 25-page document entitled "The Confidentiality of Alcohol and Drug Abuse Patient Records Regulation and the HIPAA Privacy Rule: Implications for Alcohol and Substance Abuse Programs." The document is located at www.samhsa.gov. It carefully details what can and cannot be disclosed and strongly emphasizes the patient's rights (discussed later in this chapter) and the necessity for the patient's signed informed consent (discussed in the Crisis Intervention section in Chapter 8).

Joint Commission

The Joint Commission (JC) is the leading national accrediting body of health-care organizations. Earning accreditation by the Joint Commission indicates commitment to quality on a daily basis within the entire facility. Two other goals of a JC accreditation are reducing the risk of undesirable patient outcomes and encouraging continuous improvement. Originally established to survey hospitals, the accreditation can now be achieved by long-term care facilities, mental health agencies, home health, and hospices to provide quality care, including mental health and substance abuse treatment to children, adolescents, and adults. Accredited facilities and clinics have demonstrated compliance with the highest standards of clinical care and administrative quality.

In 2004, the JC established the National Patient Safety Goals (NPSG). These goals are revised annually. Sentinel events, identifying the sources of hospital acquired infections (HAI), ensuring two-patient identifiers, and a list of "dangerous abbreviations" are among these goals.

> **Tool Box** ▶ Joint Commission Web site at:
> www.jointcommission.org
> **National Patient Safety Goals:**
> www.jointcommission.org/standards_information/npsgs.aspx

> **Critical Thinking Question**
> You have just started working on the medical unit in your hospital. You have been assigned a female patient called "Ms. X." You are curious about the fact that Ms. X is not using her real name. While reading her chart, you learn she is in an abusive relationship. You see the warning that "Ms. X's husband is not allowed in the unit at any time." When you go to meet the patient, you are shocked; Ms. X is your next-door neighbor. What do you do? What do you say to her husband? What do you say when your family asks you, "What happened?"

Responsibility

Responsibility is a key concept at all levels of nursing practice; however, responsibility does not necessarily mean independence. Responsibility for the professional RN can mean different things than it does for the LPN/LVN. Nurses are expected to know their scope of practice for their state. Responsibility means performing to the best of one's ability within the boundaries of that scope of practice. Sometimes this means knowing when to say "No." Sometimes it means calling the state governing agency to ask specific questions.

Responsible behavior for a nurse also means keeping his or her personal life in a manageable state. "Nurse, heal thyself" is not an unrealistic statement. Nurses need to be physically and emotionally prepared to be helpful to patients, and this cannot be done if one's personal health is neglected. Nobody wants to be tended by a nurse who is not sleeping well or is preoccupied with personal problems. A good rule for nurses is to follow the recommendations in their personal lives that they would give to their patients.

It is the nurse's responsibility to communicate with patients and coworkers. Nurses must be alert to changes in patients' conditions, both physical and psychological. The actions nurses perform, the observations they make, and the documentation they complete are the most effective ways to be helpful and to ensure continuity of care for patients.

Nurses also have a responsibility to their coworkers. Agencies have different ways of organizing the way nurses perform their jobs. Some agencies practice "team" nursing, and some assign primary-care patients for whom the nurse is responsible for managing care during the entire hospitalization. Some facilities use a "buddy" system to ensure help for lifting and to cover the patient load during breaks or meetings. Regardless of the system used, each nurse is in some way interdependent on other staff members.

Nurses also have a responsibility to communicate effectively with coworkers. Being familiar with the techniques of communication discussed in Chapter 2 will ensure that nurses are able to address these behaviors more assertively. The responsibility nurses have for each other professionally may be different from the kind they have for their patients, but it is every bit as important, for it ultimately affects the quality of care nurses are able to give.

Accountability

Accountability is part of working independently within his/her scope of practice. A nurse is accountable for his/her own actions. Being accountable is important in all settings, including hospital, long-term care, home care, office setting, and psychiatric facilities. It means knowing when to ask for help, finding a reference to refresh the memory, or looking up a medication that is not familiar. It means doing everything the nurse possibly can to ensure that he/she is providing the safest, most accurate care to patients. It means that when the nurse says he will follow through with an order or a request, he will do so.

> **Critical Thinking Question**
> You depend on the other staff members to come to work. What happens when you must work one or two people short? Who really suffers as a result? How do you feel when your "buddy" or helper overstays a break or mealtime? What is your response to that? How does that affect the amount of time your patients may have needed? What about your ability to perform safely when you are filling in for someone who is not there?

Abiding by the Current Laws

Good Samaritan Laws

Good Samaritan laws offer immunity for citizens who stop to help someone in need of medical help. Nurses, physicians, and other medically trained personnel may not always be protected by Good Samaritan laws. The Good Samaritan law came out of **tort** law. A tort is a "a wrongful act other than a breach of contract for which relief may be obtained in the form of damages or an injunction" (Merriam-Webster Online). The Good Samaritan law varies from state to state, so it is important to understand the implication of this law in your state. The basis for all Good Samaritan laws, however, is that a third party cannot be charged with negligence unless help is given recklessly or that person makes the situation significantly worse, according to the guidelines for that particular state.

Tool Box |▶ Link to Good Samaritan laws in other states:
www.heartsafeam.com/pages/faq_good_samaritan

Involuntary Commitment

Each state has its own regulations about people who need to be hospitalized against their will. This action is reserved for people exhibiting behavior that makes them potentially dangerous to themselves or to others. The average length of time for involuntary **commitment** is approximately 48 to 72 hours but could be more or less depending on state law. During this time, the person is observed and examined by the medical and nursing staff. The patient has full ability to exercise his or her rights under the **Patient Bill of Rights** in that state. At the end of the legal "hold," the patient chooses either to leave or to stay for further treatment. Most of the time, the patient realizes a need for help and stays.

Sometimes it is the professional opinion of the treatment team that the patient remains a threat to self or the community but that the patient cannot make the appropriate decision. This then becomes an issue of proving incompetence and becomes part of the legal system.

Voluntary Commitment

Most patients who are hospitalized for some type of mental illness are there voluntarily; that is, at some point they realized they needed help. It does not mean they will be happy to be there, of course. There remains a stigma in the United States about being hospitalized for problems relating to a person's emotions or behavior. Many times, society assumes that these disorders are weaknesses in character rather than illnesses. It can be embarrassing to be labeled "mentally ill"; this diagnosis can follow a person for life and affect his or her personal and professional relationships. Being diagnosed with a mental illness could possibly hinder a person from attaining life insurance. It is no wonder that sometimes people allow themselves to be hospitalized for a mental illness only as a last resort. Patients who agree to voluntary treatment are legally allowed to sign themselves out; this is often discouraged by the treatment staff except under certain situations, and it is possible for the staff to institute an involuntary commitment for a patient if they consider him or her to be potentially dangerous. Voluntary and involuntary commitment is discussed again in Chapter 8.

Nurses must be aware of all laws and circumstances affecting the commitment. They must maintain the physical and emotional safety of the patient during the time of hospitalization. Confidentiality is crucial. Educating the public will be helpful in continuing to eliminate the negative implications of issues surrounding mental illness.

■ Patients' Rights

In the 1960s, civil rights was at the forefront. Gaining rights for oppressed people of many backgrounds was actively sought by groups such as the American Civil Liberties Union (ACLU). It was largely due to the efforts of this group that civil rights were addressed for people in prisons and for those warehoused in institutions for the mentally ill.

By the 1980s, the Patient Bill of Rights became a requirement for people receiving care in a facility, as well as for the health-care workers providing that care. These requirements vary from state to state but are based on federal guidelines and are supported in most states. Agencies in states subscribing to a Patient Bill of Rights are to have the rights listed and displayed in a prominent place in the facility. Patients are to be informed of the implications of their rights and are to be given a copy of the Bill of Rights upon admission to the health-care facility. This also is mandated when care is provided in the home. Table 3-1 lists frequently adopted patient rights.

Table 3-1 Most Frequently Adopted Patient Rights

Patient Right	Description	Nursing Considerations
1. Treatment in the least restrictive alternative	Patients are not to be held in any stricter conditions than their behavior or diagnosis warrants.	Patients are not to be hospitalized if they can be treated as outpatients and are not to be kept in lockup if not dangerous, and so on. Check the agency protocol and physician's orders for the individual patient. You must still maintain safety for the patient and others.
2. Freedom from restraints and seclusion (except in emergencies)	Restraining can be with either physical or chemical restraints. Many areas require specific diagnosis-related restraint orders.	Be aware of the individual's diagnosis and correlating orders. • Make accurate observations and documentation about the patient's physical and behavioral response to restraint. • One guideline is to check circulatory function every half hour and to exercise and reposition the patient in restraint at least every 2 hours.
3. Give or refuse consent for medications/ treatments (including electroconvulsive therapy and psychosurgery)	All patients have the right to say yes or no to treatments that affect them. This must be *informed* consent, meaning the patient fully understands the treatment, potential outcomes, and potential effects of refusal.	Nurses can reinforce the physician's explanation of treatment. Examine the patient's understanding; if there is little or no understanding of treatment, the nurse needs to have the physician return and explain again to the patient and significant others.
4. Possess and have access to personal belongings	Anything of a personal nature that the patient wishes to remain with him or her must be given to the patient.	Carefully document any teaching about safety of personal items. If your local laws allow, have the patient sign a waiver of responsibility for personal items.
5. Daily exercise	Patient needs some form of physical activity at least once daily.	Exercise is according to patient's ability and activity order. Exercise can range from passive range of motion (PROM) to the most strenuous activity the patient can safely perform.
6. Visitors	Patient can visit with anyone he or she chooses.	Determine at time of intake who will be visiting regularly. In cases of family concern over certain people the patient may wish to visit, safety must be a key issue. At times, nurses may need to monitor visits and visitors. Carefully document the patient's emotional and physical outcome of visits.

Continued

Table 3-1 Most Frequently Adopted Patient Rights—cont'd

Patient Right	Description	Nursing Considerations
7. Writing materials	Paper, pencils, pens, and so forth must be available to patients.	Unless contraindicated for safety reasons, nurses can assist in ensuring that these items are available at all times. If safety is an issue (e.g., stabbing self or others with a sharp object), this condition needs to be noted in charting.
8. Uncensored mail	Mail must not be opened before the patient receives it.	If patient is unable to physically open the mail or if there is concern that cognitively the patient will lose a check, for example, the nurse or another agent of the facility may witness the opening of the mail. Arrangements can be made with a family member or guardian to sign checks or see to the patient's affairs if the patient is unable to do so.
9. Courts and attorneys	Legal access remains intact for anyone who is hospitalized, whether voluntarily or involuntarily.	Patients can call an attorney at any time. Nurses and agency representatives may be asked to help them. In cases when this seems inappropriate, patient, staff, and family can discuss alternatives in a family conference. Any outcomes need to be incorporated into the care plan and documented.
10. Employment compensation	Wages are not to be withheld during hospitalization.	Under certain legal conditions, compensation may be withheld for reasons other than a stay in a health-care facility. This would be confidential information but must be incorporated into the care plan and documentation.
11. Confidentiality (records, treatment, and so on)	Information about the patient is to be kept secure and private.	Discussion of the patient's condition must take place only in designated places and with designated persons. • Many states have cautioned nurses against giving *any* information regarding the patient over the telephone. In some states, a nurse can be in jeopardy of losing a license for releasing information over the phone. • Be careful of the wording in your charting. • Release information only to those people who are specifically required or legally entitled to have it.
12. Be informed of these rights	Patients must have full understanding of their civil rights while under facility care.	The nurse or the facility representative will explain in detail the meaning of these rights for the patient. Depending on your local law and agency policy, the patient may be asked to sign a document stating that these rights have been explained. Usually, a copy is then kept with the patient record and the patient keeps a personal copy.

In addition to these frequently adopted patient rights, some states have adopted a set of patient rights for psychiatric patients. These rights may include the patient's right to:

- Marry or divorce
- Sue or be sued
- Be actively involved in his or her care
- Be employed if possible
- Retain licenses (driver's license, license to practice one's profession)

> **Clinical Activity**
> Ask one of the nurses on staff: Where are patient files kept? How do you maintain confidentiality?

In 1990, the U.S. Congress passed the Patient Self-Determination Act (PSDA), which all health-care agencies must follow. PSDA includes the following patient rights:

1. The right to facilitate their own health care decisions
2. The right to accept or refuse medical treatment
3. The right to make an advance health care directive

> **Clinical Activity**
> Compare the current year and the year when the Patient Bill of Rights became effective. Interview a nurse who was working in the field prior to the bill's passage and a nurse working after the bill's passage. Determine how the Bill of Rights has affected or changed their interactions with patients.

Patient Advocacy

With the emergence of the Patient Bill of Rights, patient advocates and patient ombudsmen began speaking out for patients' needs. These individuals are either volunteers within the community or paid workers from an agency whose job is to ensure that patients, especially those considered vulnerable, are being treated in a safe, legal manner.

Everyone is responsible for reporting abuse and neglect of those who are considered vulnerable. Nurses and health-care workers have a moral, legal, and ethical responsibility to report known or suspected abuse of people who cannot care for themselves. Part of a nurse's scope of practice is to be a voice, or an advocate, for the patients under his or her care. This is the meaning of patient **advocacy.**

Sometimes the nurse is just not sure if abuse is occurring. It is usually better to err on the side of safety for a patient and to report the concern to a supervisor. In most areas, it is acceptable to contact the investigating agency directly. Regardless of the procedure a nurse chooses to report his or her concerns, always check the agency's policy and procedure for such reporting and for the documentation that is required.

Community Resources

According to the provisions of the Community Mental Health Centers Act, every community offers some form of help to people in need. This help can be in the form of hospital emergency rooms, shelters, crisis centers, or social service offices. Most communities have a list available for the asking. Clinics and hospitals provide lists to people who are at risk or who ask for the resources. Depending on the facility's policies, the nurse may be able to help patients choose a community resource to access after discharge. Be sure to provide information on fees for the services provided by the individual agencies. They vary greatly in relation to offered services, fees, and acceptable insurance. Some are free, whereas some provide assistance on a "sliding scale" or according to ability to pay. Many states have reduced resources for mental health care in the past two decades, which has contributed to many societal problems as well as frustration for nurses. This situation needs to be addressed. It is important for nurses to identify what resources are available through colleagues within their agency.

If a patient is unaware of community resources at the time of discharge, the nurse can suggest that, if the time comes, the patient can find resources online or in the local phone book. The nurse can also inform the patient that it is always acceptable to call the local hospital to request a list. Shelters for victims of abuse usually are *not* advertised; these are kept confidential to maintain safety for the people who need them.

Key Concepts

1. It is the nurse's responsibility to know the Code of Ethics and standards of nursing practice for the state in which he or she is practicing. They will vary from state to state.
2. Collaborative practice means working together with all levels of nursing and all ancillary disciplines to provide the best possible care for the patient.
3. Honesty in nursing practice and excellence in verbal and written communication are crucial to the care of the patient and to the credibility of the nurse. A nurse will be judged by correct spelling and grammar (American format) in a court case. A nurse's competency can be questioned if his or her spelling and grammar are poor.
4. Cultural considerations such as space, time, waiting, language, and touch (to name a few) are important parts of the nurse-patient relationship. They are also important in the culture of nursing. A nurse's personal beliefs may be different from the standards that are part of the culture of nurses.
5. The patient's well-being and wishes, the state Nurse Practice Act, and agency policy dictate how nurses can care for the patient in a safe and respectful manner.

CASE STUDY

1. Nurse P, LPN, had worked for Agency X, a nursing home in a small Midwestern community, for 10 years. Over the years, Nurse P gained the trust and respect of everyone she worked with or cared for on the job. Nurse P's reputation was very good in the community as well. On one particular day, a patient asked Nurse P, "Go to my purse and get my glasses, would you please?" This apparently had happened many times before, so Nurse P sensed no reason for concern. Several hours later, a family member noticed that the patient was missing an amount of cash and a wedding ring, which the patient kept in the purse "for safe-keeping." The patient recalled asking Nurse P to retrieve the glasses from the purse. Other patients and staff had also seen Nurse P in the patient's purse. The case went to small claims court. Nurse P was found guilty and was made to pay restitution. In addition, Nurse P's license to practice nursing in that state was revoked.

1. What could Nurse P have done to avoid this situation?
2. What are your thoughts about this situation? For the patient? For Nurse P? For the "fairness" of the situation?
3. What are your feelings about this situation?
4. What are Nurse P's chances of becoming licensed again? In her state? In another state? What would the situation be if this were your state?

REFERENCES

Aiken, T. D. (2004). *Legal, Ethical, and Political Issues in Nursing.* 2nd ed. Philadelphia: FA Davis.

American Nurses Association. (2001). *American Nurses Association Code of Ethics for Nurses with Interpretive Statements.* Washington, D.C.: American Nurses Publishing.

Fossett, B., and Nadler-Moodie, M. (2004). *Psychiatric Principles and Applications for General Patient Care.* 4th ed. Brockton, MA: Western Schools.

Kelly-Heidenthat, P., and Marthaler, M. T. (2005). *Delegation of Nursing Care.* Canada: Thomas Delmar Learning.

Merriam-Webster. (2012). Retrieved from www.merriam-webster.com/

National Federation of Licensed Practical Nurses. (2003). *Nursing Practice and Standards.* Raleigh, NC.

Neeb, K. (1994, October). The culture of nurses. *Nursingworld Journal, 20,* 1.

The Joint Commission
www.jointcommission.org

RAMP
www.njsna.org/displaycommon.cfm?an=1&subarticlenbr=40

Public Health Law
www.publichealthlaw.net/Reader/docs/Tarasoff.pdf

National Patient Safety Goals
www.ispn-psych.org/docs/standards/scope-standards-draft.pdf

Patient and Physician Relationship
http://depts.washington.edu/bioethx/topics/physpt.html

HIPAA
www.hhs.gov/ocr/privacy/Community Mental Health Centers Act
history.nih.gov/research/downloads/PL88-164.pdf

Tarasoff Decision
http://www.adoctorm.com/docs/tarasoff.htm

Test Questions

Multiple Choice Questions

1. The code of behavior that combines professional expectations that border on legal issues is called:
   a. Commitment
   b. Ethics
   c. Nurse Practice Act
   d. Patient Bill of Rights
2. The document that defines the scope of nursing practice in each state is called:
   a. Commitment
   b. Ethics
   c. Nurse Practice Act
   d. Patient Bill of Rights
3. The set of rules designed to protect patients and others who are described as "vulnerable" is called:
   a. Doctrine of Privileged Information
   b. Collaborative practice
   c. Nurse Practice Act
   d. Patient Bill of Rights
4. Sandra is an RN who is working with you. Sandra is from the local pool/registry and you are the staff LPN or LVN at the facility. You see Sandra charting her medications and treatments before she administers them. Choose the best therapeutic communication technique to use when approaching Sandra.
   a. "Why are you doing that?"
   b. "I am concerned about the legality and safety of charting before giving medications, Sandra."
   c. "You know it is wrong to chart before giving the medications."
   d. "You really shouldn't do that, Sandra."
5. A few hours later, Sandra gets sick and goes home. You know that she charted before giving her medications, and you saw her passing some medications. You are not sure who got their medications and who did not. Mrs. G, a patient who is alert and oriented and a reliable historian for herself, sees you and says, "That new nurse forgot my medication this morning. It's my heart medication and I need it. Would you get it for me?" You see the medication has been charted already. Your next action would be:
   a. Refuse the patient, telling her, "You're mistaken, Mrs. G. That medication is signed for, so you must have gotten it."
   b. Give Mrs. G her heart medication and assume she is right.
   c. Call the physician.
   d. Inform your supervisor of the entire situation.
6. The Health Insurance Portability and Accountability Act:
   a. Requires patients to be treated in designated regional treatment centers.
   b. Approves of patient records being transported in personal vehicles by medical staff.
   c. Allows patients to have some say in what medical information can be divulged and to whom.
   d. Prohibits all transmission of medical records electronically.
7. Mr. Ouch has just had bilateral total knee replacement. He is in your transitional care unit. He repeatedly calls out in pain, disturbing the other residents, yet he refuses to take the prescribed pain medication, stating, "You're all just trying to knock me out." You:
   a. Shut his door, leaving him alone with some privacy until he settles.
   b. Offer another pain relief technique, realizing he has the right to refuse medication.
   c. Have additional staff come to the room to assist while you administer a prescribed injection.
   d. Inform him his behavior is not appropriate and is disruptive to others, and that he needs to stop calling out.

8. The licensed vocational nurse/licensed practical nurse (LPN/LVN) knows that his or her scope of practice includes all of the following except:

a. Administering nursing care under the direction of a registered nurse (RN)
b. Documenting the patient's data
c. Independently ordering medications for the patient
d. Assisting the physician or registered nurse with more complex care and procedures

9. The patient is semiconscious and is in need of emergency surgery to relieve a subdural hematoma. The nurse knows that:

a. Emergency situations do not require prior consent.
b. He or she must obtain written consent for invasive procedures.
c. This is not a function of the LPN/LVN; the nurse should call his or her supervisor.
d. The patient must be alert in order to obtain informed consent.

10. Mr. B. is a 65-year-old attorney who has been admitted to your floor for blood work and neurological examinations. He is loud and verbally demanding of the staff. He says, "I know my rights. You nurses have to do whatever I ask. It's your job." The nurse responds:

a. "That is not one of your rights, Mr. B."
b. "You are taking time away from other patients, Mr. B."
c. "The Patient's Bill of Rights does make some provisions, Mr. B. Let me sit and talk with you about those rights."
d. "Why are you so angry, Mr. B?"

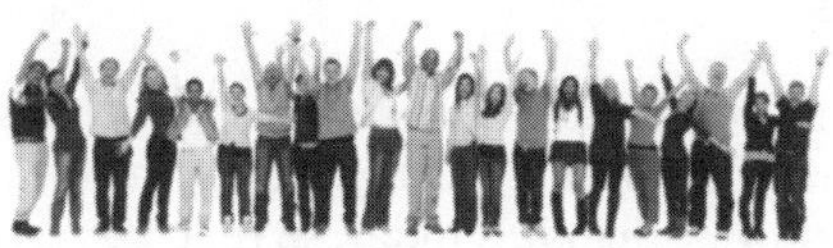

CHAPTER 4

Developmental Psychology Throughout the Life Span

Learning Objectives

1. Identify major theories of personality development from newborn through adult development.
2. Identify developmental tasks from prenatal development through death, according to the major theorists.
3. Identify possible outcomes of ineffective development, according to the major theorists.
4. Identify the five stages of grief/death according to Kübler-Ross.

Key Terms

- Accommodation
- Assimilation
- Autonomy
- Behavior
- Behavioral theorist
- Ego
- Id
- Lunar month
- Maslow's Hierarchy of Needs
- Menarche
- Operant conditioning
- Psychoanalytic
- Psychosexual
- Puberty
- Superego
- Unconscious

The study of developmental psychology encompasses the study of human growth and development, which is a specialty subdivision of psychology. This chapter covers only the very basics of human development. A sample of the main theorists in the field of child development is presented, along with others whose theories are applied more in the areas of adult personality development. For the separate developmental age groups, a chart is shown delineating the general physical and behavioral traits that are commonly seen in these age groups (pages 64-68). The characteristics may cover beliefs from several of the individual theorists you will study.

Neeb's Tip

Remember, these are only theories. Many scientific studies have been performed in the specific disciplines; however, it has yet to be proven that any one is true for *everyone* in *every* instance. Each person is unique. Individuals are subjected to different factors such as genetics and environment, which may affect development.

Each person develops at his or her own pace. While reading and learning about these theories, compare them with your personal experiences and observations, as well as with the patient assessments you will be performing. Some theorists may have more validity to you than others.

> ■ ■ ■ Critical Thinking Question
> Do other cultures use any of these developmental theories when observing human development?

■ Developmental Theorists: Newborn to Adolescence

Sigmund Freud (1856–1939)

The theories of Sigmund Freud (Fig. 4-1) are considered controversial in today's world. Sigmund Freud was an Austrian neurologist. He believed, after observing **behaviors** of children, that the personality was developed as early as age 5 years and fully developed by age 12 years. He said that the personality must develop in a certain way and at strictly defined ages and that failure to progress in this manner would certainly lead to dysfunction.

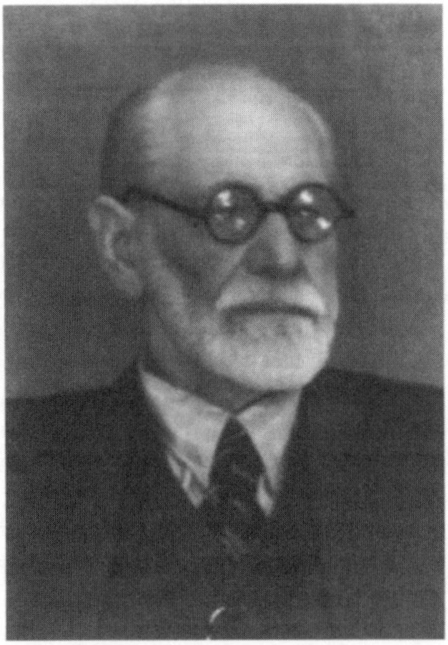

Figure 4-1 Sigmund Freud.

Bear in mind that the life span of young Western Europeans during these years was much shorter than it is today, so that 12 years of age seemed much older than it does by today's standards.

One of Freud's main tenets, or beliefs, is that behaviors resulting from ineffective personality development are **unconscious.** He believed that ineffective personality development was in some way related to the relationship of the child to the parent and that it was related to what he called **psychosexual** development.

Freud's theories have validity for some people today, but others denounce them. Although the reader is not expected to "convert" to any of the theories discussed in this text, it is necessary to have a working knowledge of the main theories of personality development. Freud is of particular interest because, in addition to his highly debated ideas, he was the first to also offer a reasonably organized method of treatment. Because he was the first publicized theorist, all other theories have evolved as a result of his. Sigmund Freud's beliefs surface in almost every topic covered in this text. All other theorists compare their theories with Freud's, either in agreement or in opposition.

Table 4-1 shows Freud's psychosexual or **psychoanalytic** stages of development. Included in the table are some of the expected behaviors Freud thought one might witness as a child passes through these ages. The last column lists some behaviors that have been suggested as outcomes of failure to progress through his idea of proper personality development. Discussion of Freud and his theories continues later in this chapter.

Erik Erikson (1902–1994)

Erik Erikson (Fig. 4-2) was a psychoanalyst and a follower of Freud. Erikson took Freud's main concepts and expanded them to include nonphysical criteria. Erikson understood that people are individuals and that no matter how young the person, everyone is different. Erikson's observations indicated a variable that was different from the psychosexual and age-specific theory offered by Freud. That variable is called an emotional component. Table 4-2 shows Erikson's Eight Stages of Development.

Table 4-1 Freud's Stages of Development (Psychoanalytic or Psychosexual Stages)

Stage of Development	Approximate Ages	Tasks/Characteristics	Examples of Unsuccessful Task Completion
Oral	Birth–18 months	Use mouth and tongue to deal with anxiety (e.g., sucking, feeding)	Smoking, alcoholism, obesity, nail biting, drug addiction, difficulty trusting
Anal	18 months–3 years	Muscle control in bladder, rectum, anus provides sensual pleasure and parent pleasing; toilet training can be a crisis	Constipation, perfectionism, obsessive-compulsive disorder
Phallic	3–6 years	• Learn sexual identity and awareness of genital area as source of pleasure; conflict ends as child represses urge and identifies with same-sex parent • Electra Complex: "Penis envy"—Daughter wants father for herself; discovers boys are different from her • Oedipus Complex: Son wants mother to himself; father is a rival	Homosexuality, transsexuality, sexual identity problems in general, difficulty accepting authority
Latency	6–12 years	Quiet stage in sexual development; learns to socialize	Inability to conceptualize; lack of motivation in school or job
Genital	12 years–adulthood	Sexual maturity and satisfactory relationships with the opposite sex	Frigidity, impotence, premature ejaculation, serial marriages, unsatisfactory relationships

Frequently, his stages are identified by the words highlighted in the column headed Developmental Tasks. Note that the developmental tasks are always listed as contradictions (i.e., trust versus mistrust) of each other. This is one way that Erikson indicated his ideas about emotional fluctuation in people.

Classroom Activity

- Describe which of the following stages you have experienced according to Erik Erikson:
  - Adolescence
  - Young Adult
  - Adulthood
  - Maturity

Clinical Activity

Select an adult patient during your clinical experience, and compare his biological age with Erikson's developmental stages. Is your patient's age appropriate to his developmental task?

- Young Adult
- Adulthood
- Maturity

Jean Piaget (1896–1980)

Jean Piaget (Fig. 4-3) was a Swiss psychologist whose outlook on development was completely different from those of his colleagues Freud and Erikson. Piaget's theory is called

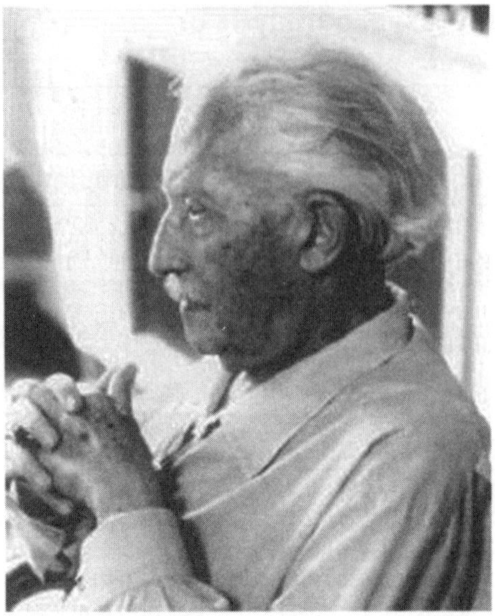

Figure 4-2 Erik Erikson.

Cognitive Development. *Cognitive* means the ability to reason, make judgments, and learn. Piaget believed that development was not as much a part of chronological age as of experiential age. Piaget was so sure of his ideas that he said they were applicable to any living organism; the catch is to make the observations and comparisons about the cognitive process according to the expected ability for that organism. Piaget believed that intelligence consists of coping with the environment (Dennis & Hassol, 1983). He believed that a person must complete each stage of development before he or she can progress to the next stage. Table 4-3 on page 56 shows the four stages of Piaget's theory of development.

Critical Thinking Question

Jamie is 2 years old. Jamie's parents are becoming frustrated because Jamie is "so naughty." They say that Jamie is always saying "No!" and "Mine!" They say that Jamie is fascinated by playing with the dirty diapers. They feel responsible for what they believe is "disgusting" behavior and wonder what they are doing "wrong." They are quick to point out that "Jamie's older sibling never did these things. Is there something wrong with us? Is there something wrong with Jamie? Please help us!"

Lawrence Kohlberg (1927–1987)

Lawrence Kohlberg (Fig. 4-4) believed in Piaget's theories, but he perceived that very young people have the ability to understand and judge right and wrong. Kohlberg's theory is therefore called the Development of Moral Judgment.

Table 4-2 Erikson's Eight Stages of Development

Stage	Approximate Ages	Developmental Tasks	Examples	Examples of Unsuccessful Task Completion
Sensory	Birth–18 months	Trust vs. mistrust	Nurturing people build trust in the newborn.	Suspiciousness, trouble with personal relationships
Muscular	1–3 years	Autonomy vs. shame and doubt	"No!"—Toddler learns environment can be manipulated.	Low self-esteem, dependency (on substances or people)
Locomotor	3–6 years	Initiative vs. guilt	Child learns assertiveness can manipulate environment—disapproval leads to guilt in the toddler.	Passive personality, strong feelings of guilt
Latency	6–12 years	Industry vs. inferiority	Creativity or shyness develops.	Unmotivated, unreliable

Table 4-2 Erikson's Eight Stages of Development—cont'd

Stage	Approximate Ages	Developmental Tasks	Examples	Examples of Unsuccessful Task Completion
Adolescence	12–20 years	Identity vs. role confusion	Individual integrates life experiences or becomes confused.	Rebellion, substance abuse, difficulty keeping personal relationships; may regress to child-play behaviors
Young Adult	18–25 years	Intimacy vs. isolation	Main concern is developing intimate relationship with another.	Emotional immaturity; may deny need for personal relationships
Adulthood	21–45 years	Generativity vs. stagnation	Focus is on establishing family and guiding the next generation.	Inability to show concern for anyone but self
Maturity	45 years–death	Integrity vs. despair	Individual accepts own life as fulfilling; if not, he or she becomes fearful of death.	Has difficulty dealing with issues of aging and death; may have feelings of hopelessness

Neeb's Tip *Caution:* Morality, the ideas that people consider to be "right" and "wrong," is highly cultural.

Kohlberg was a professor at Harvard University for many years. He developed and published his theory of moral development in 1958 as his doctoral thesis. It was based on some of the ideas of Jean Piaget. His true interest was in the mechanisms people use to justify their decisions. Although he was interested in the morality of his subjects, he was especially interested in how people support their decisions. He studied only male subjects ranging in age from 10 to 16 years. Kohlberg's theory is expressed in three levels. Each level has two sections. Table 4-4 shows these stages.

Kohlberg believed that these stages build on the learning achieved from the stage before it. Therefore, the stages must be experienced in the exact order, and one is not to backtrack, or revert to a previous stage. Part of his belief was that moral development can be promoted via formal education. In fact, there is a mild resurgence of Kohlberg's theory emerging in some classroom environments today. Kohlberg's theory has been criticized

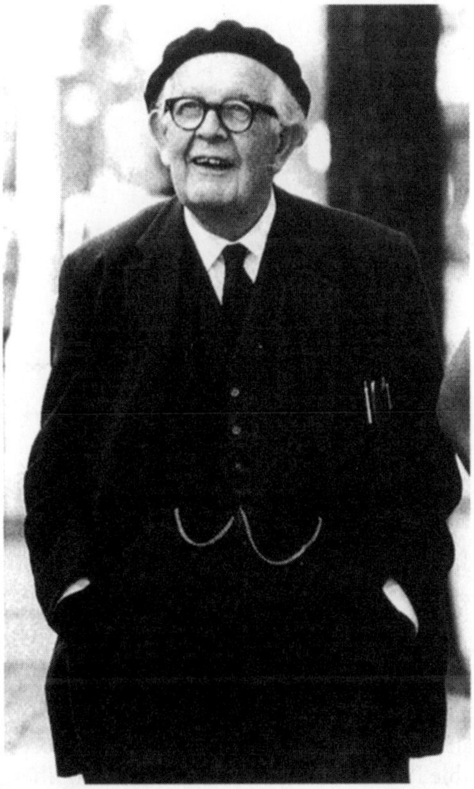

Figure 4-3 Jean Piaget.

Table 4-3 Developmental Theory of Jean Piaget

Stage	Approximate Age	Expected Ability
Sensorimotor	Birth–2 years	• Uses senses to learn about self • Schemata develop, which are plans or ways of learning to assimilate and accommodate. They include the behaviors of looking, hearing, and sucking.
Preoperational	2–7 or 8 years	2–4 years: • Thinks in mental images • Symbolic play • Develops own languages 4–7 or 8 years: • Egocentrism—sees only own point of view but *cannot* do this until age 7 or 8. With age, this ability develops.
Concrete Operational	8–12 years	• Ability for logical thought increases. • Moral judgment begins to develop. • Numbers and spatial ability become more logical.
Formal Operations	12 years–adult	• Develops adult logic. • Able to reason things out. • Able to form conclusions. • Able to plan for future. • Able to think in concepts or abstracts.

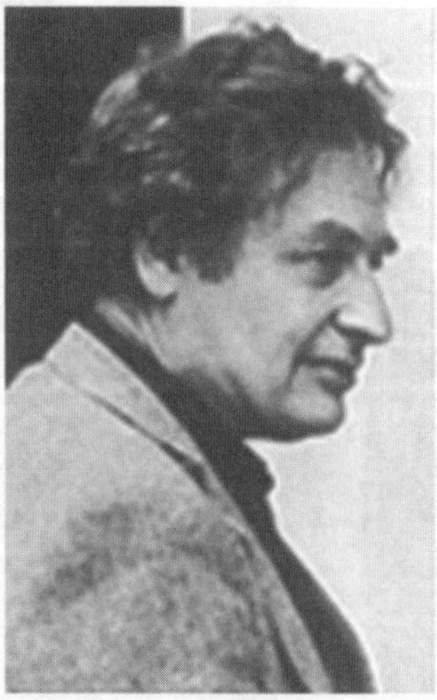

Figure 4-4 Lawrence Kohlberg.

on the grounds that it is sexist and culturally biased. It indicates that some cultures and peoples never progress to the highest level and suggests that behaviors that are acceptable in some cultures are "wrong." Kohlberg's theory also does not consider the emotional responses that daily problems and stressors can produce. Psychologist Carol Gilligan published a book in 1982 indicating that boys, girls, men, and women are all able to feel compassion and morality but that the genders process their morality from different perspectives, a variable that was not considered in Kohlberg's study.

> ■ ■ ■ Classroom Activity
> • As a class, develop a safety checklist for toddlers/preschool-age children. This checklist can be used as a tool for new parents, day-care providers, or others in your community.

■ Developmental Theorists: Adolescence to Adulthood

Sigmund Freud (1856–1939)

In addition to his five psychosexual stages of development, Sigmund Freud had a model for the components of personality. He said

Table 4-4 Lawrence Kohlberg's Theory of Development of Moral Reasoning

Stage	"Right" Behaviors	Why We Should Do "Right"	What If We Do Not Do "Right"
Level I: Preconventional			
1. Punishment and obedience orientation	*Do not do it* if it will result in punishment.	To avoid punishment and to see what one can "get away with"	I will be punished and I do not like that.
2. Concerned with having own needs met	It is "right" if I (or if *we*) get something I want out of it.	To help me get my needs and wants fulfilled	I will lose recognition for the importance of "others."
Level II: Conventional			
3. "Good boy, good girl" orientation	"Good" means living up to what is expected of us.	Self and others think we are "good."	Avoiding "blame" is more ethical than getting a "reward."
4. "Law and order"	"Right" means obeying the laws and rules.	It maintains social structure.	"Law" will have less importance than the will of "society."
Level III: Postconventional (Principled Level)			
5. Social Contact	"Right or good" is behaving according to a general consensus.	We blend together for the greatest good and the welfare of all.	May become aware that "moral" and "legal" may not be the same
6. Universal "good"	Universal rules of justice and equality for all prevail. This is the "ideal" according to Kohlberg.	Live within the universal "good" according to own conscience.	Few people reach this according to Kohlberg. Therefore, in his own manual, the latest revisions do not measure this stage.

that the personality consists of three parts: the id, the ego, and the superego. Remember that Freud believed that *all* the components of human behavior are set in the unconscious. The behaviors may appear to be very purposeful and deliberate, but in Freud's theories, they are supposedly responses to situations of which people are not aware.

Id is the part of the personality that is concerned with the gratification of self. The sayings "pleasure principle" or "if it feels good, do it!" are attitudes that arose from those who believe that all people have underdeveloped ids. These individuals promote the idea that people need to allow the id to take care of "me, myself, and I."

Ego, in Freud's world, had a different connotation from the modern-day common use of the word. Ego, as Freud taught, is the balance to id. Ego keeps id under control (in a mentally healthy individual) by responding in an unconscious form of a "now, wait a minute" attitude. For example, perhaps you had an exam that was in a subject you felt fairly confident about, so you chose to study less than you would for other exams. You went partying with friends for the weekend instead. Think about this as id behavior. As you entered the testing area, a gnawing feeling started to enter your consciousness. You sensed "butterflies" in the pit of your stomach. You saw the first question on the exam and your mind went temporarily blank. That is the ego response. It's telling you there are two sides to every situation. In this scenario, the ego is telling the id, "Hmm. Maybe you aren't quite as confident as you thought you were!" And the id says, "This test was made just for me."

The third part of the personality theory of Sigmund Freud is the superego. The **superego** could be called the "killjoy" of the personality. It is the conscience. It is the part of the personality that allows people to determine what is right, wrong, good, and bad. The values exhibited by the superego are not to be confused with the same terms used by Lawrence Kohlberg; according to Freud, having these values is not a matter of choice or of learning.

A person who is well-adjusted, or mentally healthy, has all three components of the personality, according to Freud. Freud would expect anyone in whom any of the components is absent or out of balance to display maladaptive behaviors. Defense mechanisms have been associated strongly with Freud's theories. Discussion of these defense mechanisms and maladaptive behaviors is found in later chapters of this book.

Karen Horney (1885–1952)

Karen Horney (Fig. 4-5) was a psychoanalyst and one of the very few early female theorists. Her ideas were very close to those of Freud; however, she believed that the causes of abnormal behaviors or mental illness were related to ineffective mother-child bonding. Karen Horney developed the **psychoanalytic** social theory where she strongly believed that a person's childhood contributed and influenced a child's personality in later life. Horney believed that safety and security are important factors in a child's life. Without it in their earlier years, difficult behaviors could be the results. Horney emphasized that it is the responsibility of the parents to provide that safe and secure environment (Dewey, 2007).

Ivan Pavlov (1849–1936) and B. F. Skinner (1904–1990)

Pavlov and Skinner worked on "conditioning," or manipulating, behaviors. They are called **behavioral theorists** because they believed that working with different behaviors and different stimuli could obtain different responses. Behavior modification is a direct result of their work.

Pavlov (Fig. 4-6) worked on involuntary responses. His well-known study was carried out with dogs, steaks, and a bell. When the dogs saw a choice piece of meat, they salivated in preparation for eating it. Pavlov incorporated the ringing of a bell when the meat was presented so that, in time, the researcher rang

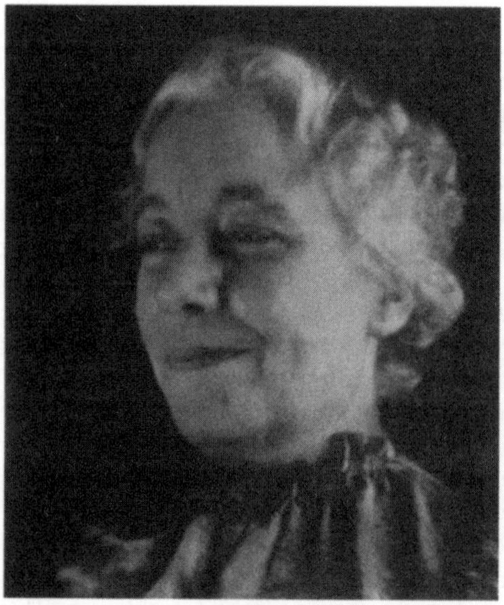

Figure 4-5 Karen Horney.

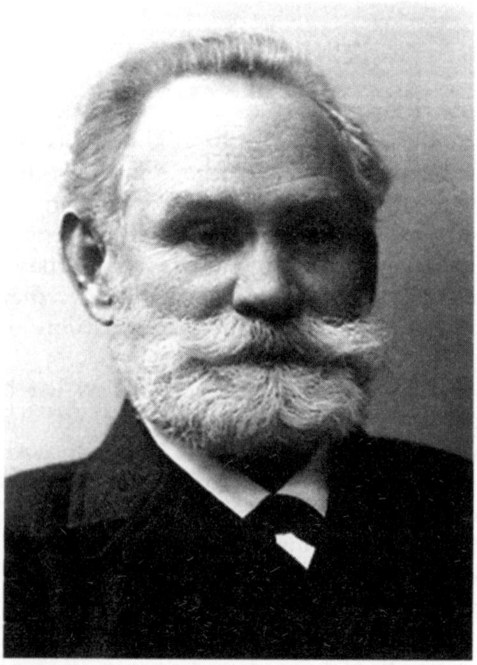

Figure 4-6 Ivan Pavlov.

the bell and the dogs' association of meat with the sound of the bell stimulated the salivation response. This was a great breakthrough in the study of causes of behavior and ways in which behavior can be manipulated.

B. F. Skinner (Fig. 4-7) worked on **operant conditioning**, which is based on voluntary responses. Operant conditioning, very simply stated, means taking a behavior and operating on it by changing the variables or conditions surrounding the behavior. Skinner is known for the "Skinner boxes" in which he kept the animals he studied. These so-called boxes were cages big enough for the animal to move around in and contained an apparatus for the animal to operate voluntarily in response to different stimuli. There are three main parts to Skinner's theory: response, stimulus, and reinforcer. Table 4-5 defines these parts.

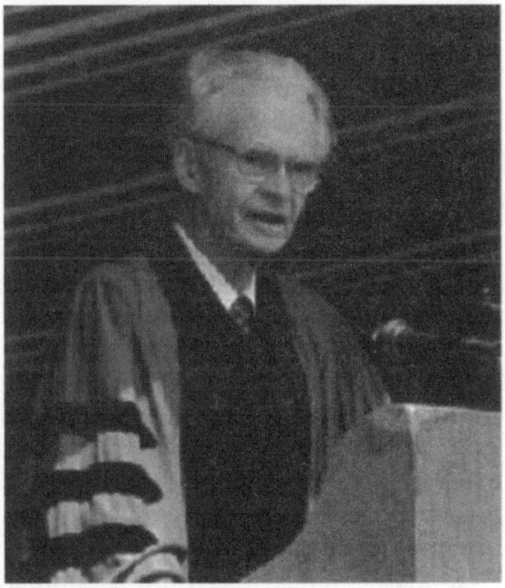

Figure 4-7 B. F. Skinner.

Skinner's theory led to the development of behavior modification. It is possible to "modify" or change any behavior by using appropriate stimuli and reinforcers to obtain the desired behavior.

Both positive and negative behaviors can be changed. Today, it is generally believed that positive reinforcing is the most effective way of changing a behavior. Pointing out the positive qualities in a person or patient or focusing on the abilities (positive) rather than the disabilities (negative) seems to yield the best results. For instance, pretend that the behavior a supervisor wants to operate on is getting a particular coworker to arrive to work on time. The supervisor has two possible paths to follow: One is positive reinforcing; the other, negative reinforcing.

EXAMPLES

Negative: "Nurse M, you are routinely late for work. This is very difficult on your patients and on the rest of the staff. One more instance of being late, and you will be fired."

Positive: "Nurse M, you are still occasionally late for work. I have noticed, however, that you have been late only three times this month. If you continue to improve your timeliness, I will be able to give you a raise at your next review."

Table 4-5 Operant Conditioning: B. F. Skinner

Skinner's Theory	Explanation
Response	Any movement or observable behavior that is to be studied. The response is measured for frequency, duration, and intensity (e.g., chicken rings bell in cage).
Stimulus	The event that immediately precedes or follows the operant behavior. The object is to find the stimulus that gets the chicken to ring the bell (e.g., food, noise, boredom).
Reinforcer	A variable that will cause the operant behavior to repeat predictably or increase in frequency. Sometimes this is called a "reward." The reinforcer has to be meaningful to the person whose behavior is being "operated" on (e.g., chicken pecks bell and food drops into tray; when chicken wants food, it knows that pecking the bell will produce food).

The positive reinforcement method seems to give some dignity and positive self-regard to the employee. It allows the employee to understand the consequences and to make choices about being late. It will then be up to the supervisor to follow through with whichever consequences are earned by Nurse M. In the 1960s, positive reinforcement was used with chickens as a form of entertainment on New Jersey's Atlantic City boardwalk.

Abraham Maslow (1908–1970)

Abraham Maslow (Fig. 4-8) is one of a group of theorists described as person-centered, patient-centered, or humanist. Person-centered theories involve observing and treating the whole person. Nursing is highly centered in the person-centered and behaviorist theories. One of the main ideals embraced by the nursing profession is **Maslow's Hierarchy of Needs.** This hierarchy, or orderly progression of development, takes in the physical components of personality development as well as the emotional components. Self-esteem is a tenet of humanistic psychology.

Maslow's Hierarchy of Needs has five levels. Maslow said that one must pass through these stages in order and that it is not possible for a person to move up to the next level until the previous level has been mastered. Many times this hierarchy is depicted as a large triangle or a staircase to help visualize the progression from the "basic" needs to the "higher" needs of people (Fig. 4-9). The steps are as follows:

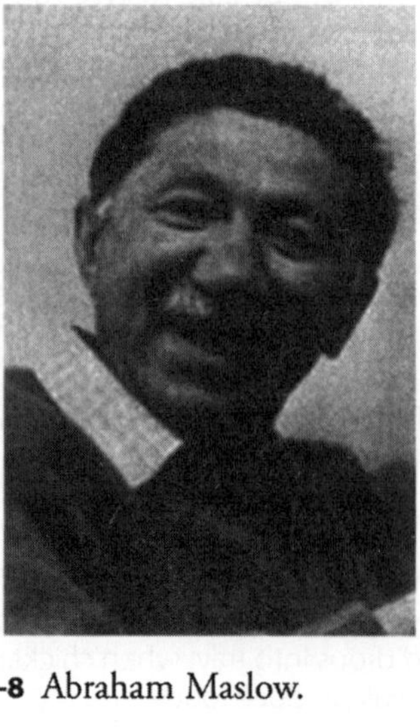

Figure 4-8 Abraham Maslow.

1. Physiological needs
2. Safety and security
3. Love and belonging
4. Self-esteem
5. Self-actualization

Physiological Needs

These are elements people need to survive: food, water, oxygen, clothing, absence of extremes in temperature, ability for body excretions, and sexual activity. These are considered necessary for life to continue. Without food, clothing, and a shelter that is clean and of a comfortable temperature, an individual could die; without sexual activity, the species could die. The physiological needs can be considered needs for survival. When preparing a plan of care for a patient, if the physiological needs are not categorized as a priority, he/she will not survive. Can the patient proceed to the next level of the hierarchy pyramid without water or fluids? Can the patient survive without oxygen? Can the patient survive without elimination? These are the questions that a nurse must ask when doing a patient assessment. Being able to identify what takes priority can assist the nurse while taking the National Council Licensure Examination (NCLEX) as well as providing patient care. Maslow's theory is an important component of the nursing discipline.

Safety and Security

It is important that people feel safe and free of fear. When individuals feel comfortable that their physical needs are being met, they begin to feel a sense of safety that they can maintain their survival. Bear in mind that having these basic needs met does not necessarily mean living in wealth or with steady employment. People who live on the street for whatever reason learn to survive and are proud of their ability to survive in conditions that most people would consider deplorable. For some people, street life is a

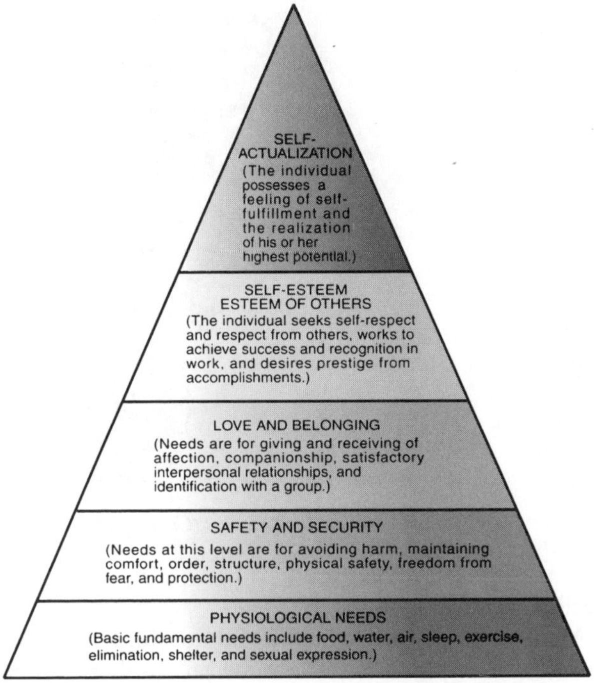

Figure 4-9 Maslow's Hierarchy of Needs. *(From Townsend (2011): Essentials of Psychiatric Mental Health Nursing, 5th ed. Philadelphia: F.A. Davis Company, with permission.)*

choice, and they meet the criteria of Maslow's hierarchy.

Love and Belonging

It is a popular belief within psychology that loneliness is a major cause of depression. Quotes such as "Man does not live by bread alone" and "No man is an island" have implied this for many years, and it is now being borne out scientifically. People need to feel loved, appreciated, and part of a group. The opening song in the television comedy "Cheers" expresses the importance of everyone knowing each other's name and being happy that you are there. The focus of that sense of love and belonging may change over the life span. For babies and young children, the love needs to come from parents or other caregivers; in adolescence and adulthood, the focus may change to a significant life partner or a peer group, or both. Regardless of the developmental stage of life, people need to feel loved.

Self-Esteem

The "higher" needs begin with the idea that "If I am loved by someone, there must be something special and good about me." Finding that "something" and learning to accept, appreciate, and acknowledge one's positive traits is the goal of the fourth need of Maslow's hierarchy: esteem or self-esteem.

Self-esteem is the ability to be confident that one is a person with good qualities and that others know and appreciate these qualities. This sounds easier to achieve than it often is. When someone compliments a person on a new piece of clothing, a haircut, or a job well done, what is that person's usual response? "Oh, this old thing? Do you really think so? I think it's way too short now" or "It was nothing, really" are responses people often give. In addition to the effect it has on effective communication, responding in this manner does not show positive self-esteem. One of the most difficult things for people to do is to learn to say "Thank you" when given a compliment. "Thank you" not only acknowledges the other person's positive regard for a quality one possesses, but it reinforces to one's "self" that "Yes, I did do that well and I do deserve the recognition." Unfortunately, people sometimes interpret this simple response as "false pride" and consider it to be in poor taste to acknowledge themselves in a positive manner. Women have been socialized this way for years, and although there has been some improvement over the past 20 years, there is much work yet to be done in this area.

Self-Actualization

The fifth and final rung on Maslow's hierarchy ladder is called self-actualization. This means achievement, taking risks, and working to one's individual potential. The self-actualized person is a problem solver. Situations can be creatively dealt with when a person is confident enough to stretch the limits of ability. Taking the risk to stretch boundaries by joining the nursing profession is an example of seeking out self-actualization. Even though it may not feel comfortable yet, it is a process for self-improvement.

Gender differences have been a subject of discussion since the beginning of time. Men and women have always said that they just do not understand each other. Proof of that exists now. Scientists can truthfully, confidently, and nonjudgmentally say that "Yes, there are differences in the way men and women think, communicate, and process life." Psychologist Carol Gilligan studied this phenomenon (Gilligan, 1982). She hypothesized that one of these fundamental differences appears to affect Maslow's hierarchy: women tend to value relationships as a basic need, and men tend to value achievement as a basic need. This is not an issue of right or wrong; no value statement is being made. It is important, however, that nurses who are observing and collecting data on their patients understand that differences in patient attitudes and responses to treatment may be related to gender.

Carl Rogers (1902–1987)

Carl Rogers (Fig. 4-10) was also a person-centered or humanistic psychologist. Although he believed that all people need to be "prized and loved," his theory is a bit different from Maslow's. The phrase associated with Carl Rogers is "unconditional positive regard." Rogers believed that each individual may have different ideas about life and the world

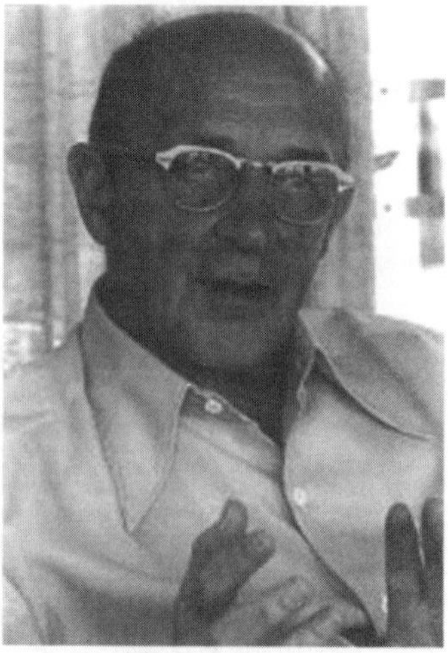

Figure 4-10 Carl Rogers. *(Courtesy of Bonnie Drumwright, PhD, Gold River, CA.)*

he or she lives in. He did not think it was appropriate to put a value on another person's perception of the world, so he said that every person deserved to be treated with respect and "unconditional positive regard" just by virtue of being a human being.

He also differed from Maslow in the area of self-actualization. Rogers believed that self-actualization is the basic motivator for people and that all people have a built-in desire to achieve their capabilities.

Nursing practice is based very strongly in Rogers' theory. His eight steps to being a helping person are listed in Table 4-6.

Carl Jung (1875–1961)

Although he broke from some of Freud's ideas, Carl Jung (Fig. 4-11), a Swiss psychologist, also believed in the effects of the unconscious mind. He included in his definition of "unconscious" both repressed personal experiences and representations of universal human experiences, those experiences all people have. He used different terminology to describe the various parts of human personality, and he believed that healthy personalities are a balance between the conscious and the unconscious. "Self" to Jung meant the deep, inner part of people. He believed that males and females are different organisms

Table 4-6 Rogers' Eight Steps

Empathy	"Walk in another's shoes."
Respect	Care for patient as a *person,* not just a patient.
Genuineness	Helper is a sincere/authentic role model.
Concreteness	Identify patient's feelings by careful listening and stereotyping.
Confrontation	Discuss discrepancies in behavior.
Self-Disclosure	Share self, as is appropriate to situation.
Immediacy of Relationships	Helper selectively shares own feelings.
Self-Exploration	The more we explore ourselves, the greater/better the coping/ adapting.

Source: Prochaska, J. O. (1984). Systems of Psychotherapy. Pacific Grove, CA: Brooks-Cole.

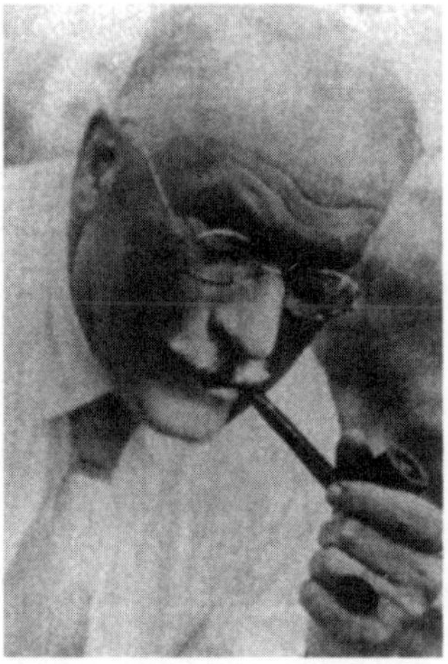

Figure 4-11 Carl Jung.

but that each contains part of the other. The human endocrine system shows that men have traces of female hormones and women have traces of male hormones. To Jung, it logically followed that this fact affects the way each person develops his or her personality. Therefore, he used the term "anima" to describe the feminine tendencies in men and the term "animus" to describe the male characteristics in women.

"Mask" is a word Jung used to define the part of the personality that one presents socially. It hints at the idea that one's innermost self may be different from his or her public self.

Stages of Human Development

Nurses are entrusted with caring for people of all ages. Many nursing program mission statements refer to the concept that nursing must cover a continuum of experiences throughout the life span. It becomes the nurse's responsibility to have a working knowledge of the main physical and behavioral changes that can be expected within certain age groups. It is also important to have some idea of the complications that might occur if developmental tasks are not completed successfully. This is called the study of developmental psychology. Table 4-7 identifies the life stages, some of the expected major physical development, expected behavioral development, and possible outcomes of failure to meet certain developmental tasks. This chart incorporates traits from all the theorists identified in this text. It is not a substitute for knowing the concepts of the individual theorists.

Life is an accumulation of experiences. Some of those are positive and some are not. Each person has to deal with gains and losses as he or she travels through life. Patients may be in different stages of loss with their illness. Each age group has its own set of gains and losses. Learning to deal with these ups and downs early in life can make the more significant experiences less difficult to cope

(Text continued on page 68)

Table 4-7 Overall View of Human Development

Life Stage	Age Range (ages vary somewhat according to theorist)	Expected Physical Development	Expected Behavioral Development	Potential Outcome of Ineffective Development
Prenatal	Conception through 10th **lunar month** (lunar month = 28 days)	• Cells differentiate (specialize) by the end of the first trimester. • Intrauterine conditions of mother may affect prenatal development.	• Fetus kicks and may respond to stimuli such as familiar voices, music.	• Threats to mother's health of primary concern (e.g., smoking, drugs, malnutrition); mother's prenatal habits seem to have a strong influence on the developing baby. • Alcohol consumption during pregnancy of special concern; can lead to a condition called fetal alcohol syndrome (FAS), which can cause physical anomalies as well as cognitive, emotional, and behavioral complications in child.
Newborn	1st month of life	• May have flattened nose, unevenly shaped head, bruises from the passage through the birth canal; these physical characteristics will change over the first month of life.	• Bonding (e.g., touching, talking) of parents and baby is said to be crucial to development of trust. • Sucking reflex • Can see 7–10 inches • Likes bright colors • Likes to be talked to • Prefers female voices • Likes touch, cuddling, rocking, and the like • Will not be "spoiled" by this attention • Can hold head up for a few seconds • Follows light with eyes	• Angry crying • Mistrust • Withdrawal • Stress, which slows further development

Table 4-7 Overall View of Human Development—cont'd

Life Stage	Age Range (ages vary somewhat according to theorist)	Expected Physical Development	Expected Behavioral Development	Potential Outcome of Ineffective Development
Infant	2nd month–$1^1/_2$ years of life	Infants are all very much alike (physically and developmentally) until the age of 10 months.	2–4 months: • Begins to laugh • Follows people's movements with eyes 5–7 months: • Holds head erect • Turns head toward voices • Babbles/coos • Drinks from a cup 8–10 months: • Sits up alone • Says "mama," "dada"; understands "no" and "bye-bye"	• Poor parent-child relationship can lead to mistrust and poor self-concept. • Failure-to-thrive syndrome • Separation anxiety
Toddler	$1^1/_2$–3 years	• Long trunk • Short legs • Brain about $^3/_4$ of full size in order to be able to support future growth and development • Walking	• Toilet training • Learning sex roles by copying behaviors of same-sex parent • Self-centered • Does not share • Wants things now • Both boys and girls learning **autonomy** (independence) by using the word "no" • **Assimilation**, which is taking in and processing of information via the senses • **Accommodation**, which is the ability to adjust to new information or situations	• Anger • Regression • Reversion to infant-age behaviors

Continued

Table 4-7 Overall View of Human Development—cont'd

Life Stage	Age Range (ages vary somewhat according to theorist)	Expected Physical Development	Expected Behavioral Development	Potential Outcome of Ineffective Development
Preschool (Early Childhood)	3–6 years	• Medical and dental examinations important • Nutrition can be challenging; children are starting to pick and choose their favorite foods; time to start teaching good nutrition. • Lead poisoning still a threat: it tastes sweet and may still be found in some older plumbing or in old paint layers in housing units.	• Cognitive development is a primary activity; many questions; "Why" a frequently used word. • Socializes • Play important for self-expression and anxiety relief • Reading is the best parent-child activity. • Aggressive behavior (roughhousing) • Active imagination possibly leading to nightmares • Mixed feelings about going to school	• Enuresis—the involuntary bed-wetting in preschool and school-age children who have been toilet trained; often due to poor personal relationships • Encopresis—involuntary bowel movements in the same population as enuresis
School Age	6–12 years	• Body thinning out and growth slowing temporarily • Forming friendships with same-sex friends • Losing baby teeth and gaining permanent teeth • By age 6, brain almost full size; neurological system develops from head down • By age 6 or 7, vision at its peak • Vision and hearing screening usually begun by the time the child enters school • Agility increases	• Learning to share • Peer group activities important • Beginning to show acceptance of moral issues by questions and discussions • Reversibility: the ability to put things in an order or sequence or to group things according to common traits	• Shyness and/or fear of school if trust and autonomy have not developed fully; may be a result of not being included in peer groups; has been defined as a "silent prison" • Gangs—can be the result of negative types of peer groups • Stuttering—repetitive or prolonged sounds or speech flow that is interrupted; seems to happen four times more often in boys: may be stress-related

Table 4-7 Overall View of Human Development—cont'd

Life Stage	Age Range (ages vary somewhat according to theorist)	Expected Physical Development	Expected Behavioral Development	Potential Outcome of Ineffective Development
School Age—cont'd		• Scoliosis (lateral curvature of the spine) screening possibly encouraged • Late childhood (10–11 years old)—beginning of sexual development, especially in girls, who now are maturing about 2 years ahead of boys • Colds frequent, due to social habits		• Accidents—the leading cause of death in children; teaching safety to families and children is important. • Child abuse/neglect noted more frequently; all health-care personnel have the duty to report abuse or suspected abuse (discussed in more detail in Chapters 5 and 22).
Adolescent	12–18 years	• Growth spurt (musculoskeletal system) • Endocrine system maturing (hormones) • Secondary sex characteristics developing (facial and underarm hair, males' shoulders broaden, females' hips broaden and breasts develop) • **Puberty**—individual is capable of reproducing • **Menarche**—female's first menstrual period, which happens around age 11–15 (it is important to know that nutrition and exercise affect this)	• Learning independence • Learning self-sufficiency • Learning new social roles • Mood swings • Boredom • Introspection • Preoccupation with body image • Own "language" • Peer group very important—teens need intimacy • Possible experimentation with alcohol, drugs, sex • Communication between parent and adolescent crucial • Talking on phone/internet for hours	• Anorexia/bulimia frequent dangers for males as well as females; usually from white, middle-class families • Males who mature later seem to have the hardest time adjusting. • Suicide a major concern for this age group, usually because of feeling unimportant and not being taken seriously by adults

Continued

Table 4-7 Overall View of Human Development—cont'd

Life Stage	Age Range (ages vary somewhat according to theorist)	Expected Physical Development	Expected Behavioral Development	Potential Outcome of Ineffective Development
Young Adult	18–35 years	• Body usually in optimal physical condition	• Intimacy the main task to accomplish • Schooling and career planning important • Marriage and family decisions made	• Problems with developing intimacy • Difficulty leaving parent's homes
Adult	30–60 years	• Gradual decline in hearing and visual acuity • Body beginning to shorten somewhat as musculature and bone structure change • Lung and cardiac capacity beginning to decrease somewhat	• Generativity, or passing down values and skills to the next generation (personally and professionally)—a major task of the adult	• Disappointment with own achievements/next generation • Stress demands from different generations
Older Adult	60 years–death	• Visual and hearing acuity continue to decline • Body becomes susceptible to an increasing number of physical and emotional illnesses	• Acceptance of limitations on independence and physical ability • Acceptance of the idea of death and beginning to prepare for it • Acceptance of retirement • Increases in stress throughout the life span	• Fear of death and dying • Difficulty with retirement—identity is often associated with career • Depression relating to aging, loss of friends, and so on

with. Overuse of defense mechanisms (see Chapter 7) can be curtailed with effective stress-management techniques, which can be learned very early in life. It is important for nurses to understand the developmental stages throughout life, and this includes the end of life. The process of death and dying is one that all people will face at some point.

Classroom Activity

- As a class, develop a teaching plan that could be used with children who are experiencing the divorce of their parents. The checklist should be detailed enough to accommodate age-appropriate communication and information. The class might prefer to do a separate checklist for each developmental group.

Death and Dying

Losing a loved one at any age or for any reason is a difficult experience. Separation, loss, and grief are human conditions that are unavoidable. Today's world presents conflicting phenomena. People have a better quality of life and better health care than ever before. Because of this, the average life expectancy is 78.7 years (CDC–National Center for Health Statistics).

On the other hand, people exist in a fast-paced and competitive society, which causes high levels of stress and encourages people to make unhealthy choices in their diets and lifestyles. This results in people dying of myocardial infarctions in their 30s and 40s. Automobile accidents and recreational activities are taking the lives of children at higher numbers than ever before. According to the Centers for Disease Control and Prevention (CDC), violence is a global cause of death. Even though people know intellectually that they will die, they often struggle with death as if it is unexpected. We have been called a "death-denying society."

Psychologist Dr. Elisabeth Kübler-Ross (Fig. 4-12), who died in 2004 at age 78, was a leader in the study of the *process* of death and dying. She made her reputation by learning about the activities of the mind and body at and around the time of death. Her initial studies were based on only 200 subjects, all of whom had cancer; yet her theory has survived and has spanned more than 40 years.

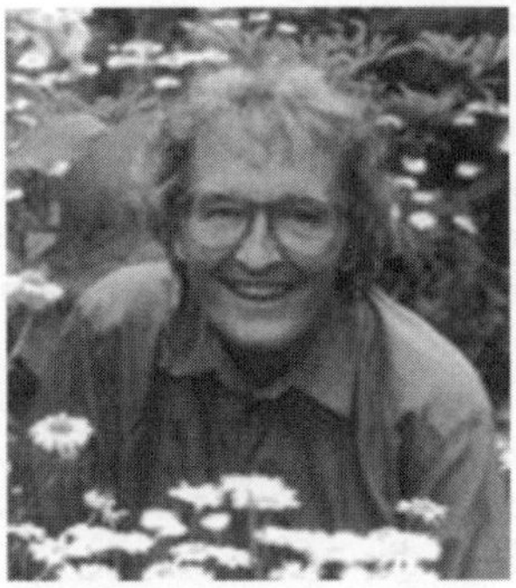

Figure 4-12 Elisabeth Kübler-Ross. *(Courtesy of Ken Ross, Scottsdale, AZ.)*

Her idea implies that the end result of experiencing the five stages of grief or dying is the ability to die in peace and with dignity. These stages apply to the dying people and those they leave behind and to other major losses in life. These stages are listed in Table 4-8.

Death, and the activities that accompany it for the dying person and those left behind, is not only physiological; it is also deeply rooted in cultural and spiritual tradition. Just as every person is unique in life, so will the rituals surrounding the activities of death be very personal and individual.

Dr. Kübler-Ross emphasized the importance of communicating throughout the dying process. People who are in comas or in the end stage of death may not be able to respond to verbal cues or participate in conversation, but it is widely believed that they continue to hear

Table 4-8 Five Stages of Grief/Death and Dying by Dr. Elisabeth Kübler-Ross

Stage	Key Words	Expected Behaviors
Denial	"Not me!"	Refuses to believe that death is coming; states "That doctor doesn't know what he/she is talking about!"
Anger	"Why me?"	Expresses envy, resentment, and frustration with younger people and/or those who are not dying
Bargaining	"If I could have one more chance . . ."	May become very religious or "good" in an effort to gain another chance at life or more time to live
Grief/Depression	Realizes that "bargaining" is not working and death is approaching	Becomes depressed, weepy; may "give up," quit taking medications, quit eating, and so forth
Acceptance	"OK . . . but I don't have to like it!"	Enters a state of expectation; may begin to call family members near; needs to complete "unfinished business"; prepares spiritually to die

what is going on in their environment. For this reason, nurses must be careful in talking to the patient and the family, even immediately after the patient's death. Again, people from some cultures and religions believe that the "spirit" or "soul" remains in the room for a period of time after death. Regardless of the belief system, it is a sign of respect to the patient and the significant others to include the patient in the conversation and continue to speak in terms of the reality of the situation.

Neeb's Tip Dr. Kübler-Ross' theory also emphasizes the fact that hearing is the last sense to leave a person before death.

Children go through the same stages as adults; and as with adults, they may need special help to come to terms with losing a loved one. The help nurses give to younger patients must be age-appropriate. Infants and toddlers may not be able to understand what happened, but they do sense the change. Keep their routine as normal as possible. Provide them with physical closeness and a safe environment.

Children from 2 to 6 years of age may have the sense that death is reversible. How often do they see cartoon characters "die" and then immediately return to animated life? When the reality that grandmother or grandfather is not coming back to life is understood, it is important that the child understands that he or she did not cause the death of the loved one.

Children ages 6 to 12 are at varying degrees of understanding. It is important to allow and encourage children to talk about their feelings. Recent incidents of violence involving this age group have provided the opportunity for grief counselors to intervene with children who have survived the ordeals.

Teens are bridging the gap from childhood to adulthood and may respond to grief and loss as an adult at times and then as children. Provide structure, routine, and an environment in which they may freely express their thoughts and feelings.

When caring for dying patients, the nurse needs to be aware of the existence of and state's recognition of an advance directive or "living will" (where the wishes of the dying person are placed on a legal document, signed by the person while competent, and witnessed), and the family's wishes. Advance directives also identify who the decision maker(s) will be if the person is unable to speak for him/herself.

Euthanasia (sometimes called "mercy killing") is illegal in the United States, but "physician-assisted suicide" (also called aid in dying) is now legal in some states. These topics will continue to be debated. Competent adults have the right to decline any medical treatment even if it hastens death. All of these can bring out strong emotions for families and the nurse who is caring for people at the end of their lives. Nurses need to be educated about the ethical and legal considerations around providing end of life care.

The nurse's responsibilities at the patient's death vary from state to state. For instance, in some states nurses are allowed to pronounce the death of a patient; in other states this must be done only by a physician. Death is defined differently from state to state. Physical signs such as vital signs, skin color and temperature, presence or absence of activity on electroencephalogram (EEG) and electrocardiogram (ECG), and the ability to be viable, or to live without mechanical assistance, are criteria used by states to define death. It is the nurse's responsibility to know the legal definition of death in the state in which he or she is working.

Critical Thinking Question

Your patient is in a monogamous homosexual relationship and is in the final stage of life. Death is imminent, but the patient is still alert and oriented. Family and partner are in the room. The patient asks you to ask the physician to "put me to sleep." The patient's partner weeps but supports the request; the family members threaten to sue if the physician does "any such thing." What are your thoughts and feelings about this request? What will you do to help the patient? The family? The partner? What if this were your parent or child who was about to die? What would you think and feel then?

Key Concepts

1. There are many theories about personality development in human beings. Although they are only theories, there are strong indications of validity in all of them. The licensed practical nurse (LPN) and the licensed vocational nurse (LVN) must have a working knowledge of some of the more commonly accepted theories of human development throughout the life span.
2. Dr. Elisabeth Kübler-Ross developed a theory of five stages that people go through when they are grieving or dying. Although others have presented theories on this topic, hers remains the most commonly accepted theory in nursing.
3. Each person is an individual and will go through stages of development or grief at his or her own pace. These theories are guidelines to help nurses understand what patients may experience as they go through certain stages in their lives.

CASE STUDY

Mr. Y, a 24-year-old construction worker, suffered a traumatic brain injury after falling from scaffolding when his safety equipment failed. He was comatose for 8 days. During this time, family and friends kept a constant vigil. His wife was 6 months pregnant and fearful about having to raise the baby alone. Many conversations were held in his room while he was in the coma. When he awakened from the coma, he was able to tell most of what was said. He wondered why "nobody answered me when I talked to you." He especially wanted to reassure his wife that "Nothing would keep me from seeing that baby!"

1. What suggestions could a nurse have made to the family of this patient regarding patients who are comatose?
2. How can a nurse help the patient who has concerns about "memories" he or she acquired while in a coma (e.g., what is real and what is not, what things might have been said in confidence, and so forth)?

REFERENCES

Barry, P. D. (2002). *Mental Health and Mental Illness.* 7th ed. Philadelphia: JB Lippincott.

Barger, R. N. (2000). *A Summary of Lawrence Kohlberg's Stages of Moral Development.* Notre Dame, IN: University of Notre Dame.

Centers for Disease Control and Prevention. National Center for Health Statistics. (n.d.). Retrieved from www.cdc.gov/nchs/fastats/lifexpec.htm

Centers for Disease Control and Prevention. (n.d.). Retrieved from www.cdc.gov/violenceprevention/globalviolence/index.html

Dennis, L.B., and Hassol, J. (1983). *Introduction to Human Development and Health Issues.* Philadelphia: WB Saunders.

Dewey, R. (2007). *Karen Horney's theory.* Retrieved from www.intropsych.com/ch11_personality/karen_horneys_theory.html

Gilligan, C. (1982). *In a Different Voice: Psychological Theory and Women's Development.* Cambridge, MA: Harvard University Press.

Kübler-Ross, E. (1969). *On Death and Dying.* New York: Macmillan.

Lickona, T. (1991). *Educating for Character: How Our Schools Can Teach Respect and Responsibility.* New York: Bantam.

Test Questions

Multiple Choice Questions

1. A 4-year-old patient comes into the clinic with her father. She is being checked for a recurring ear infection. As you prepare her to see the physician, she says to you, "I love my Daddy. I'm going to marry him like Mommy someday!" Which one of Freud's stages of development is she most likely demonstrating?
a. Genital
b. Oral
c. Anal
d. Phallic

2. Patient Y is 20 years old. Y is a perfectionist and very routine-oriented. Freudian theorists would say that Patient Y did not successfully complete which of the following stages of development?
a. Genital
b. Oral
c. Anal
d. Phallic

3. Patient Y (from question 2) is being treated by a behavioral psychologist. When Patient Y begins to miss meals and activities because of the need to complete routines perfectly, the staff is to intervene. Patient Y failed to come to dinner on your shift. You go to check on the patient and see Y carefully placing personal items in a special place in the bathroom. Your best response to Y from a behavioral and therapeutic background would be:
a. "Y, where were you at dinner tonight?"
b. "Y, you blew it. You didn't come to dinner and you know what that means: no pass for the weekend."
c. "Y, I am just here to remind you it is dinnertime."
d. "Y, it is not appropriate to miss dinner. What is the consequence of that, according to your care plan?"

4. In prenatal development, cell differentiation is normally completed by the end of the:
a. First trimester
b. Second trimester
c. Third trimester
d. First lunar month

5. The infant mortality rate is highest mothers who are:
a. Over 35 years old
b. Over 30 years old
c. Under 20 years old
d. Under 15 years old

6. The term *anima* from Carl Jung's tl describes:
a. Male characteristics in women
b. Feminine characteristics in men
c. Male characteristics in men
d. Feminine characteristics in wom

7. According to Erikson's theory, the opmental task stage a 3- to 6-year-needs to accomplish is:
a. Identity
b. Industry
c. Intimacy
d. Initiative

8. Infants seem to be very much alike (developmentally) until the age of:
a. 2 months
b. 6 months
c. 10 months
d. 12 months

9. A toddler's ability to take in or ack edge changes in the environment is called:
a. Adjustment
b. Assimilation
c. Accommodation
d. Autonomy

10. The parents of a 2-year-old arrive a hospital to visit the child. The chil the play room and ignores the pare during the visit. This 2-year-old bel indicates:
a. The child is withdrawn
b. The child is more interested in p with other children
c. The child has adjusted to the ho ized setting
d. A normal pattern

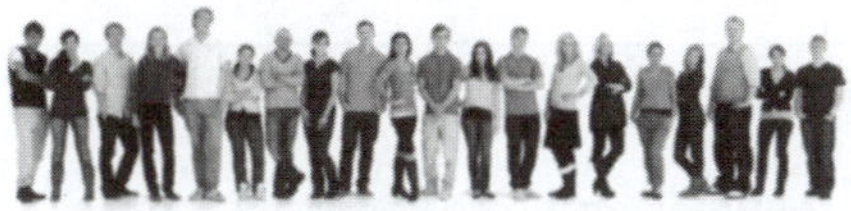

CHAPTER 5

Sociocultural Influences on Mental Health

Learning Objectives

1. Define culture.
2. Identify factors to consider when assessing culture and ethnicity.
3. Differentiate between religion and spirituality.
4. Define ethnicity.
5. Identify parenting styles.
6. Differentiate between abuse and neglect.
7. Define stereotype.
8. Define prejudice.
9. Define homelessness.
10. Identify some possible reasons for homelessness.
11. Identify nursing care for people who are homeless.

Key Terms

- Abuse
- Culture
- Ethnicity
- Ethnocentrism
- Homeless
- Parenting
- Prejudice
- Religion
- Stereotype

Many professionals in the field of psychology believe that social and cultural environments have a great influence on the way people develop and process life. They believe that positive or negative social and cultural experiences early in life result in similar positive or negative behavior and beliefs in adulthood.

Neeb's Tip Part of the nurse's role is to learn about traits that are common among people and those that are different. It is important to understand people's customs and beliefs to avoid unrealistic expectations of patients.

Culture and ethnicity are among the topics that are said to have the greatest influence on people throughout their life span.

■ Culture

Culture is a term that is often misused. Culture is a shared way of life, the combination of traditions and beliefs that make a group of people bond together (also see Chapter 3). Culture is not based on one's color of skin or country of origin. For example, in the 1960s, a group of young people who were speaking out against the politics and morals of their parents began living in groups (Fig. 5-1). The area they chose to start this movement was the Haight-Ashbury district in San Francisco. They called themselves "hippies," and they shared a way of life that consisted of experimenting with drugs; living together without being married (or "free love," as it was termed); dressing in ripped, dirty clothing; not cutting their hair; and doing just about everything else that was opposite to the values of the "older generation." This group believed

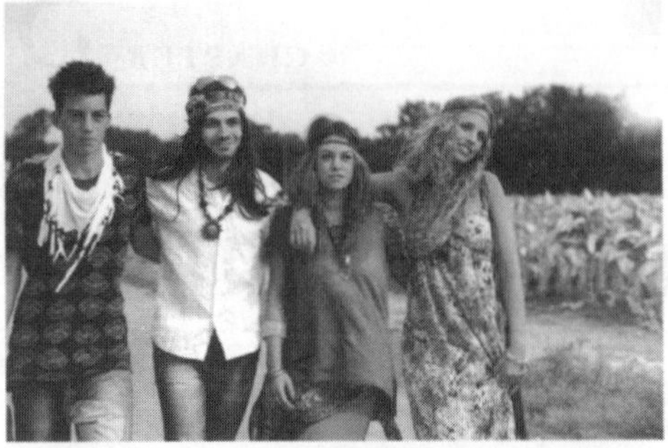

Figure 5-1 The hippies of the 1960s represented their own unique culture.

in loving everyone, regardless of race, creed, and color—as long as the individual embraced the beliefs of the group. The group's symbols were the daisy and the peace sign, and "flower power" and "power to the people" represented some of the ideals they followed. Much to the chagrin of the over-30 age group, these young people fit the definition of a "culture." It was called a "subculture" or "counterculture" at the time. Today, the "goth" statement many youth are making may be equated to the statements of their parents or grandparents in the 1960s.

Neeb's Tip Nurses may discover that when it comes to being knowledgeable about other cultures, they have been living in a glass jar—only seeing other cultures but unaware of how to interact with them.

Bringing cultural competence to patient care is a primary responsibility of the nurse. Culturally diverse nursing care takes into account the following areas: communication, space, social organization, time, environmental control and biological variation according to the Transcultural Assessment Model developed by Giger and Davidhizar (Giger, 2013). Culturally diverse care means the nurse is adapting care in a manner congruent with the patient's culture.

Tool Box | Transcultural Nursing Assessment Tool
www.culturediversity.org/assesmnt.htm

Clinical Activity
While preparing a care plan for an assigned patient, ask the patient about his or her culture. Determine if any of the patient's traditions or beliefs have been included in the plan of care.

A psychoanalyst named Karen Horney (see Chapter 4) proposed the theory that some cultural traditions and beliefs cause disturbances in personal relationships and that this can lead to some forms of emotional disturbances. Today, one can look at other groups who have a shared belief system and a shared way of life. Madeleine Leninger, a nurse theorist, also realized the importance of transcultural nursing. Leninger established the Culture Care Theory. It was while caring for children that she found how their behavior needs were related to their culture; without understanding each of these cultures, functioning as a health-care provider was difficult (Leininger, 2006)

Clinical Activity
As a class, formulate a list of 10 questions you can use during your clinical experience while doing assessments on someone of a different culture or alternative lifestyle. Questions are subject to the instructor's approval.

Religious beliefs are often included in discussions of culture; however, it is important to note that the religion is *not* usually the culture. For people who practice Judaism or Islam, the relationship between their religious beliefs and their cultural beliefs is so entwined that it is hard to separate those traits. However, the hippie group mentioned earlier contained people raised in many different religions.

Religion is the belief in a higher power. This belief system can be very strong—so strong that people have fought wars over religion and even now continue to wage war in the name of religion. Rituals or worship services are usually

Box 5-1 Cultural Assessment—Questions to Ask

- Where was the patient born? If the patient is an immigrant, how long has he or she been in this country?
- What is the patient's ethnic affiliation? How strong is the ethnic identity?
- Who are the patient's major support people? Does patient live in an ethnic community?
- Who in the family takes responsibility for health concerns and decisions?
- Are there any activities in which the patient may decline to participate because of culture or religious taboos?
- Does the patient have any special food preferences, or food refusals because of culture or religion?
- What are the patient's primary and secondary languages, and speaking and reading abilities?
- What is the patient's religion, what is its importance in daily life, and what are current practices?
- What is the patient's economic situation? Is income adequate for his or her needs?
- What are the patient's health beliefs and practices?
- What are the patient's perceptions of the health problems and expectations of health care?

Source: Gorman and Sultan (2008). Psychosocial Nursing for General Patient Care, 3rd ed. Philadelphia: F.A. Davis Company.

Critical Thinking Question

Your patient is from a different country and speaks only minimal English. Your translator has seen the patient and has gone over the hospital routines, rules, and patient's rights. The patient's mother insists on staying in the room 24 hours a day and refuses to let you perform assessments and care for the patient. The patient is in pain, but the mother will not allow pain medication to be given. The patient will not accept the food from the hospital. You smell food cooking and enter the room to find the mother cooking on a hot plate, which is a fire code violation. What can you do in this situation?

included in organized religions. Religion is often the subject of stereotype. A **stereotype** is a fixed notion or conviction about a group of people or a situation.

Classroom Activity

- Interview a person whose religion is different from your own. You may use the interview format from Chapter 6. Present the interview results orally or in writing to the class. Discuss what you thought you knew about the religion prior to the interview. Discuss what you learned after the interview. Review literature on that specific religion and compare the information from the interview.

Native Americans are an example of a group that worships different gods or spirits. Of course, it is improper to categorize all Native Americans into one large group; there are many nations and many tribes, each with its own set of beliefs. One belief is that certain numbers are sacred to some Native Americans, and they may attribute special qualities to the four directions of north, south, east, and west.

Spirituality and religion are extremely important to some patients and unimportant or nonexistent to others, although both are different. Nurses must be comfortable talking to patients about their religious and spiritual needs without pushing personal values on patients. A patient's success at recuperating from an illness or a surgical procedure may be deeply tied to his or her spirituality. Nurses who are not comfortable in these situations should offer to call the chaplain in the facility or a spiritual leader of the patient's choice.

Religions involve items considered sacred. Such items may include books (e.g., Bible, Koran), jewelry (brooch, pin, or cross), the person's dress (headwear, loose-fitting clothing), or other type of personal effects. It is generally believed that patients should be allowed to keep these items when possible. In situations in which a patient may be in poor mental health and possession of these items is of actual or potential danger to the patient or others in the area, it may be necessary to remove the items. If that becomes necessary, enlisting the assistance of a representative from the particular religion may be helpful.

Tool Box |▶ Religion Diversity
www.bbc.co.uk/religion/religions/

Classroom Activity
- Have a culture awareness day presentation. Describe the following traditions for your religion or culture:
  - Foods
  - Music
  - Weddings
  - Death practices
  - Myths

Ethnicity

Ethnicity defines one's more personal traits and identifies a person with his or her shared heritage. Language, country of origin, and skin color are parts of one's ethnicity. There can be different ethnic groups within a culture. For example, a blonde, blue-eyed woman exhibits physical characteristics of her ethnic background. However, these characteristics say little about her culture; that would require speaking to her and obtaining some information. People are generally very proud of their culture and ethnicity. Many communities have festivals that celebrate their different cultures and ethnic groups. These festivals do much to educate the community about the various people living together in it. Sometimes one can learn a lot about a group of people from the kind of food they eat, and these celebrations are usually overflowing with foods of the particular group.

Neeb's Tip Education can help eliminate **prejudice**, which is judging a person or situation before all the facts are known. Prejudice is a destructive behavior; it is hurtful and it shuts the door on the enrichment of the society.

Laws in the United States are intended to minimize displays of prejudice relating to race, creed, gender, age, and so on. Unfortunately, it is impossible to legislate the beliefs of individual people. Nurses are in a perfect position to teach and model interpersonal relationships and, it is hoped, to make great strides in eliminating prejudgment of others.

Health care may not be completely free of guilt in the area of race. A study was conducted at Emory University School of Medicine in Atlanta, Georgia (Todd et al., 2000). For 40 months, researchers studied 217 patients who sought treatment for long bone fractures. Of these patients, 127 were black and 90 were white. Patients with this type of fracture usually require some type of pain medication. The study showed that, even though the injuries and pain levels were similar, 43% of the black patients received no pain medication, compared to 26% of white patients. The study could not determine the exact rationale for the outcome. Did some patients refuse medication? Did some not ask? Was it a cultural choice? Did medical staff make assumptions about drug misuse in some people? Nurses should be wary of statistics and be careful about silent stereotypes.

Critical Thinking Question
Should a patient's identification bracelet specify if the patient has insurance coverage? If the patient does not have any coverage, will the care be the same as if the patient had coverage?

The hurt of prejudice has led to an emergence of **ethnocentrism,** which is when people believe that their particular ethnic or religious group has rights and benefits over and above those of others. Gangs, supremacist groups, and terrorist groups may have had their roots in hate and prejudice.

Sadly, society is reminded of the plight of the Jewish people, who lived through the horror of concentration camps. The United States shows the scars of the inhumane treatment of the African and African American people, who have been fighting for their civil rights for over 200 years. And it remains a topic of debate today. The validity of affirmative action is being questioned and, in fact, being called by some a form of discrimination against other people. In 2008 the citizens of the United States elected their first African American president, which gave many hope that some social scars will heal. Religion, culture, and ethnicity, as well as prejudice caused by any of those characteristics, are personal and deeply felt by members of the respective groups. It is important to keep the lines of communication open. People learn by sharing with each other, so it is much better to ask a person about something than to make an assumption about it. Making such an assumption is stereotyping, which can end a helping relationship between nurse and patient.

Many mental health professionals believe that people raised in an atmosphere of prejudice and stereotype tend to become angry, hateful, and aggressive adults. There is no proof that *all* people who are subjected to prejudice and stereotype develop into adults with such negative attitudes. This is one of the dangers in reading statistics on these topics: Statistics can be very misleading and can in fact support the negative stereotypes.

Classroom Activity

- Interview a person who is from a culture different from your own. You may use the interview format from Chapter 6. Present the results orally or in writing. This will reinforce the information presented in Chapter 6, as well as provide first-hand information pertinent to this chapter.

Box 5-2 Enhancing Cultural Sensitivity

- Know your own attitudes, values, and beliefs.
- Be aware of your own ethnocentrism.
- Be aware of your own prejudices that may influence your assessment.
- Maintain an open mind and seek out more information about your patient's culture, beliefs, and values.
- Communicate your interest about the patient's beliefs and values.
- Approach the patient as an individual. Avoid assuming that all people from one cultural background hold the same beliefs.

Source: Gorman and Sultan (2008). Psychosocial Nursing for General Patient Care, 3rd ed. Philadelphia: F.A. Davis Company.

Nontraditional Lifestyles

The definition of "family" is changing (Fig. 5-2). Gay marriage and civil unions have opened very active debates. In June 2013, the U.S. Supreme Count knocked down the Defense of Marriage Act to pave the way for federal recognition of same sex marriages. Same-sex marriages are now legal in many states. It is becoming more common in schools and clinics for children to have "two mommies" or "two daddies." People with lesbian, gay, bisexual, and transgender (LGBT) lifestyles are "out" in the open and living life as normally as the more traditional father/mother/children families of decades earlier. All age groups are affected. However, despite signs of increased acceptance, LGBT individuals as well as their families may still struggle with facing being "different."

People have been leading different lifestyles all along but were far less comfortable professing it in years past. Aging happens to all, regardless of lifestyle preference. By the year 2030, according to the National Gay and Lesbian Task Force, there will be approximately four million gay elders requiring social services and living in long-term care facilities. How will that change the way nurses provide care? Overtly, probably very little; good nursing care will remain good nursing care. However, nurses may need to learn to alter their communication style to ask for and accept people's preferences for roommate, type of clothing to wear, or activities to attend. Activities may cross gender barriers in a different way than they do today. Who shares bathrooms may become a different priority. Clearly, in the not too distant future, nurses practicing in clinics and long-term care or assisted living facilities can expect some changes in the clientele as well as the way in which those people will require assistance.

Additionally, more individuals are choosing to start and raise families as single parents. Parents are adopting children from other countries, other ethnicities, and other races. One family may now include parents and siblings with assorted skin tones and languages. The global family is rapidly and constantly evolving.

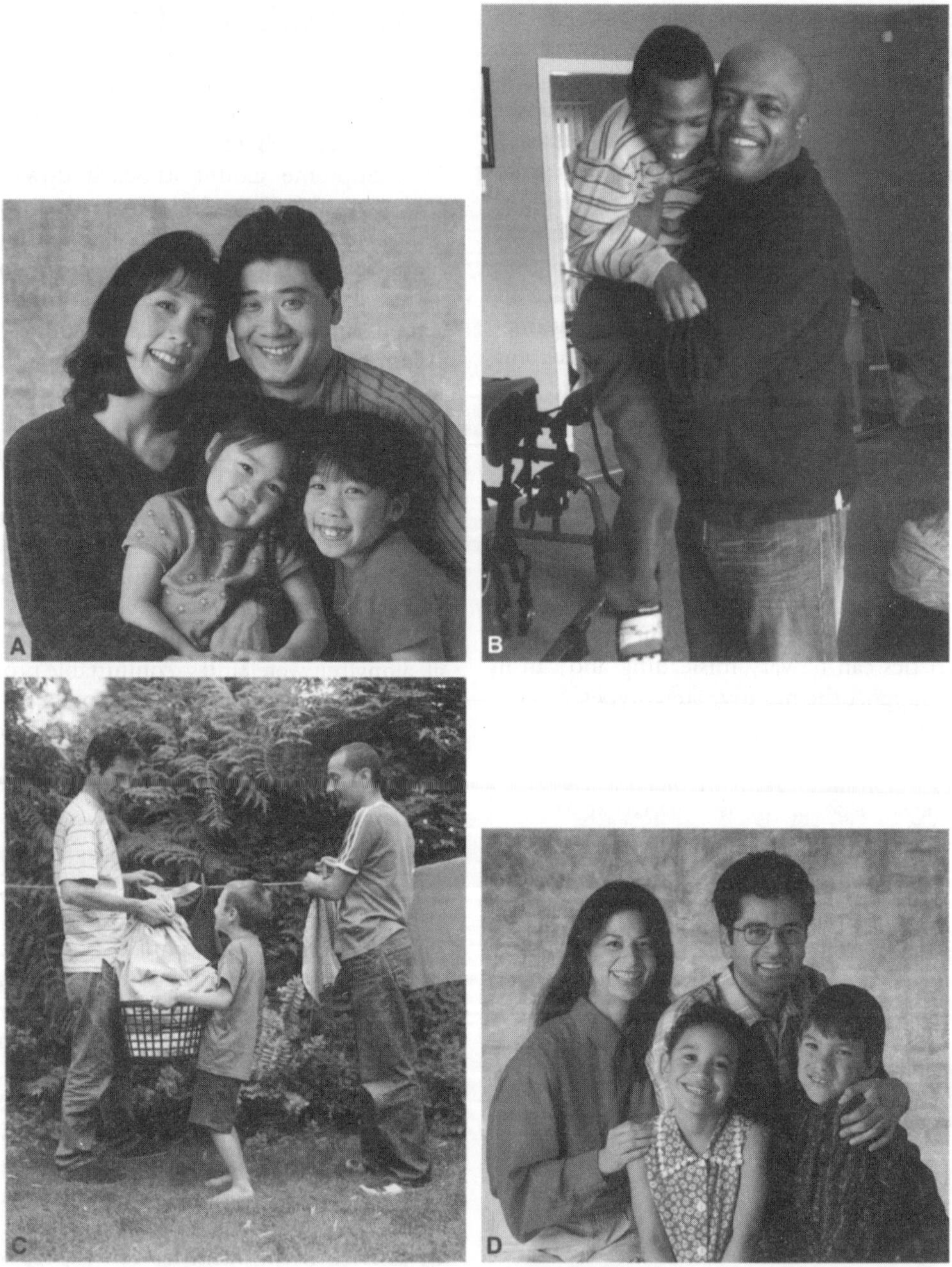

Figure 5-2 The definition of "family" is changing. A, Traditional family, with a mother, father, and their biological children. B, Single-parent family. *(Courtesy of Robynn Anwar.)* C, Gay couple and child. *(Photograph by Creatas.)* D, "Blended" family, in which each spouse has his or her own children, whom they bring into a new family.

■ Homelessness

Homelessness is not a mental illness (Fig. 5-3). It receives brief mention in this text because many of the people in the United States who are **homeless** also have some threat to their mental health.

The picture of the homeless population is as varied as those who have homes. Some people are working full-time but are homeless. They might be victims of the economy, foreclosures, or other situations not related in any way to having a mental illness. Since 2008, tent cities have appeared across America (Fig. 5-4). A small number of people choose to live on the streets. Others have been forced to live on the street or in a shelter as a result of forces out of their control.

Many more of the homeless are suffering from a variety of mental illnesses. Some people are homeless as an indirect result of the health-care delivery system. Approximately one-third of the homeless population in the United States is mentally ill, with many more having substance abuse issues (Mental Health Association of Colorado). The rise in homelessness is linked to the rising cost of rental housing and poverty (National Coalition for the Homeless, 2009). Because of the diagnosis, the availability of benefits for the mentally ill, and the nature of the illnesses, people with certain illnesses have a difficult time trying to live independently with their illness. They end up out of work, out of money, and out of a home. They may be noncompliant with their medications, have no access to getting refills, lose the medication, or have it stolen on the streets. A large number of people who use community-based mental health services are the poor, especially the homeless poor (Barry, 2002). Tragically, many of the homeless are also veterans. Services are available through Veterans Affairs, but the person may have challenges in how to access them.

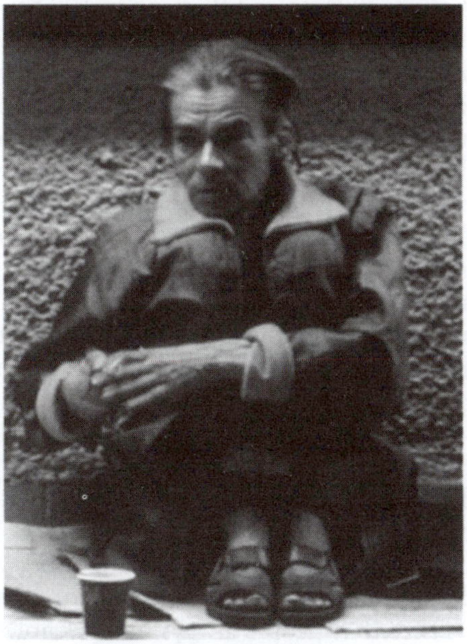

Figure 5-3 Homelessness is not a mental illness, but many homeless people face threats to their mental health. *(Courtesy of Telecom Pioneers, Nova 5 Chapter #5, Brooklyn, NY.)*

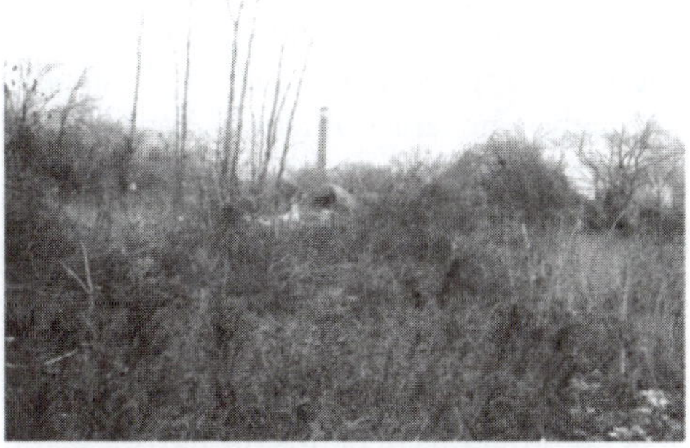

Figure 5-4 Tent city for the homeless in Camden, New Jersey. *(Courtesy of Robynn Anwar.)*

> ■ ■ ■ Critical Thinking Question
> You are the only source of income for your family. You are laid off because of a merger of two agencies. How long can you survive with no income? How will you pay for insurance? Jobs are not plentiful; the outlook for comparable employment in the near future is bleak. How close are you to living on the street? What will be the plan of action for you and your family?

In the 1950s, deinstitutionalization led to the discharging of people who were technically able to be "in the community" but who were not always able to cope with the stresses of caring for themselves, caring for their families, and maintaining employment. For some mentally ill people, this kind of pressure and competition is the factor that keeps them ill. The Urban Institute Study of 2000 estimates there are approximately 3.5 million people annually who are homeless. Approximately one-third of those are children (Box 5-3.)

In 1987, the Health Resources and Services Administration–Health Care for the Homeless (HRSA–HCH) was formed to provide information and help create plans to help the homeless. The problem is that funding of federal programs depends on statistics, and it is extremely difficult to get accurate numbers because they change markedly approximately every 2 months (*Society Magazine,* 1994).

Patients may be brought to a facility through the emergency department or by a law enforcement agency. Sometimes medication is given to stabilize the patient, and he or she is returned to the community; other times the patient is admitted to a medical unit. Unfortunately, sometimes the mental health issue is overlooked because of the health-care provider's focus being on physical health.

Box 5-3 Homeless in America. Who Are They?

Group	Approximate Percentage
Families with children (2007)	23%
Children under the age of 18 (2003)	39%
People between the ages of 25–34 (2004)	25%
People ages 55–64 (2004) 6%	
Single females (2007)	65%
Single males (2007)	35%
Veterans of wars (served in the armed forces)	40%
African American (2006)	42%
Caucasian (2006)	38%
Hispanic (2006)	20%
Native American (2006)	4%
Asian (2006)	2%

Note: These numbers are approximations and will vary according to the study and the area of the country.

Source: National Coalition for the Homeless (2009). *Who is Homeless?* Retrieved from http://nationalhomeless.org/factsheets/who.html.

Shelters of varying types exist in many cities. They are funded and staffed in different ways. For example, some are church funded and some rely on grants and underwriting by large businesses. Some are completely operated by volunteers and some have some paid staff. Depending on the resources available, shelters for homeless people provide anything from meals and overnight shelter to health care, dental care, and assistance with job placement.

Often, however, behavioral conditions exist in such shelters. Homeless people may be required to stay drug- and alcohol-free and to show proof that they are compliant with medications or some other criteria to help them return to an improved lifestyle.

What techniques do nurses need to help patients who may be homeless and physically or mentally compromised?

1. Treat the whole person, not the homelessness.
2. Treat the person as any other patient.
3. Maintain all patient rights.

■ Economic Considerations

A study by Eron and Peterson in 1982 found that the lower the socioeconomic status, the higher the incidence of abnormal behavior in U.S. society. That statement, however, is not completely accurate. The study showed that the statement applies more strongly to patients with schizophrenia than it does to those with mood disorders. The implication is that there are always other variables besides socioeconomic status. For example, people who live in poverty or underprivileged circumstances will very likely have greater stressors than will people of higher socioeconomic status. So, is it the lack of money or increased stress that leads to the disorder? Such questions make it very difficult, if not impossible, to make absolute statements about the correlation between disease and any variable. Behaviorists emphasize that people always have a choice. If the foregoing statements about poverty and illness were completely true, then it would follow that *all* people in that same circumstance would be mentally ill.

However, this is simply not the case. What variable causes some people to be ill and others not to be ill? Is it choice? Is it genetic? Is it learned behavior? This is part of the intrigue of the study of the mind.

Abuse

Abuse is misuse of a person, substance, or situation. Sometimes people say that they cannot be abusing because they know what they are doing. This is not true. Anyone who misuses or overuses a person, a substance, or a situation (such as gambling or power) is displaying abusive behavior.

Some individual forms of abuse are discussed in Chapter 22. Abuse in general is a growing phenomenon in society. People debate about whether a higher incidence of abuse exists now or whether people are just talking about it more openly. Violence is a learned behavior. It is well documented that in the majority of physical abuse situations, the abuser was abused at some point.

When it comes to substance abuse, the findings are not quite as conclusive. Some studies indicate that this type of abuse may be genetic, learned, or possibly due to a chemical imbalance in the body. A phenomenon called the "addictive personality" is defined as grouping abuse disorders together. It is important for nurses to understand that there may be more than one cause for a particular mental health problem. Good communication and data-collecting skills will help the nurse find potential causes for each patient's mental health problem.

Poor Parenting

What is a "good" parent? Is it the parent who lets the child do anything the child wants? Is it the parent who buys all the newest fads for the child? Is it the parent who teaches strict values and ethics? Maybe it is the parent who is with the child at all times. **Parenting** is the method of raising children that is used by parents or other primary caregivers. Parenting is a learned behavior; it is not an innate skill. So, how do parents *learn to be* parents? Typically, one tends to parent based on the way he or she was parented. That means all the cultural and religious values that have been planted in one parent's belief systems are brought out in the open and blended with those values from the other parent's upbringing. Then, it is up to the parents to take one day at a time and learn from their mistakes. Sometimes parenting is learned from friends and neighbors. Sometimes schools, health-care facilities, and communities offer classes for parents.

> **Critical Thinking Question**
>
> You are home one evening and you hear the 18-month-old child of your upstairs neighbors. The child has been crying for 3 hours. You have heard no footsteps in the apartment. The answering machine picks up each time you attempt to call. You become concerned and call the building supervisor to open the apartment. When you get in, you find unsanitary conditions, and the parents are not in the apartment. You look outside and see the parents several apartments down, partying with friends. What are your responsibilities? How will you respond to the parents? Whom will you notify? The parents tell you to mind your own business. What will you say to them? What will you do if it happens again?

Reactions to altered parenting styles are varied. Again, there is no "perfect" situation or guarantee of being "good" parents. Parenting is stressful. No matter what patients are concerned about during their hospitalization, it is almost certain that their children will be a paramount focus of attention. Nurses can help parents not only through the stress of being hospitalized and apart from their children, but also with the stresses of parenting in general by helping parents choose healthy lifestyles. Good nutrition, moderate exercise, and "adult time" apart from the children can be effective stress relievers.

Diana Baumrind (1971) has classified three different types of parents. They are described as follows:

1. *Authoritarian parent:* This parent sets up very strict rules. The child has little or no voice in family decisions. This style of parenting is evidenced by novelty clothing imprinted with the saying, "Because I'm the Mommy/Daddy, that's why!" This authoritarianism can lead

to a rebellious, hostile child who may enter adulthood angry, violent, unwilling to obey laws, and unable to make consistent decisions.

2. *Authoritative parent:* This style of parenting has firm, consistent rules and limits, while allowing for discussion and occasional flexibility of those rules according to special circumstances. Children are allowed some freedom, within set limits, and some voice in decisions. Researchers think that this is the preferred style of parenting. It offers a balance between rules and responsibilities, which allows the child to learn to make appropriate choices and accept the outcomes of those choices.
3. *Permissive parent:* This is the type of parent many adolescents wish they had. This style of parenting provides little structure and few guidelines. The child is not sure of his or her boundaries. If one does not learn boundaries, it becomes difficult to learn how to control oneself and how to behave in certain situations. Permissive parents can be in danger of being accused of neglect. The parent acts as the child's friend rather than the parent of the child.

■■■ Clinical Activity

Choose someone you know who is a parent. This can be a family member, friend, neighbor, or anyone you feel comfortable with. Using the parenting definitions of Diana Baumrind, identify what basic parenting style you think this parent uses.

■■■ Key Concepts

1. Culture, ethnicity, sexual orientation, and religion are deeply rooted human experiences. They are not "good" or "bad"; they are different for each individual or group of individuals who claim membership in that culture, ethnic group, or religion.
2. People have many more similarities than they have differences. It is important for nurses to concentrate on the similarities among people and to be comfortable asking questions about the background of their patients and coworkers. Role modeling cooperative relationships can be very helpful in teaching others about cultural sensitivity.

CASE STUDY

Harold is a 76-year-old nursing home resident. He has type 1 diabetes and gives himself his own insulin. He has the diagnosis of paranoid schizophrenia but has been asymptomatic for 1 year. Harold is also a severe alcoholic, and he periodically leaves the nursing home against medical advice and is gone for 2 to 3 days. He has friends "on the street" because, before being institutionalized, that is where he lived. Harold goes to the local shelter for meals and knows he can go to the hospital to get his insulin. He has no family in the vicinity who can participate in his care. He no longer meets the criteria for skilled-care nursing. A decision must be made about his future, as he will no longer be eligible to remain in this nursing home. Harold wishes to be his own advocate and is found to be legally capable of making his own decisions. The outcome for this patient is that he chooses to "take my chances" and return to the streets. He has not been seen again by any of the nursing home staff. No further information is available about this patient.

1. Considering Maslow's Hierarchy of Needs, how would you classify Harold?
2. What are the arguments both for and against his decision to leave the nursing home?
3. Do you consider Harold to be mentally healthy and competent? Why or why not?

REFERENCES

Barry, P.D. (2002). *Mental Health and Mental Illness.* 7th ed. Philadelphia: J. B. Lippincott.

Baumrind, D. (1971). Current patterns of parental authority. *Developmental psychology* (monograph 1), *4,* 1–103.

Cummins, H.J. (June 22, 2003). Coming out, moving on. Minneapolis, MN: *Star Tribune.*

Eron, L.D., and Peterson, R.A. (1982). Abnormal behavior: Social approaches. In M.R. Rosenzweig and L.W. Porter (Eds.), *Annual review of psychology 33,* 231–65.

Galanti, G. (1991). *Caring for Patients From Different Cultures—Case Studies From American Hospitals.* Philadelphia: University of Pennsylvania Press.

Giger, JN. (2013). *Transcultural Nursing.* St Louis: Mosby.

Gorman, L.M., and Sultan, D.F. (2008). Cultural considerations. In *Psychosocial Nursing for General Patient Care.* 3rd ed., pp. 49–56. Philadelphia: F.A. Davis.

Kaplan, B.J. (November 2002). Gay elders face uncomfortable realities in LTC. *Caring for the Ages,* American Medical Directors Association (November 2002), Vol. 3, No. 11.

Leininger, M. (2006). Part one: Madeleine M. Leininger's theory of culture care diversity and universality. In M. Parker (Ed.), *Nursing Theories and Nursing Practice.* 2nd ed., pp. 309–320. Philadelphia: F.A Davis.

Martin, M.L. (2000). Ethnicity and Analgesic Practice: An Editorial. *Annals of emergency medicine, 35,* 77–81.

Mental Health Association of Colorado. *Homelessness.* www.mhacolorado.org/file_depot/0-10000000/Homelessness.pdf

Merriam-Webster. (2012). *Merriam-Webster; an Encyclopedia Britannica Company.* Retrieved from www.merriam-webster.com/dictionary/homeless

National Coalition for the Homeless. (2009). *Who is homeless?* http://nationalhomeless.org/factsheets/who.html

Purtilo, R., and Haddad, A. (2002). *Health Professional and Patient Interaction.* 6th ed. Philadelphia: W.B. Saunders

Social science and the citizen: Counting homeless (1994, November/December). *Society Magazine.*

Todd, K.H., Deaton, C., D'Adamo, A. P., and Goe, L. (2000). Ethnicity and analgesic practice. *Annals of emergency medicine, 35,* 11–16.

Test Questions

Multiple Choice Questions

1. The concepts of space, time, and waiting are:
   a. Religious
   b. Cultural
   c. Economic
   d. Ethnic

2. The condition of judging a person or situation before all the facts are known is called:
   a. Hatred
   b. Abuse
   c. Prejudice
   d. Stereotype

3. Homelessness is being blamed, in part, on:
   a. Deinstitutionalization
   b. Access to community services
   c. Mental illness
   d. All of the above

4. Nurses who care for patients who are homeless understand that in the United States:
   a. Homelessness is classified as a mental illness.
   b. Approximately one-third of the homeless are mentally ill.
   c. All the homeless have some form of mental illness.
   d. People must be mentally ill to choose to be homeless.

5. A patient is admitted with the diagnosis of paranoid behavior. The patient claims to be of a religion requiring the wearing of very heavy necklaces. You research the religion and determine this to be true, but the patient has been seen violently flinging a necklace at his or her roommate. Your best nursing action is:
   a. Call an assistance code.
   b. Remove all religious items.
   c. Do nothing: it is his or her religious right.
   d. Enlist the assistance of a religious representative to negotiate removal of the item(s) in question.

6. Parents accompany their ill 8-year-old child to the clinic. The child was diagnosed last month with type 1 diabetes and is insulin dependent. The parents admit they are not administering the insulin, as their religious beliefs do not allow foreign substances in any form for any reason. A check of the patient's chart clearly indicates that diabetes teaching had been done with this family unit at last month's visit. Your initial nursing action is:
   a. Report the parents for child endangerment, as nurses are mandatory reporters.
   b. Inform the parents that this child could die without the required insulin.
   c. Leave the room and call a doctor or RN to the room stat.
   d. Collect information pertaining to what the religion would allow and facilitate discussion with the doctor.

7. When collecting data during an intake interview, the nurse understands: *(select all that apply)*
   a. Most homeless people are unemployed.
   b. Culture is a shared belief system.
   c. Prejudice exists within the health-care delivery system.
   d. There is no correlation between mental illness and the condition of homelessness.

8. The most common reasons for homelessness include: *(select all that apply)*
   a. Economic setbacks
   b. Lack of ambition and laziness
   c. Major health expenses
   d. Desire to live independently
   e. Mental health

9. Language, country of origin, and skin color define:
   a. Religion
   b. Culture

c. Ethnocentrism
d. Ethnicity

10. Diana Baumrind describes authoritative parenting as:
a. The child has little or no voice in any of the family's decisions.
b. The parents are always reminding the child that they are the parents.
c. The child has a minimum amount of guidelines.
d. The child has rules and has limits set.

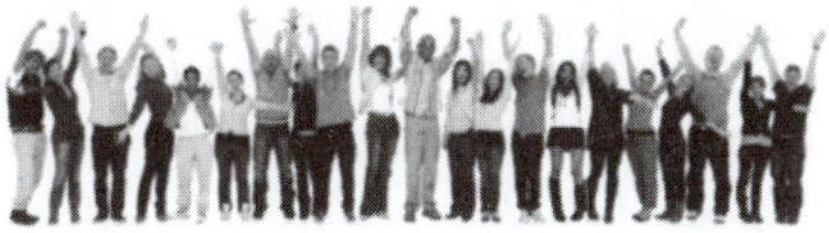

CHAPTER 6

Nursing Process in Mental Health

Learning Objectives

1. Define the role of the LPN/LVN in the five steps of the nursing process.
2. Identify the components of a mental health status assessment.
3. State the need for the nursing process in mental health issues.
4. State the concepts of patient interviewing.
5. Prepare a patient interview.
6. Collaborate in creating a nursing process for a given, hypothetical patient.
7. State the concepts of patient teaching.
8. Prepare and implement a teaching exercise.

Key Terms

- Affect
- Awareness
- Data collection
- Evaluation
- Formal teaching
- Implementation
- Informal teaching
- Judgment
- Memory
- Mood
- North American Nursing Diagnosis Association (NANDA)
- Nursing diagnosis
- Nursing Interventions Classification (NIC)
- Nursing Outcomes Classification (NOC)
- Nursing process
- Orientation
- Patient interview
- Patient teaching
- Plan of care
- Scope of practice
- Subjective
- Thinking/cognition

The **nursing process** is a tool used throughout all areas and levels of nursing (Fig. 6-1). The nursing process is a formula for nurses to provide individual patient care and learn how to organize and implement that care in a systematic, universal way. The nursing process also allows the nurse to determine if the plan and interventions produce a favorable outcome for the patient. In preparing to care for the patient with the use of the nursing process, the nurse will need to incorporate critical thinking to arrive at the planned outcome. It is part of the culture of nurses to be part of a positive outcome.

Scope of practice, determines that the registered nurse (RN) and the licensed practical

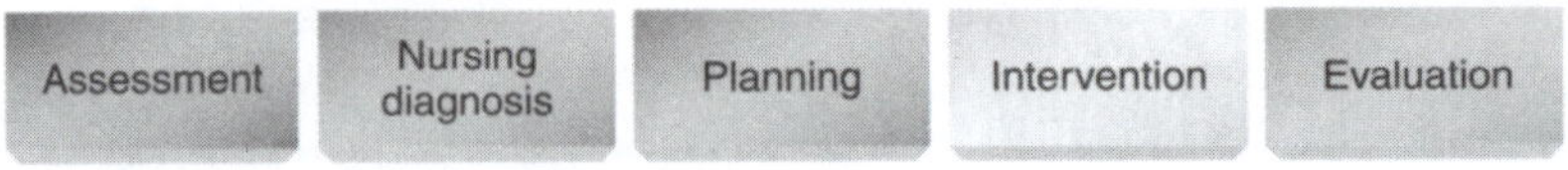

Figure 6-1 Steps in the nursing process.

nurse/licensed vocational nurse (LPN/LVN) play different roles in the nursing process. In the early 1950s, Hildegard Peplau (Chapter 1) hypothesized that nurses are a tool best utilized in relationship to the patient and the environment and in collaboration with other nurses and health-care professionals. She stressed the phases of a working relationship that included a termination phase where nurses prepare both themselves and their patients for termination of the relationship. Her model is still widely used in nursing process and nursing practice today.

Neeb's Tip LPNs/LVNs should know and understand their scope of practice in order to provide safe and effective health care.

In the early 1970s, the American Nurses Association (ANA) developed Standards of Practice for RN and LPN/LVN prepared nurses. The association differentiated between the RN's role and the LPN's role in the nursing process. Individual state Nurse Practice Acts and Boards of Nursing may also offer their own interpretation of the ANA guidelines relating to the role and scope of practice for the LPN/LVN prepared nurse in the nursing process. The following provides step-by-step implementation of the nursing process.

Step 1: Assessing the Patient's Mental Health

Assessment is the first step in the nursing process. The role of the LPN/LVN in Step 1 is to *assist* with the assessment. The registered nurse is responsible for the initial assessment when the patient is admitted or transferred in a facility. **Data collection** is made during every contact a nurse has with a patient. It is essential to the well-being of the patient and in assisting the medical team in making the best choices concerning that person. Nurses collect data about the patient and his or her condition. In most cases, this is accomplished with the help of a form that is used by the facility. Nurses also use nonverbal communication skills to assess the patient's attitude, tone of voice, facial expression, and so on. The problem with many of these generic forms is that they are written in closed-ended format. They are very impersonal and may not reflect the specific information needed about that patient.

It is during the data collection/assessment part of the nursing process that the mental status exam is performed. The mental status exam is a series of questions and activities that check eight areas: the patient's (1) level of **awareness** and **orientation,** (2) appearance and behavior, (3) speech and communication, (4) **mood** and **affect,** (5) **memory,** (6) **thinking/cognition,** (7) perception, and (8) **judgment.** These examinations are of varying lengths and formats, but they all assess the patient's mental capabilities.

Table 6-1 lists areas to be included in a mental status examination. It also suggests the type of assessment made and ideas for questions or commands used by members of the health-care team to make the assessments, as well as some parameters for responses of a person with normal and abnormal mental functioning.

Tool Box |▶ Mental Health Status Examinations Components
www.ncbi.nlm.nih.gov/books/NBK320/

There are many ways to improve the quality of data collection. Two ideas for improving data collection in the form of interviews are listed here. Remember, this is not an exhaustive list of reasons to interview patients. For the purposes of this text, the

Table 6-1 Mental Health Status Examination

Area of Assessment	Type of Assessment	Suggested Methods of Assessment and Normal Parameters	Alterations to Normal Assessment
Appearance	Objective and **subjective** observations such as dress, hygiene, posture; and about the patient's actions and reactions to health-care personnel.	Clean, hair combed; clothing intact and appropriate to weather or situation. Teeth in good repair. Posture erect. Cooperates with health-care personnel.	Displays either unusual apathy or concern about appearance.
Behavior	Objective	Cooperates with health-care personnel.	Displays uncooperative, hostile, or suspicious-type behaviors toward health-care personnel.
Level of Awareness	Subjective and objective assessment of the patient's degree of alertness (wakefulness).	Awareness is measured on a continuum that ranges from unconsciousness to mania. "Normal alertness" is the desired behavior. There is usually a standard guideline for helping with this assessment, but subjective observations can be documented as well, if the patient cannot stay awake for even short intervals or is overly active and has difficulty staying in one place for any period of time.	Outcome is not within normal limits if the patient is difficult to arouse and keep awake or finds it difficult to feel calm.
Orientation	The degree of patient's knowledge of self.	Orientation measures the person's ability to know who he or she is, where he or she is, and the day and time, usually within 1 or 2 days of the actual day and time. Measurement techniques are accomplished by asking the patient, "What is your name?" "Where are you right now?" and "Tell me what the day and date are." Asking "Who is the president of the United States?" is used here as well. Nurses frequently document this as "oriented ×3," but it is best to also write down the objective data on which this routine answer is based.	Abnormal results of orientation are the patient's inability to correctly answer questions pertaining to the patient or to commonly known social information.

Continued

Table 6-1 Mental Health Status Examination—cont'd

Area of Assessment	Type of Assessment	Suggested Methods of Assessment and Normal Parameters	Alterations to Normal Assessment
Thinking/ Content of Thought	Subjective assessment of what the patient is thinking and the process the patient uses in thinking.	Formal testing may be undertaken by the psychologist or psychiatrist to determine the patient's general thought content and pattern. Nurses may contribute to the assessment of thought by documenting statements the patient makes regarding daily cares and routines.	Behaviors including flight of ideas, loose associations, phobias, delusions, and obsessions may become apparent. These alterations in "normal" thought processes are defined and discussed in future chapters that relate to specific illnesses.
Memory	Subjective assessment of the mind's ability to recall previously known recent and remote (long-term) information.	Recent memory: Recall of events that are immediately past or up to within 2 weeks before the assessment. One measurement technique is to verbally list five items. After 1 minute, patient should be able to recall 4–5 of those items. Continue with assessment and at 5 minutes, patient should be able to recall 3–4 of the items. Remote memory: Recall of events of the past beyond 2 weeks prior to assessment. Patients are often asked questions pertaining to where they were born, where they went to grade school, and so on.	Inability to accurately perform recent or remote recall exercises within parameters; may indicate symptoms of delirium or dementia.
Speech and Ability to Communicate	Objective and subjective assessment of aspects of patient's use of verbal and nonverbal communication.	Patient can coherently produce words appropriate to age and education. Rate of speech reflects other psychomotor activity (e.g., faster if patient is agitated). Volume is not too soft or too loud. Stuttering, repetition of words, and words that the patient "makes up" (neologisms) are also assessed.	Limited speech production; rate of speech is inconsistent with other psychomotor activity. Volume is not appropriate to situation (speaks at a very loud volume even when asked to speak more quietly). Stuttering, word repetition, or neologisms may indicate physical or psychological illness.

Table 6-1 Mental Health Status Examination—cont'd

Area of Assessment	Type of Assessment	Suggested Methods of Assessment and Normal Parameters	Alterations to Normal Assessment
Mood and Affect	Subjective and objective assessment of the patient's stated feelings and emotions. Affect measures the outward expression of those feelings.	Mood is the stated emotional condition of the patient and should fluctuate to reflect situations as they occur. Facial expression and body language (affect) should match (be congruent with) stated mood. Affect should change to fluctuate with the changes in mood.	Mood and affect do not match (e.g., facial expression does not change when stating opposite feelings).
Abstract Thinking/ Judgment	Subjective assessment of a patient's ability to make appropriate decisions about his or her situation or to understand concepts.	Give patient a "proverb" to interpret, such as "You can't teach an old dog new tricks." Patient should be able to give some sort of acceptable interpretation such as "old habits are hard to break" or "it is hard to learn something new." *Or* give the patient a situation to solve (judgement). For example, ask the patient what he or she would do if a small child were lost in a store. An appropriate response might be "to call the manager" or "to try to calm the child."	Patient cannot interpret the sayings in an acceptable manner. Patient cannot complete problem-solving questions appropriately. The patient might answer very literally, "Dogs can't learn anything when they get old" or "I would go through the child's pockets to see if there were any phone numbers in them."
Perception	Assesses the way a person experiences reality. Assessment is based on the patient's statements about his or her environment and the behaviors associated with those statements. Nurses and health-team members must document this often-subjective information in objective terms.	All five senses are monitored for interaction with the patient's reality. Patient's *insight* into his or her condition is also assessed.	Presence of hallucinations and illusions. These are discussed further in Chapter 15. Individuals who are not within normal boundaries of judgment or insight will not be able to state understanding of the origin of the illness and the behaviors associated with it.

word *interview* pertains to any nurse-patient interaction that requires a nurse to obtain specific information from a patient. The **patient interview** is usually the primary method of data gathering. It is important to collect data about the whole person. Data related to thoughts and feelings are as important to any nurse-patient interview as the physical data collected.

> **Critical Thinking Question**
> Pick a student partner to interview. Select any topic and develop a 5-minute interview. Write it twice: once with only closed-ended questions and aggressive statements, and once with only open-ended questions and assertive statements. Compare the two versions. How was it different as the interviewer and how was it different for the interviewee?

> **Classroom Activity**
> - Group activity: Discuss the normal parameters presented and your perception of what is normal in light of the mental health status examination.

1. Intake/Admission Interview

Most facilities have developed standard interview forms that suit their particular needs. The forms are written in a very matter-of-fact way and are usually in a closed-ended format (Chapter 2). Patients who are frightened, angry, or just too ill at the moment may easily refuse to answer those closed-ended questions. The patient may have heard the questions before and feel frustrated by what he or she perceives to be inefficiency or poor communication among the staff when the same questions are repeated. This can set up both the nurse and the patient for a difficult time. It is up to the nurse to rephrase the questions in an open-ended format that will seem more individualized to the patient.

EXAMPLE

Standard form: "Do you smoke or use alcohol? _____ YES _____ NO."

Nurse interviewer: "I am required to provide you with information about the hospital's policies on the use of tobacco and alcohol." This statement might then be followed by the standard closed-ended question, "Do you use any tobacco or alcohol?"

Questions can be changed from the closed-ended type to open-ended in most cases. Practice and patience on the part of the nurse interviewer will make this a more profitable experience for both the nurse and the patient.

2. Helping Interview

The helping interview is used to determine or isolate a particular concern of the patient and to help the patient learn to help herself or himself (Fig. 6-2). Patients may trust nurses because nurses have built a rapport with them and are usually more easily accessible than physicians. It is always important to remember, though, not to help to the point of interfering with the patient's ability to help herself or himself.

Consider a situation in which the patient is not progressing according to a "normal" postoperative course. The nurse notices the patient weeping and senses that a need is not being met. The nurse can use this opportunity and observation to begin obtaining information

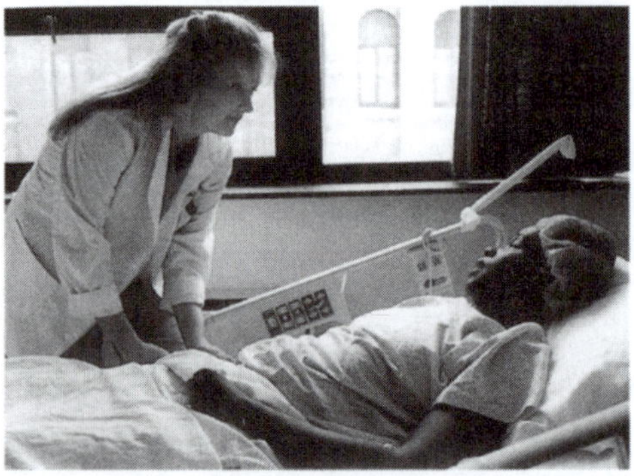

Figure 6-2 The helping interview allows the nurse to determine a patient's special needs and concerns. *(From Williams and Hopper (2011). Understanding Medical-Surgical Nursing, 4th ed. Philadelphia: F.A. Davis Company, with permission.)*

from the patient that may help explain the delayed postoperative progress.

Guidelines for Nurse-Patient Helping Interview

1. *Be honest:* Tell the patient the purpose of the interview.
2. *Be assertive:* If the interview is mandatory (e.g., intake, preoperative), the patient must understand that it is required. Contract for a mutually acceptable time to conduct the interview so that the patient will be aware of the time involved.
3. *Be sensitive:* Sometimes the questions are very difficult or embarrassing for the patient to answer. The nurse should assure the patient that he or she understands the patient's feelings and that the information shared by the patient is part of the patient's medical record. Only the patient, the patient's designee, and people who are involved in his or her caregiving will have access to this information.
4. *Use empathy:* The nurse should let the patient know that he or she is interested in what is being said and that the nurse is there to be helpful. Acknowledge the patient's feelings but do not judge the patient.
5. *Use open-ended questions:* Personalize the questions as much as possible. Use this time to discuss and clarify as much information as you can to avoid having to repeat parts of the interview later.

■ Step 2: Nursing Diagnosis: Defining Patient Problems

Processing the collected data is a function of the registered nurse, according to the ANA. Once data is collected, **nursing diagnoses** are identified. Nursing diagnoses are a universal language on which the interventions are based. There are different models or theories of nursing diagnosis that may be used and recommended by your work setting. These include nursing diagnoses published by the **North American Nursing Diagnosis Association (NANDA).**

> **Tool Box** |▶ Nursing Diagnoses:
> http://www.nanda.org

It is the registered nurse's responsibility to assimilate the data that has been collected and choose one or more potential nursing diagnoses for the patient. The LPN/LVN needs to understand the function of the nursing diagnosis. In collaborative nursing practice, LPN/LVNs can make suggestions and offer rationales to the RN that may be incorporated into the patient's **plan of care.**

An emerging format for writing a diagnostic statement for a patient's plan of care is the P.E.S. Model. The components of this model are: P, the problem or need; E, the etiology or cause; and S, the signs, symptoms, or risk factors. The nurse blends these components into a "neutral" statement that avoids value-laden or judgmental language. The nursing diagnosis is not a medical diagnosis as used by physicians. Rather it is a common language among nurses to help clarify the patient's needs (see Appendix E, Assigning Nursing Diagnoses to Client Behaviors).

■ Step 3: Planning (Short- and Long-Term Goals)

The LPN/LVN role is again as a partner in care planning. The ANA believes that the RN has the primary responsibility for this step of the nursing process. Planning care involves setting short-term and long-term goals from the patient's perspective, not from the nurse's perspective. It is for this reason that the patient and significant others must be involved in the plan of care. Recovery will happen much more quickly if the patient plays an active role in decision making and does not have the impression that treatment is being done *to* or *for* him or her but rather collaboratively *with* the person.

Prioritizing the goals is the second part of planning care. This is one area in which the patient and the nurse might not see things the same way. Nurses and patients look at the same problem from two different perspectives, and the patient's priority may be quite different from the nurse's priority. Whenever possible, the patient's priority should be considered. When there is a threat to life or health that is a direct response to the patient's priority, however, the nurse must intervene and explain the reason that the patient's wishes will have to wait a while.

The aim of selecting goals that will improve mental health status is to keep the mind-body connection intact. It is estimated that about 95% of physical healing is related to a positive mental attitude (PMA). It will be of great help to the patient if the nurse is able to detect alterations in that mental attitude and set goals with the patient to maintain the best outlook and strongest possible effective coping skills. In planning the patient's goals, there should be a short-term and long-term goal for the patient. Both goals should be realistic and measurable with a target date for them to be completed.

■ Step 4: Implementations/ Interventions

The LPN's role is to assist with identifying and carrying out the specific steps that will help the patient reach the goals. Nurses are able to provide input about new interventions that may be helpful, and the LPN/LVN is often the person who begins to help adapt certain procedures to assist the patient. A nurse may use this opportunity to conduct some new patient teaching or to reinforce prior teaching. Relaying information about **implementation** (putting the care plan into action) and patient progress to the RN will provide the information the team needs to offer the best possible care for the patient. Nurses also need to understand and specify the rationale (reason) for the implementations that are selected and be prepared to explain them to patients and families provided the patient consents to their involvement. Table 6-2 provides information about the nursing process.

States differ in the role the LPN plays in outcome statements or performing an **evaluation** of interventions. In much the same way NANDA developed problem or nursing diagnostic standards, work is being done to standardize outcome statements. **Nursing Interventions Classification (NIC)** is a comprehensive standardized language. It provides a number of direct and indirect intervention labels with definitions and possible nursing actions. The interventions address general practice and specialty areas (Doenges and Moorhouse, 2003).

■ ■ ■ Clinical Activity

If your clinical affiliates will allow, arrange to shadow a nurse from the mental health unit. Write a summary of the following experience:

- Observations of the nurse-patient relationship
- Communication style
- Understanding
- Patient responses

Table 6-2 The Nursing Process

Assessment	Nursing Diagnosis (NANDA)	Planning	Implementation/ Intervention	Evaluation
Subjective/ Objective	Relates to the assessment data to determine how the nurse will plan for the care needed.	Planning the patient's outcome: Short-term goals Long-term goals Must be: Measurable and realistic with target dates.	Defines what actions the nurse/health-care provider will provide. The nurse/health-care provider should be able to provide a rationale for each action/treatment provided.	Patient's outcome. The nurse/health-care provider can determine if the plan and the interventions provide the expected outcome. Determine which interventions can be terminated.

Tool Box |▶ The nursing process is a systematic approach in providing care.
http://nursingworld.org/EspeciallyForYou/What-is-Nursing/Tools-You-Need/Thenursingprocess.html

Critical Thinking Question
Your state Nurse Practice Act allows you, the LPN/LVN, to oversee care and function as a charge nurse, as long as a registered nurse is on call. Your medical patient has gone out on a 3-hour pass with relatives and returns to your agency refusing to perform the guidelines as stated in the care plan. Your patient is argumentative but answers questions appropriately. Your data collection includes fruity odor on breath, mood swings, and hunger. You need to re-evaluate and revise the care plan but are unable to make contact with the RN on call. What would you consider to be appropriate nursing diagnoses? What interventions can you perform and still remain within your state's scope of nursing practice?

Patient Teaching

Many implementations or interventions that are helpful to the patient involve **patient teaching.** Frequently, facilities have special teams or departments to carry out certain teaching (e.g., diabetes education), but teaching is becoming a bigger part of a nurse's responsibility. This is true at all levels of nursing preparation. The doctor is still responsible for the initial information given, but the nurse does the "fine-tuning" required to send patients home safely. Nurses teach about medications, coping strategies, adaptive equipment, and anything else the patient requires, not only for the period of hospitalization, but also for the time when the patient leaves the facility. Individual states and facilities set the guidelines regarding teaching responsibilities for doctors and nurses.

Everyone needs a little help to get started with teaching, regardless of what sort of teaching will be done. Like the forms used for the patient interviews, the facility may use standardized classes or teaching sheets. This practice helps ensure that continuity exists in teaching and that the critical information has been given to the patient. There are some legal ramifications to teaching as well. Even with standardized teaching tools, nurses still need to be aware of some principles of teaching and learning. Nurses have an advantage in teaching because, with the exception of nursing diagnosis, the same format they learned for nursing process can be used for setting up a teaching plan.

Teaching in any form is most effective when it is started as soon as possible after admission. Nurses teach patients in different ways. Teaching falls under the categories of either **formal teaching** or **informal teaching.**

Formal teaching is any situation in which a class is scheduled or a specific objective must be met. The instructor is often a staff nurse who has worked in the specific area being taught. Formal teaching involves a nurse instructor and one or more patients. Usually a preset curriculum is used in these classes. The time to teach in the formal setting will most likely be limited by the facility according to staffing needs, because the nurse instructor probably also has a patient assignment. Examples of formal teaching include diabetic teaching and back-care classes.

Classroom Activity
- Divide the class into groups of five. Each group should provide a presentation of the steps in the nursing process using different learning styles.

Informal teaching, or adjunctive teaching, happens anytime, anywhere, whenever the patient needs information. The patient may see the nurse in the hall, or the nurse may notice that the patient is working with the colostomy bag in his room or reading the exercise pamphlet. These are excellent times to reinforce what the patient has learned or to make gentle suggestions for improving his or her technique.

Clinical Activity
Review the medication chart of your assigned patient and provide an informal teaching about one of the medications. Write the outcome of the informal teaching.

Principles of Learning

Nurse-teachers need a basic understanding of the principles of learning and teaching. Some of these principles are listed here:

1. Each person learns differently. Some people process information visually, others by hearing, and still others by hands-on (tactile) learning.
2. Each person learns at his or her own pace. The larger the class, the more levels of ability the nurse will have to work with. Some patients catch on more quickly than others.
3. People learn best when the information is *meaningful* to them. Nurses should think of their own education: The things they are interested in are the things they work harder at. Subjects that they do not like seem to be hard or boring, yet they are required for graduation. Patients may not see the importance of the class that they may be required to attend as a criterion for discharge.
4. Learning is most effective when the information is presented in small segments. This may be dictated by the facility, but when the nurse can be flexible, it is best to present only as much as the patient can absorb.
5. *Success breeds success:* Positive reinforcement will help the patient succeed at learning the required task. The stronger the positive reinforcement, the greater the learning. Once patients have been successful, they will want to continue to learn.

Neeb's Tip Active listening enables the nurse to focus on the patient's strengths.

Principles of Teaching

1. *Know the patients:* What are their abilities? What is their prior level of knowledge? What are the cultural or language differences of the patients in the class?
2. *Know the material:* It is not as important to give a perfect lecture or demonstration as it is to be able to interpret the questions patients may have. Sometimes the nurse-teacher will need to adapt the care plan to meet a particular patient's need. A nurse-teacher who is not comfortable with the material will be less helpful to the patient than one who can individualize the curriculum to the various needs of the class.
3. *Have a teaching plan:* A good teaching plan will improve a nurse's confidence and delivery of the material. A teaching plan is constructed in much the same way as the nursing process. A very simple format, such as APIE for the nursing process, may be easily transformed into a teaching format. An example of the APIE format follows.
   - A = Assessment. What is the need for the teaching? Who are the patients? How much time is available? Assessing the need to teach can be as simple as one or two statements. For example, "Good afternoon, everyone. My name is Sandy. This is the class about bipolar care, and it is open to anyone diagnosed with bipolar disease." Assessment can also be enhanced by the use of a pre-test or questions to the class to determine their past knowledge in this area.
   - P = Plan. In true nursing process, this is often called the goal. Nurse-teachers need to ask themselves a few questions, such as: What do you plan to accomplish in the session? How do you think you will do it? Again, this can be accomplished in one or two statements. For example, "This is the first in a series of three classes, and the task for today is to learn about the different types of appliances and equipment you have available to you." What is accomplished in the first session is considered as a short-term goal and the accomplishments in the third session will be the long-term goal.
   - I = Implementation. This is the step-by-step method nurse-teachers use to accomplish the plan. It is similar to the implementation portion of the nursing process. The nurse-teacher will have as many or as few steps as

needed. In prepared curricula, the steps are written out, but it may or may not be necessary to perform each step. This will depend on the patient group. Chances are good that a class or skill will never be taught exactly the same way twice. There will, however, be critical items that nurses need to cover with all patients to meet legal and safety issues.

- E = Evaluation. In a teaching plan, nurses evaluate the patient's learning as well as the teaching performance. Some questions that nurse-teachers need to reflect on for this part of the teaching plan are: How do you know the patient has grasped the concepts and skills from the class? What do you look for? Do you need to ask for a return demonstration? Does it need to be perfect? How did you do? Did you achieve the plan? Did you have enough time? Too much time? What will you do differently next time? How did your students evaluate the session? Evaluation criteria may change from time to time as well.

4. *Be flexible:* To the extent that the facility's program allows, be familiar enough with the material to be able to build in extra practice time for the tactile learners, extra videos for the visual learners, or time to review verbally for the auditory learners. Be able to teach in several different styles.
5. *Be able to evaluate the learning:* In health teaching in the facility, evaluation can be in the form of a question-answer session, a short quiz, or a return demonstration.
6. *Plan to allow a few minutes after the class for questions:* Even though the nurse may ask for and welcome questions during the session, there are always people who are not comfortable asking questions in a group. These people will want your time in private, so allow some time to clarify their concerns at the time or to set up a time to help individuals later in the day.

Once the plan has been developed, the nurse needs to think about how to implement the teaching. This requires familiarity with some commonly used methods of teaching.

Teachers tend to teach according to the method of learning they prefer. For instance, if nursing students prefer lecture classes, they probably feel most comfortable teaching in a lecture format. If a specific nursing instructor was particularly helpful to a nurse as a student, the nurse may prefer to role-model that teacher's methods when teaching patients. No teaching method is better or worse than any other method. What makes the difference is the learning style of the patients and the rapport that nurses build with them. Because classes in facilities generally have more than one "pupil," the nurse-teacher will need to be able to use different methods of presenting. Because people's personalities are different, each group will have a different dynamic and each class will be different.

The typical methods used in health teaching are lecture and demonstration.

1. *Lecture:* This is a method designed for information giving. It is unilateral; the nurse talks, and the patients listen. It is interactive only when there is some form of question-answer period or brainstorming. Lecturing is an excellent method of introducing a topic to patients and giving them some theory. It is a way to explain the significance so the material becomes meaningful.

In preset programs, the lectures are usually prepared in either text or outline form, so the nurse-teacher has to invest minimal time researching, writing, or setting up for the lectures. Lecture classes may include videos, slides, or charts. Learning from the lecture method is traditionally evaluated through quizzes or question-and-answer sessions. Because not all patient participants are comfortable answering in a group, it may be difficult to assess how much learning each individual achieves.

Neeb's Tip Not everyone has the same learning style.

2. *Demonstration:* Demonstration is an excellent technique to follow in an

introductory lecture. For visual and tactile learners, it is a preferred method of learning.

In prepared programs, the demonstration outline will be provided. The nurse-teacher is responsible for having the equipment ready for each patient. In diabetic teaching, for example, the nurse needs to have ready the syringes, sterile saline for injection, gloves, injection pad, and any other equipment that the agency uses.

Demonstrations are effective because, after the initial demonstration, the nurse-teacher can have the individual perform a return demonstration. One-on-one help can be provided if needed. This allows the nurse to make more objective assessments of the patient's learning and therefore predict the patient's ability to safely perform the technique after discharge. It also allows the nurse to individualize the technique or provide options to the patient.

Evaluation for this method of teaching is usually the return demonstration. The nurse watches each patient perform the technique at a level that is safe for the patient to perform when at home and not under the guidance of the health-care professional. If a home care nurse is assigned to the patient, patient teaching continues; the nurse also teaches the family or significant others.

Additional Patient Teaching Tips

- It is customary to assess eye contact and to equate eye contact with interest and attentiveness. It is important for the nurse-teacher to remember that this is a cultural behavior. Not all cultures believe that eye contact is a positive thing; indeed, many cultures consider direct meeting of eyes a sign of blatant disrespect for people who are older or in a position of respect or authority. Nurses and teachers are respected in those cultural groups, and it would be a mistake on the part of the nurse to assume that the lack of direct eye contact is a sign of disinterest in or disrespect for the material.
- *Be honest:* Nobody said a nurse must have all the answers. If a nurse-teacher does not know something, he or she should admit it. The nurse should look up the information and either bring it to the individual who asked or bring it to the next session of the class.
- *Have fun!* Teaching can be a very rewarding part of nursing. There is no better way to reinforce nursing knowledge than to teach it to someone else. It is one way of being generative, and it is one way in which nurses can keep the nursing culture alive.

■ Step 5: Evaluating Interventions

In this final step of the nursing process, the LPN/LVN plays an assisting role. The LPN/LVN's observations and documentation about the effect of the interventions on the patient and progress in attaining the goal are of great importance. Accuracy in verbal and written reporting of the patient's progress will help determine whether the interventions are helpful or whether they need to be re-evaluated and changed. In some instances, some of the interventions can be terminated, depending on the patient's progress (DeWit, 2009)

Nursing Outcomes Classification (NOC) is also a standardized language, which provides outcome statements; a set of indicators describing specific patient, caregiver, family, or community states related to the outcome; and a five-point measurement scale to facilitate tracking patients across care settings. It can help demonstrate patient progress even when outcomes are not fully met. NOC also is applicable in all care settings and specialties (Doenges and Moorhouse, 2003).

■ ■ ■ Critical Thinking Question

Select a topic to teach the class. This can be any topic with which you are comfortable. You have 10 minutes (classroom instructor may choose own time limit) to teach your topic. Develop a teaching plan. Teach your topic. Evaluate your teaching. What would you do differently the next time?

Key Concepts

1. Nursing process is an example of collaborative nursing practice. RNs are primarily responsible for the steps of the nursing process; LPN/LVN-prepared nurses assist in data collection, planning, implementing, and evaluating the nursing process.
2. The nursing process format can be used by other health-care disciplines to create a care plan.
3. Nurses are conducting more interviewing and teaching on a daily basis. Entry-level nurses need a basic knowledge of both skills. Individual states and facilities set the guidelines for teaching within the scope of the nurse's practice.
4. Nursing process is a helpful tool for preparing a teaching plan.
5. The ANA has set guidelines that dictate the roles of the RN and the LPN/LVN in collaborating in the nursing process.
6. New models for collaborative nursing and nursing outcome statements are being developed.

CASE STUDY

Mark is a 15-year-old student who has recently quit attending his high school classes. Mark has always been a straight-A student who participated in many social and athletic activities at his school.

Today, Mark's friend Tony brings Mark to the clinic that is part of your community's hospital. Tony tells you, "Mark got in with a bad group. He's been doing' the stuff real bad. He's been doing the needles and the smoking. He's been with me for two days, man, and he's real sick. Help him."

You and the physician undertake an assessment of Mark and find that he has yellowing of his sclera. He has a fruity odor on his breath and is vomiting copiously. Mark's level of consciousness is guarded; he is in and out of coherence and is not a reliable source of information about himself at this time.

The physician notifies Mark's parents and explains that Mark may have several conditions, including but not limited to serum hepatitis.

Meanwhile, you continue to admit Mark to the hospital for further testing and medical care. He is placed in enteric isolation as a precaution. An IV is started and you begin to explain the hospital routines to Mark. After you tell him that he must remain in his room for now and that his visitors will be limited during the time of the isolation precautions, he becomes angry. He conveys to you that this is "an invasion of his privacy" and that "you nurses are all part of the conspiracy."

1. How would you start the nursing process for this patient?
2. Describe some questions you would ask as part of the mental status exam

REFERENCES

DeWit, S. (2009). *Fundamental Concepts and Skills for Nursing.* 3rd ed., pp. 48–55. Philadelphia: Elsevier.

Doenges, M.E., and Moorhouse, M.F. (2012). *Application of Nursing Process and Nursing Diagnosis: An Interactive Text for Diagnostic Reasoning.* 4th ed. Philadelphia: F.A. Davis Company.

Martin, D.C. (1990). *The Mental Status Examination.* Retrieved from http://www.ncbi.nlm.nih.gov/books/NBK320/

Townsend, M.C. (2012). *Psychiatric Mental Health Nursing,* 7th ed., Philadelphia: F.A. Davis Company.

Nursing Process

http://nursingworld.org/EspeciallyForYou/What-is-Nursing/Tools-You-Need/Thenursingprocess.html

Mental Status Exam

www.dshs.wa.gov/manuals/socialservices/sections/MSE_GUIDELINES.shtml

Patient Teaching

www.upmc.com/patients-visitors/education/pain-control/pages/default.aspx

Test Questions

Multiple Choice Questions

1. The nursing process is a method for:
   a. Systematic organization and implementation of patient care
   b. Documenting patient needs
   c. Differentiating the RN role from the LPN/LVN role
   d. Data collection

2. You are assisting in collecting data on a new patient in your unit. The physician suspects alcohol abuse. You want to learn the patient's history and frequency of alcohol use. Your best choice for collecting these data might be to ask:
   a. "Do you use alcohol?"
   b. "How often do you get drunk?"
   c. "How many times a week would you say you drink alcohol?"
   d. "Why do you use alcohol? It's bad for you."

3. When conducting patient teaching, the best method to evaluate the success of the patient is:
   a. Lecture
   b. Redemonstration
   c. Implementation
   d. Assessment

4. The mental status exam takes place in what part of the nursing process?
   a. Assessment
   b. Plan
   c. Implementation
   d. Evaluation

5. Which of the following are components of the planning part of the nursing process? *(select all that apply)*
   a. Short-term goals
   b. Long-term goals
   c. Subjective
   d. Objective
   e. Evaluation

6. According to ANA, the RN is the primary person for developing this part of the care plan:
   a. Nursing diagnosis
   b. Implementation/interventions
   c. Evaluation
   d. Assessment

7. Which of the following is/are part of the principles of teaching? *(select all that apply)*
   a. Being flexible
   b. Evaluate the learning
   c. Teach without a teaching plan
   d. Know the patient

8. The Mental Health Status Examination includes: *(select all that apply)*
   a. Memory
   b. Judgment
   c. Mood and tone
   d. Mood and affect
   e. Level of awareness and orientation

9. NANDA is responsible for:
   a. Interventions
   b. Implementation
   c. Appearance
   d. Nursing diagnosis

10. Dianne was sitting in her hospital bed holding the orange given to her to practice her insulin injections. When the nurse entered the room, Dianne asked when she was going to inject herself instead of the orange. This statement indicates that Dianne is ready for:
    a. Discharge to home
    b. More time injecting the orange
    c. Informal teaching
    d. Formal teaching

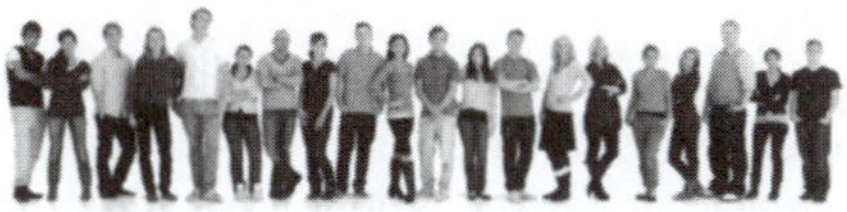

CHAPTER 7

Coping and Defense Mechanisms

Learning Objectives

1. Define coping.
2. Differentiate between effective and ineffective coping.
3. Define defense (coping) mechanisms.
4. Identify main defense mechanisms.

Key Terms

- Adaptation
- Coping
- Defense mechanisms
- Effective coping
- Ineffective coping

■ Coping

"Deal with it." "Get a grip." "Don't make a mountain out of a molehill." These are pieces of advice that most people have heard or have given at some point. But what do they mean? What is coping? **Coping** is the way one adapts to a stressor psychologically, physically, and behaviorally. It is the ability one develops to deal consciously with problems and stress.

Neeb's Tip — As a health-care provider, it important to realize that coping is individualized.

Individuals have different methods of coping or dealing with their stressors. What makes some people very successful at handling stress and others not successful at all? What allows some people to have a drink or run to reduce their stress and causes others to become addicted to the same behavior? The answers to these questions are, of course, complex.

Cultures, religions, and individual belief systems seem to be the lead factors in this mystery. Personal choices also play a supporting role. It is not the value of a behavior that nurses observe; it is the desired outcome that is important. The short-term and long-term goals of a change in behavior emphasize demonstration of specific effective coping skills. Biology plays a role in coping in the presence of some psychiatric disorders. What is an effective coping skill, and how do nurses observe and measure it?

Tool Box |▶ Managing Stress
www.webmd.com/balance/stress-management/stress-management-topic-overview

Effective coping skills are those that are specifically identified to offer healthy choices to the patient. For example, it is very common to see patients use a variety of coping mechanisms to help deal with hospitalization. Hospitalization is a stressful experience for patients and families, with so many unknown and unfamiliar things, noises, and interruptions. The patient may not understand the illness or the implications of the treatment plan. Mealtimes may be different from the routine at home. The patient's plans are disrupted, financial status is altered, and there is a possible temporary loss of independence. Effective coping can be more challenging to a one-income family. Allowing the patient and his or her family members to be active participants in the treatment plan will increase the patient's ability to use effective coping skills (Fig. 7-1). The patient should be included in the decision making as to which new behaviors are acceptable and which ones are not. Practicing these new behaviors in a safe place, such as a hospital or organized group setting, is the secret to success. This will probably require a lifestyle change for the patient, and it will be hard work. As the saying goes, "Old habits die hard," but old habits can die and healthy new ones can replace them. This process of effective coping is sometimes called **adaptation**. Allowing the patient to "practice" the new coping techniques will promote confidence and decrease the stress that can accompany change. The patient will adapt to the stress by using the new tools. Chapters 8 & 9 will introduce the reader to other interventions that can be used for coping effectively with stress.

Clinical Activity
Assist in a group session and provide instructions and demonstrate a relaxation technique. Ask for feedback after the session.

One of the most helpful actions a nurse can take is to actively listen to the patient's thoughts and feelings about the stressor and

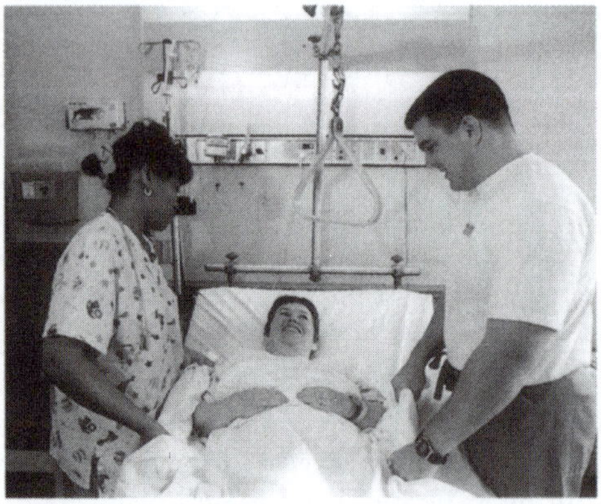

Figure 7-1 Involving patients and their families in the treatment plan can go a long way toward reducing the stress of hospitalization. *(From Williams and Hopper (2011). Understanding Medical-Surgical Nursing, 4th ed. Philadelphia: F.A. Davis Company, with permission.)*

then provide information that will reinforce the patient's positive feelings. Providing honest, positive feedback about the patient's progress in a given lifestyle change will let the patient know that others are noticing the hard work that he or she has done.

Neeb's Tip
Think about when you are verbalizing your thoughts and feelings and thinking, "Just listen to me and validate what I am saying." This is no different from what the patient expects when expressing his or her thoughts and feelings.

Often, the dividing line between effective and ineffective coping is in the degree of tension and the past experience with it. For instance, a little worry or anxiety can be a positive thing. A bride making preparations for her wedding is stressed, but the expectation is that the outcome will be positive. Most of the time when there is a little tension, people are more alert and ready to respond. The "fight or flight" mechanism can actually help people adapt to a new situation. Too much worry begins to cloud the consciousness and interferes with a person's ability to make appropriate choices and recall the new adaptive tools he or she has learned (Fig. 7-2). For example, a bride can become paralyzed with all the decisions to be made and then become unable to proceed, demonstrating ineffective coping (see below).

Ineffective coping is when the techniques people try are not successful or are hazardous. People often allow themselves to fall into habits that give them the illusion of coping. For example, a person might have a drink every time an experience is frustrating. People usually have difficulty understanding that they are using ineffective methods of coping. Ineffective coping is one's rationale for his or her behavior. These habits are called defense mechanisms.

Critical Thinking Question
Imagine that you are admitted into the hospital with an undetermined illness. Describe how it would affect you financially, as a student, and as a parent, and the stress each situation would create.

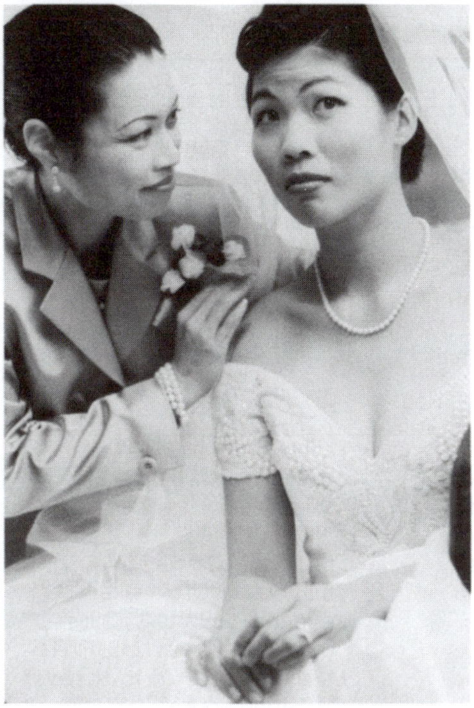

Figure 7-2 A little anxiety can be positive in some situations.

Defense Mechanisms

Defense mechanisms are mental pressure valves. Defense mechanisms give the illusion that they are helping to alleviate a person's stress level, when in reality they mask the stress and may actually end up increasing it. Defense mechanisms come out of the ego mechanism of Freud's theory of personality. Although they appear to be very purposeful, they exist, for the most part, on the unconscious level.

The purpose of defense mechanisms is to reduce or eliminate anxiety. Surprisingly, when used in very small doses, they can be helpful. It is when they are overused that they become ineffective and can lead to a breakdown of the personality. Again, people are not born with these behaviors; they are learned as responses to stress. Many times, they are developed by the time people are 10 years old.

Because the main purpose of defense mechanisms is to decrease anxiety, people tend to have their own repertoire of them and to use them (unconsciously) over and over. Periods of high stress are not the times to try something new, so the psyche uses the old "standbys" to get over yet another hump in life. Some of the commonly used defense mechanisms are shown in Table 7-1.

Classroom Activity

- List three situations that were very uncomfortable for you. What defense mechanisms did you use? How will you respond to each of these situations in a more effective manner?
- List three situations in which you observed someone else using defense mechanisms. How can you help him or her to cope in a more effective manner?

Critical Thinking Question

Nurse D, LVN, has been routinely calling in "sick" on his weekends to work. This has created a hardship for the patients and the staff. On Monday, Nurse D reports for the assigned work shift but is called to the nurse manager's office. The nurse manager informs Nurse D of the pattern that has developed in his attendance and gives him a chance to explain the situation. Nurse D says, "Well, I am a single parent and I need to take care of my children. You should assign single people without families to work the weekends. If you cared a little more about your employees, we wouldn't have to call in so often."

Nurse D is quiet for a second and then says with a shaky voice, "You make me so nervous that I've started needing a couple of drinks at night so I can sleep. I could quit drinking any time, if you'd just let me have my weekends off."

What defense mechanisms do you hear Nurse D using? How many of them have you used? If you were the nurse manager, what would you say to Nurse D? Using three of the suggested nursing diagnoses listed in Appendix E, complete a nursing process for Nurse D.

Classroom Activity

- In a group, watch a television newscast as assigned by the instructor. Pick one topic. Each group should watch its assigned newscast at the assigned time.
  1. Identify all of the defense mechanisms you can within that news interview.
  2. In what ways do hearing defense mechanisms change the way you may listen to and process what you hear in the media?

Table 7-1 Commonly Used Defense Mechanisms

Mechanism	Description	Examples
Denial	• Usually the first defense learned and used. • Unconscious refusal to see reality.	• The alcoholic states, "I can quit any time I want to." • Is *not* consciously lying.
Repression	• An unconscious burying or "forgetting" mechanism. • Excludes or withholds from people's consciousness events or situations that are unbearable. • A step deeper than "denial."	Demonstrating emotions toward a person, but unable to identify the specific reason.
Dissociation	• Painful events or situations are separated or dissociated from the conscious mind. • Could be described as an out-of-body experience.	• Patient who had been sexually abused as a child describes the situation as if it happened to a friend or sibling. • Police visit parent to inform parent of death of child in car accident. Parent tells police, "That's impossible. My child is upstairs asleep. You must have the wrong house."
Rationalization	Substituting acceptable reasons for the true reasons for personal behavior because admitting true reasons is too threatening.	• "I failed the test because the teacher wrote bad questions." • "The patient kept interrupting me so I got distracted and he caused me to make a mistake."
Compensation	Making up for something a person perceives as an inadequacy by developing some other desirable trait.	• A small boy who wants to be a basketball center; instead becomes an honor roll student. • The physically unattractive person who wants to model instead becomes a famous designer.
Reaction Formation (Overcompensation)	Similar to compensation, except the person usually develops the *opposite* trait.	• The small boy who wants to be a basketball center becomes a political voice to decrease the emphasis of sports in the elementary grades. • The physically unattractive person who wants to be a model speaks out for eliminating beauty pageants.
Regression	• Emotionally returning to an earlier time in life when there was far less stress. • Commonly seen in patients while hospitalized. *Note:* Everyone does not go back to the same developmental age. This is highly individualized.	• Children who are toilet trained beginning to wet themselves. • During serious illness, a patient exhibits behavior more appropriate for a younger developmental age, such as excessive dependency.

Table 7-1 Commonly Used Defense Mechanisms—cont'd

Mechanism	Description	Examples
Sublimation	Unacceptable traits or characteristics are diverted into acceptable traits or characteristics.	• Burglar teaches home safety classes. • Person who is potentially physically abusive becomes a professional sports figure. • People who choose to not have children run a day-care center.
Projection	Attributing feelings or impulses unacceptable to oneself to others.	• Wife tells patient's nurse, "My husband is worried about going home." (Wife is the one who worried.) • Young soldier is fearful of upcoming deployment and says, "Those other guys are a bunch of cowards."
Displacement	The "kick-the-dog syndrome." Transferring anger and hostility to another person or object that is perceived to be less powerful.	Parent loses job without notice; goes home and verbally abuses spouse, who unjustly punishes child, who slaps the dog.
Restitution (Undoing)	Makes amends for a behavior one thinks is unacceptable. Makes an attempt at reducing guilt.	• Giving a treat to a child who is being punished for a wrong-doing. • The person who finds a lost wallet with a large amount of cash, does not return the wallet, but puts extra in the collection plate at the next church service.
Isolation	Emotion that is separated from the original feeling.	"I wasn't really angry; just a little upset."
Conversion Reaction	Anxiety is channeled into physical symptoms. *Note:* Often, the symptoms disappear soon after the threat is over.	• Nausea develops the night before a major exam, causing the person to miss the exam. • Nausea may disappear soon after the scheduled test is finished.
Avoidance	Unconsciously staying away from events or situations that might open feelings of aggression or anxiety.	"I can't go to the class reunion tonight. I'm just so tired, I have to sleep."
Scapegoating	Blaming others	"I didn't get the promotion because you don't like me."

■■■ Key Concepts

1. Stress and people's responses to it are very individualized. People are not stressed by the same things, nor do they deal with their stress in the same ways.
2. Defense mechanisms are believed to be part of the ego of Freud's description of personality. They are based in the unconscious, for the most part, but they can appear to be very deliberate.
3. Use of defense mechanisms for a short period can be helpful. The mechanisms act like a pressure valve and allow the psyche to put the stress into perspective. If the patient then deals with the problem, the outcome can be an effective coping technique; if not successful, the patient's anxiety level may increase.

REFERENCES

Gorman, L.M., and Sultan, D.F. (2008). *Psychosocial Nursing.* 3rd ed. Philadelphia: F.A. Davis.

Townsend, M.C. (2012). *Psychiatric Mental Health Nursing.* Philadelphia: F.A. Davis.

Test Questions

Multiple Choice Questions

1. A person who always sounds as though he or she is making excuses is displaying:
   a. Denial
   b. Fantasy
   c. Rationalization
   d. Transference

2. The alcoholic who says, "I don't have a problem. I can quit any time I want to; I just don't want to" is displaying:
   a. Denial
   b. Fantasy
   c. Dissociation
   d. Transference

3. Your young male patient who tells you that he may not be big enough for the basketball team, but says "that's no problem because I'm a 4.0 student and on the principal's list" is displaying:
   a. Denial
   b. Transference
   c. Dissociation
   d. Compensation

4. Mr. V becomes angry that Mrs. V spent the whole day shopping with her friends. Upon her return home, he hits her and tells her, "It's your own fault. Stay home once in a while!" Mr. V is displaying:
   a. Repression
   b. Regression
   c. Dissociation
   d. Projection

5. You overhear someone jokingly repeating the social cliché, "Stop Smoking, Lose Weight, Exercise, Die Anyway" as he orders a big burger and super-sized fries. That cliché is an example of:
   a. Rationalization
   b. Repression
   c. Regression
   d. Rebellion

6. Yesterday, Tara became drunk and inappropriate at a family function. Tara's 16-year-old daughter was embarrassed and in tears. Today, Tara bought two expensive concert tickets for her daughter and a friend. This is an example of:
   a. Denial
   b. Undoing
   c. Symbolization
   d. Conversion

7. Shirley, a 70-year-old woman, went to a photo shoot for a portrait. As soon as the photographer began to photograph Shirley, she started to display signs of regression by: *(select all that apply)*
   a. Posing as a young adolescent
   b. Posing as her mother
   c. Pouting when poses were suggested by the photographer
   d. Stopping the session to make two ponytails, one on each side of her head

8. After receiving disappointing news about a job promotion, John stated, "I didn't get the promotion because I write with my left hand." This is an example of:
   a. Avoidance
   b. Regression
   c. Projection
   d. Denial

9. Effective coping skills are described as:
   a. Being able to make choices that are healthy and individualized
   b. The excessive usage of any defense mechanism
   c. Imitating the coping behavior of others
   d. Working on the problem until totally exhausted

10. The use of defense mechanisms is related to what part of Freud's personality theory? *(select all that apply)*
    a. Id
    b. Ego
    c. Superego

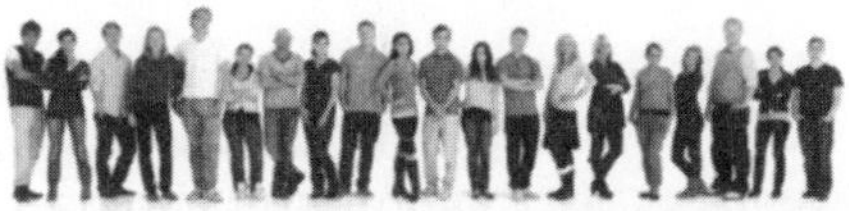

CHAPTER 8

Mental Health Treatments

Learning Objectives

1. Describe a therapeutic milieu.
2. Identify classifications of psychotropic medications.
3. Identify uses, actions, side effects, and nursing considerations for selected classifications of psychotropic medications.
4. Describe psychoanalysis.
5. Describe behavior modification.
6. Identify the nurse's role in counseling.
7. Describe three types of counseling.
8. Describe electroconvulsive therapy and the nurse's role in it.
9. Identify the five phases of crisis and the nurse's role in them.
10. Define and discuss terrorism as it relates to mental health in today's world.

Key Terms

- Akathisia
- Antidepressants
- Antimanic agents
- Antiparkinson agents
- Antipsychotics
- Behavior modification
- Cognitive
- Counseling
- Crisis
- Dystonia
- Electroconvulsive therapy (ECT)
- Hypnosis
- Milieu
- Monoamine oxidase inhibitors (MAOI)
- Person-centered
- Psychoanalysis
- Psychopharmacology
- Rational-emotive therapy (RET)
- Stimulants
- Tardive dyskinesia

People who have alterations to their mental health have special needs. When emotional health is threatened, many other daily activities can be altered as well. **Cognitive** ability (the ability to think rationally and to process those thoughts) can be decreased. Emotional responses can be decreased or even absent in some conditions. These alterations can be extremely frightening to a patient who may already feel unable to control his or her life; this can lead to a deepening of the mental disorder or even the development of another disorder.

Neeb's Tip Accurate and timely observations and data collection by the nurse may be the instrument that keeps the patient from traveling a swift downward spiral.

Patients can develop a sense of helplessness and hopelessness about themselves and their conditions. Nurses can be the tools that help the patient regain control. A nurse may be observing the patient's treatments and therapies or may be an active part of them. Either way, the nurse will be making observations about the patient's reactions and participating in the plan of care. This chapter discusses some of the more frequently used methods for treating alterations in mental health.

■ Psychopharmacology

Since the introduction of the phenothiazines in the 1950s, the number of medications available for treating patients who have mental health disorders, comprising the field of **psychopharmacology**, has increased greatly. The reasons for using medications are twofold: First, the medications control symptoms, thus helping the patient to feel more comfortable emotionally. Second, the medications are usually used in connection with some other type of therapy. The patient is generally more receptive and able to focus on therapy if medications are also used. Several classifications of psychoactive drugs (also referred to as psychotropics) are discussed below; however, there are far too many drugs to discuss each one individually in this text. In most cases, only the most common information is presented about a medication. Nurses should consult a pharmacology or drug reference book for more specific information before administering these medications or instructing patients on their use.

> **Tool Box** |▶ What is psychopharmacology?
> www.ascpp.org/resources/information-for-patients/what-is-psychopharmacology/

Antipsychotics (Neuroleptics/ Major Tranquilizers)

Action: Typical **antipsychotic** agents act on the central nervous system (CNS). Their main action is to block the dopamine receptors. Dopamine is a neurochemical that the human body contains naturally. However, if it is overproduced or utilized incorrectly, it can cause someone to exhibit psychotic behavior. Atypical antipsychotic agents block both serotonin (a neurochemical) and dopamine.

Uses: Antipsychotics are used to treat psychotic behavior such as schizophrenia and other disorders. The antipsychotic will treat schizophrenia and other acute or chronic psychotic behavior including violent or potentially violent behavior. Antipsychotics are classified as typical or atypical. Typical antipsychotic agents treat the positive symptoms of schizophrenia, such as hallucinations, delusions, and suspiciousness. Atypical antipsychotic agents reduce the negative symptoms of schizophrenia, such as flat affect, social withdrawal, and difficulty with abstract thinking. (See Chapter 15 for further discussion of these symptoms.)

Side Effects: Antipsychotics have many unpleasant side effects. Sometimes people are reluctant to take these medications because they are afraid that the side effects will be worse than the illness. Some of these side effects are photosensitivity (especially with Thorazine), darkening of the skin from increased pigmentation, anticholinergic effects such as dry mouth, and a group of side effects called extrapyramidal symptoms (EPS). There is less risk of EPS with the atypical agents, but early observation and reporting of any possible EPS are crucial to minimizing these effects on the patient. The EPS include:

1. *Drug-induced parkinsonism (pseudoparkinsonism).* Symptoms appear 1 to 8 weeks after the patient begins the medication. The major symptom is akinesia (muscle weakness), shuffling gait, drooling, fatigue, mask-like facial expression, tremors, and muscle rigidity.
2. ***Akathisia.*** Symptoms appear 2 to 10 weeks after the patient starts taking the medication. Symptoms are agitation and motor restlessness, and they seem to appear more frequently in women. There is no absolute reason for this, but it is suggested that it may be due to hormonal interaction with the medication.
3. ***Dystonia.*** Symptoms appear 1 to 8 weeks after the patient starts taking the medication. Symptoms manifest as bizarre distortions or involuntary movements of any muscle group. Tongue, eyes, face, neck (torticollis), or any larger muscle mass can become tightened into an unnatural position or have irregular spastic movements.

4. *Tardive dyskinesia (TD).* Symptoms appear within 1 to 8 weeks after the patient starts taking the medication. The frequently seen manifestations are rhythmic, involuntary movements that look like chewing, sucking, or licking motions. Frowning and blinking constantly are also common. TD is irreversible.

Neuroleptic malignant syndrome (NMS) is an uncommon but potentially fatal reaction to treatment with neuroleptic medications. Symptoms include muscle rigidity, hyperpyrexia, fluctuations in blood pressure, and altered level of consciousness. Early recognition and immediate medical care are important. Some antipsychotics, such as Clozaril, are known to cause serious blood dyscrasias and require regular monitoring of blood counts.

Contraindications: Antipsychotics should be used carefully in patients who are hypersensitive to medications or who have brain damage or blood dyscrasias.

Nursing Considerations:

- Careful teaching by doctors and nurses can help the patient to understand that these are very strong medications.
- The possibility of seizures increases in patients who require antipsychotic medications.
- Observe for any sign of EPS or NMS and carefully monitor blood work for abnormal results.
- Careful instruction to the patient and family regarding wearing a wide-brimmed hat, covering all exposed skin, and using a sunscreen when in the sun will help lessen chances of the patient's suffering sunburn, especially if the patient is using Thorazine.
- Temperature extremes should be avoided.
- Patients should be taught to avoid alcohol.
- Over-the-counter (OTC) medication and other products should not be taken without doctor approval.
- It is important to instruct the patient not to alter the dose without first discussing it with the doctor.
- Occasionally, the patient might experience some gastric distress with oral antipsychotics, so give them to the patient with food or milk.

Antipsychotic medication should be discontinued slowly. If medication is ordered once daily, teaching patients to take the medication 1 to 2 hours before going to bed works well and promotes sleep. Antacids decrease the absorption of antipsychotics, so these types of medications should be taken 1 to 2 hours *after* oral administration of antipsychotics.

Box 8-1 provides some of the most commonly used antipsychotic agents.

Also see Chapter 15, Table 15-6, Comparison of Side Effects Among Typical and Atypical Antipsychotic Agents.

Antiparkinson Agents (Anticholinergics)

Action: **Antiparkinson agents** (also called anticholinergics) (Fig 8-1) inhibit the action of acetylcholine. Acetylcholine increases as dopamine decreases at its receptor sites (the cholinergic effect). When the amount of acetylcholine available to interact with dopamine is decreased, there is a better balance between the two neurochemicals, and the symptoms of parkinsonism decrease.

Uses: Antiparkinson agents help decrease the effects of drug-induced and non–drug-induced symptoms of parkinsonism that often occur with antipsychotics.

Side Effects: Blurred vision, dry mouth, dizziness, drowsiness, confusion, tachycardia, urinary retention, constipation, and changes in blood pressure.

Contraindications: Patients with known hypersensitivity should not use these medications.

Box 8-1 Commonly Used Antipsychotic Agents

Typical: Thorazine (chlorpromazine), Haldol (haloperidol), Stelazine (trifluoperazine), Mellaril (trioridazine), Loxitane (loxapine), Prolixin (fluphenazine), Moban (molindone), Navane (thiothixene), Serentil (mesoridazine), Trilafon (perphenazine);
Atypical: Risperdal (risperidone), Clozaril (clozapine), Seroquel (quetiapine), Zyprexa (olanzapine), Geodon (ziprasidone), and Abilify (aripiprazole)

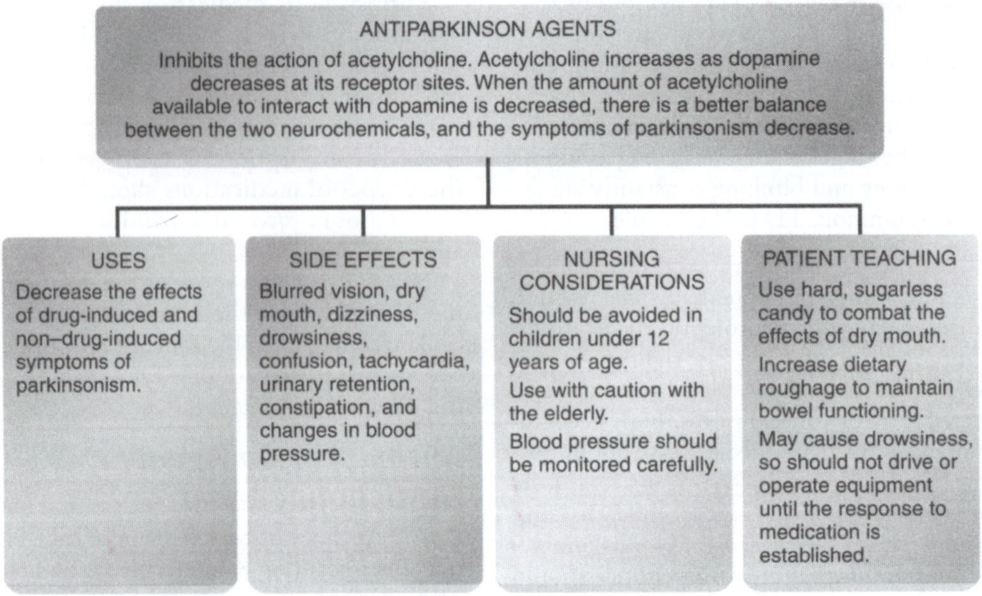

Figure 8-1 Antiparkinson agents.

People with glaucoma, myasthenia gravis, peptic ulcers, prostatic hypertrophy, or urine retention should not take these medications. These agents should be avoided in children under the age of 12 years and used with caution with the elderly.

Neeb's Tip Assess if your patient has glaucoma.

Nursing Considerations:

- Monitor blood pressure carefully (at least every 4 hours when beginning treatment).
- Encourage using hard, sugarless candy or saliva substitute to combat the effects of dry mouth.

Box 8-2 provides some of the most commonly used antiparkinson agents.

Box 8-2 Commonly Used Antiparkinson Agents

Akineton (biperiden), Cogentin (benztropine), Artane (trihexyphenidyl), Mirapex (pramipexole), Benadryl (diphenhydramine)

Antianxiety Agents (Anxiolytics/ Minor Tranquilizers)

Action: Antianxiety agents depress activities of the cerebral cortex (Fig. 8-2).

Uses: Antianxiety agents decrease the effects of stress, anxiety, and mild depression. They can be used preoperatively to help promote sedation.

Side Effects: The use of antianxiety agents can cause physical and psychological dependence. Other side effects include drowsiness, lethargy, fainting, postural hypotension, nausea, and vomiting. If discontinued abruptly, severe side effects, including nausea, hypotension, and fatal grand mal seizures, can occur anywhere from 12 hours to 2 weeks after the drug is stopped.

Contraindications: Patients with known hypersensitivity should not use these medications. People with a history of chemical dependency are not good candidates for this classification of drug because of the potential for addiction.

Nursing Considerations:

- Nurses should monitor blood pressure before and after giving this medication

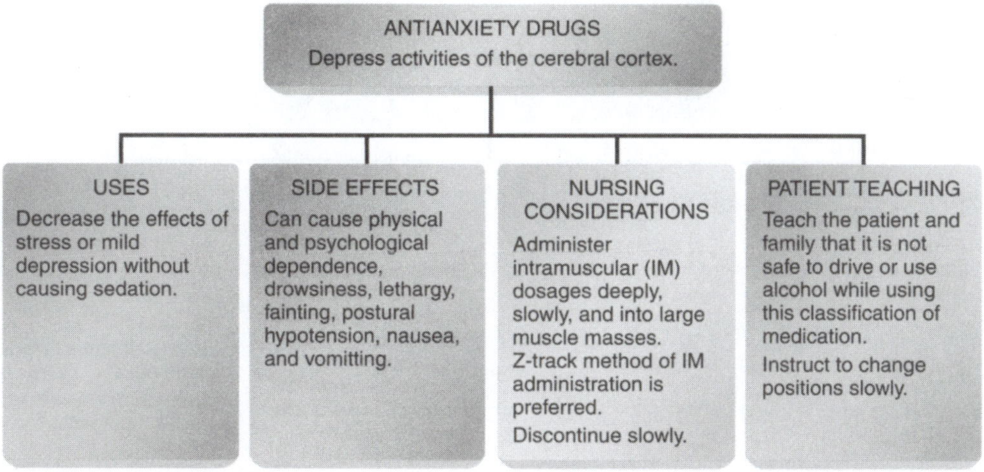

Figure 8-2 Antianxiety drugs.

and monitor for signs of orthostatic hypotension, especially if taking tricyclics (Townsend, 2012).

- The patient should rise slowly from sitting or lying positions to prevent a sudden drop in blood pressure.
- When possible, these types of drugs should be given at bedtime to help promote sleep, minimize side effects, and allow a more normal daytime routine.
- Administer intramuscular (IM) dosages deeply and slowly into large muscle masses. The Z-track method of IM administration is preferred.
- It is important to teach the patient and family that it is not safe for the patient to drive or use alcohol while using this classification of medication.

Box 8-3 provides some of the most commonly used antianxiety agents.

Box 8-3 Commonly Used Antianxiety Agents

Xanax (alprazolam), BuSpar (buspirone), Librium (chlordiazepoxide), Serax (oxazepam), Klonopin (clonazepam), Valium (diazepam), Ativan (lorazepam), and Atarax or Vistaril (hydroxyzine)

Antidepressants (Mood Elevators)

Antidepressants have several subgroups and different drug references that subdivide the antidepressants differently. There are similarities and differences among the subgroups (Fig. 8-3). Antidepressants generally take several weeks to see a change in mood.

Selective Serotonin Reuptake Inhibitors (SSRIs) (Bicyclic Antidepressants)

Action: These drugs increase the availability of serotonin, which is decreased in the brains of depressed individuals.

Uses: Treatment of depression, anxiety, obsessive disorders, impulse control disorders.

Side Effects: Potential for increased suicidal tendencies, sedation, dry mouth, agitation, postural hypotension, headache, arthralgia, dizziness, insomnia, confusion, and tremors.

Contraindications: Patients with known hypersensitivity should not use these medications. People using **monoamine oxidase inhibitors (MAOIs)** or who are within 14 days of discontinuing MAOIs should not use these medications. People using certain herbal preparations including but not limited to St. John's wort, ginseng, brewer's yeast, vitamin B_6, and ginkgo biloba should not use SSRIs without consulting their physician.

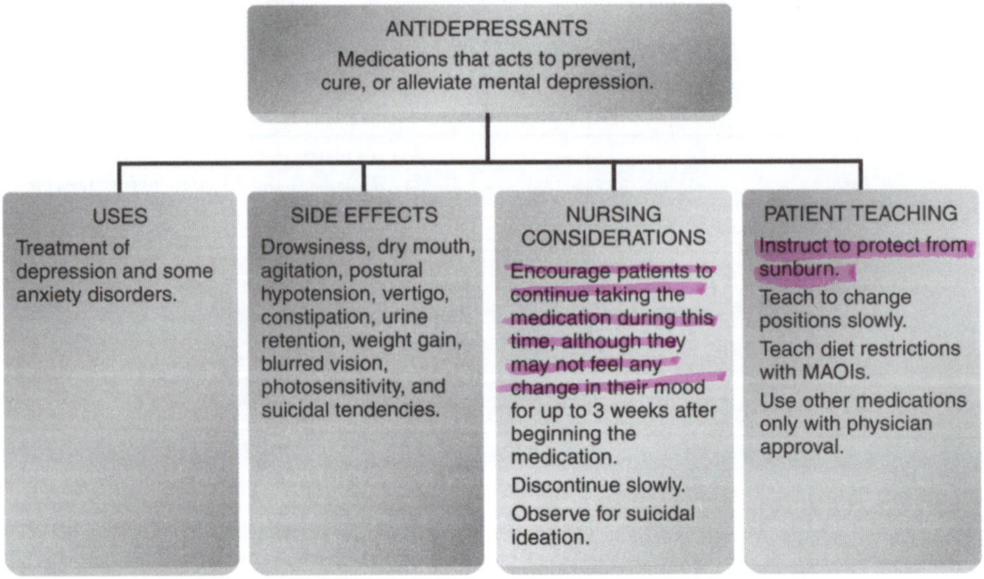

Figure 8-3 Antidepressants.

Note: In October 2004, producers of SSRIs were required by the F.D.A. to place a boxed-in warning on the medication container cautioning about the danger of increased risk of suicidal tendencies in children, adolescents, and young adults while taking this medication.

Nursing Considerations:

- Do not abruptly discontinue the medication, except under the supervision of a health-care provider. Serotonin syndrome, which includes altered mental status, restlessness, tachycardia, and labile blood pressure, can occur with abrupt discontinuation as well as when SSRIs are combined with some other medications.
- Caution should be used with driving or activities that require alertness.
- Alcohol and CNS depressants should be avoided.
- Hard, sugarless candy or saliva substitute can be used to treat dry mouth.
- The patient should change positions slowly to avoid a sudden drop in blood pressure.
- Monitor the patient for suicide ideation.

Box 8-4 provides some of the most commonly used SSRI agents.

Box 8-4 Commonly Used SSRI Agents

Celexa (citalopram), Prozac (fluoxetine), Zoloft (sertraline), Luvox (fluvoxamine), Paxil (paroxetine), Lexapro (escitalopram)

Tricyclic Antidepressants

Action: These drugs increase the level of serotonin and norepinephrine, thereby increasing the ability of the nerve cells to pass information to each other. Patients with depressive disorders generally have decreased amounts of these two neurochemicals.

Uses: Treatment of symptoms of depression, including (but not limited to) sleep disturbances, sexual function disturbances, changes in appetite, and cognitive changes.

Side Effects: Sedation, lethargy, dry mouth, constipation, tachycardia, postural hypotension, urine retention, blurred vision, weight gain, and changes in blood glucose.

Contraindications: Patients with known hypersensitivity should not use these medications. Women who are pregnant or breastfeeding and individuals with kidney disease, liver disease, or a recent myocardial infarction should not take these medications. Anyone who has asthma, seizure disorders, schizophrenia, benign prostatic hypertrophy, or alcoholism should use tricyclic antidepressants with extreme caution.

Nursing Considerations:

- Patients should not stop using these medications abruptly.
- Medications (including over-the-counter medications such as cold preparations) that contain antihistamines, alcohol, sodium bicarbonate, benzodiazepines, and narcotic analgesics can increase the effects of tricyclic antidepressants.
- Nicotine, barbiturates, and the hypnotic chloral hydrate decrease the effect of the tricyclic antidepressant.
- Serotonin syndrome can occur if combined with St John's wort.

Box 8-5 provides some of the most commonly used tricyclic antidepressant agents.

Tetracyclic Antidepressants (Heterocyclic Antidepressants)

The actions, uses, contraindications, side effects, and nursing considerations for the tetracyclic antidepressants are similar to those for SSRIs.

Box 8-6 provides some of the most commonly used tetracyclic antidepressant agents.

Box 8-5 Commonly Used Tricyclic Antidepressant Agents

Elavil (amitriptyline), Tofranil (imipramine), Pamelor or Aventyl (nortriptyline), Asendin (amoxapine), Norpramin (desipramine), Anafranil (clomipramine), Sinequan (doxepin), Surmontil (trimipramine), Vivactil (protiptyline)

Box 8-6 Commonly Used Tetracyclic Antidepressant Agents

Ludiomil (maprotiline), Wellbutrin or Zyban (bupropion), Remeron (mirtazapine), Desyrel (trazodone)

Serotonin Norepinephrine Reuptake Inhibitors (SNRIs)

Action: These drugs increase the availability of serotonin and norepinephrine, which are decreased in the brains of depressed individuals.

The uses, contraindications, side effects, and nursing considerations for the SNRI antidepressants are similar to those for SSRIs.

Box 8-7 provides some of the most commonly used SNRI agents.

Monoamine Oxidase Inhibitors (MAOIs)

Action: Monoamine oxidase inhibitors (MAOIs) prevent the metabolism of neurotransmitters by an enzyme, monoamine oxidase. Too much monoamine oxidase can lead to destructive, psychotic behaviors.

Uses: MAOIs are generally used for patients with varied types of depression who have not been helped by other antidepressants.

Side Effects: Postural hypotension, photosensitivity (sunburn potential), headache, dizziness, memory impairment, tremors, fatigue, insomnia, weight gain, and sexual dysfunction.

Contraindications: Patients with known hypersensitivity should not use these medications. MAOI medications should be given carefully to patients who have asthma, congestive heart failure, cerebrovascular disease, glaucoma, blood pressure conditions, schizophrenia, alcoholism, liver or kidney disorders, or severe headaches, as well as to those who are over 60 years old or pregnant. There are many drug-drug interactions that may occur if MAOI agents are combined with other medications. Other prescriptions and over-the-counter products should be taken only after consulting a doctor or a pharmacist.

Nursing Considerations:

- Teach patients to avoid foods containing the amino acid tyramine, a precursor of norepinephrine, while taking these

Box 8-7 Commonly Used SNRI Agents

Serzone (nafazodone), Effexor (venlafaxine), Cymbalta (duloxetine) medications. MAOIs block the metabolism of tyramine, resulting in increased norepinephrine. A hypertensive crisis may occur. Foods containing significant amounts of tyramine include

- Aged cheese (cheddar, Swiss, provolone, blue cheese, parmesan)
- Avocados (guacamole)
- Yogurt, sour cream
- Chicken and beef livers, pickled herring, corned beef
- Bean pods
- Bananas, raisins, and figs
- Smoked and processed meat (salami, pepperoni, and bologna)
- Yeast supplements
- Chocolate
- Meat tenderizers (MSG), soy sauce
- Beer, red wines, and caffeine

Box 8-8 provides some of the most commonly used MAOI agents.

Alternative Treatments for Depression

People are seeking alternatives to the prescription antidepressant drugs available through traditional western medicine. Some reasons they seek alternatives include cultural preferences, cost of medications, insurance issues, and unpleasant side effects they may experience with the medications they have used.

One such alternative is a chemical called SAMe ("sammy"). SAMe is a combination of an amino acid (methionine) and ATP. It is used as an antidepressant and sold in the United States as a dietary supplement. Other alternative forms of therapy are explored in Chapter 9.

The nurse's role is the same with these alternative choices as it is with prescription medications. Nurses must encourage their patients to discuss the use of supplements with their physicians and to provide as much information as possible to allow the patient to make safe, informed choices.

Box 8-9 provides nursing considerations for all antidepressants.

Antimanic Agents (Mood Stabilizing Agents)

Lithium carbonate was the drug of choice for treatment and management of bipolar mania for many years. In recent years, several other **antimanic agents** (Fig. 8-4) have become treatment options. Other medications being used as mood stabilizers include some anticonvulsants and calcium channel blockers.

Lithium Carbonate

Action: The exact action of lithium is not completely known at this time. It is not metabolized by the body. One hypothesis about the action of lithium is that there seems to be a connection between lithium and constancy of sodium concentration, which might help regulate and moderate information along the nerve cells, thus preventing mood swings. Another possibility is that lithium increases the reuptake of norepinephrine and serotonin, thereby decreasing hyperactivity.

Uses: Lithium is used for the manic phase of bipolar disorder and sometimes for other depressive or schizoaffective disorders.

Side Effects: Side effects can be numerous. Some of the more common ones are thirst and dry mouth, nausea and vomiting, abdominal pain, and fatigue.

Box 8-8 Commonly Used MAOI Agents

Nardil (phenelzine), Parnate (tranylcypromine), Marplan (isocarboxazid)

Box 8-9 Nursing Considerations for All Antidepressants

- Reinforce the teaching that these medications take several weeks to become effective. Encourage patients to continue taking the medication during this time, although they may not feel any change in their mood right away.
- All antidepressant medications should be tapered gradually rather than abruptly discontinued to prevent withdrawal symptoms.
- It is imperative that all patients receiving antidepressant medications be monitored for suicide potential throughout treatment.

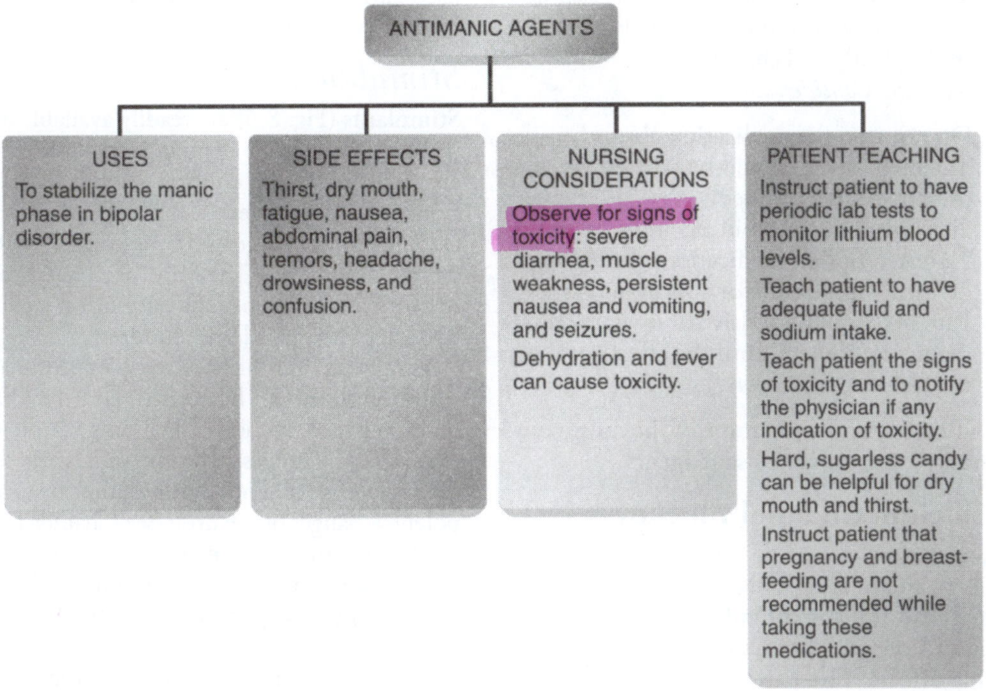

Figure 8-4 Antimanic agents.

Contraindications: Consistent with those of the other categories listed earlier.

Nursing Considerations:

- Encourage patients to keep all appointments for blood work and evaluation of drug effectiveness. Therapeutic serum levels are between 0.5 and 1.2 mEq/L for most patients (1.0 to 1.5 in acute mania). Symptoms of lithium toxicity begin to appear at blood levels greater than 1.5 mEq/L. Signs of toxicity include severe diarrhea, persistent nausea and vomiting, muscle weakness, tremors, blurred vision, slurred speech, and seizures.
- Lithium crosses the placenta and milk barriers, so women of childbearing years may need to be counseled regarding the effects of this drug on their pregnancy and breastfeeding.
- Dehydration and fevers can cause increased danger of toxicity.
- Adequate fluid and sodium intake are essential. Patients should not decrease their dietary intake of salt (unless instructed to do so by the physician) and should be taught to inform the physician immediately if they are ill.
- Hard, sugarless candy can be helpful to decrease dry mouth and thirst.

Box 8-10 provides some of the most commonly used forms of Lithium

Anticonvulsants

Action: The action of anticonvulsants in the treatment of bipolar disorder is not clear.

Uses: These drugs stabilize the manic episodes in bipolar disorders.

Side Effects: Nausea, vomiting, indigestion, drowsiness, dizziness, prolonged bleeding, headache, confusion.

Contraindications: Patients with known hypersensitivity or with bone marrow suppression should not use these medications. Caution

Box 8-10 Commonly Used forms of Lithium

Eskalith, Lithonate, Lithane, Lithobid (all are lithium carbonate)

should be used with patients with renal, cardiac, or liver disease. Caution should also be used with the elderly and children.

Nursing Considerations:

- Do not stop the medication abruptly.
- The medication should be tapered when therapy is discontinued.
- Teach patients to avoid alcohol.
- Nonprescription medications should not be used without doctor approval.
- Patients should not drive or operate dangerous equipment until the effects of the medication are known.

Box 8-11 provides some of the most commonly used anticonvulsant agents.

Calcium Channel Blockers

The action, uses, side effects, contraindications, and nursing considerations are similar to those for anticonvulsants. Postural hypotension and bradycardia are additional side effects. The patient should rise slowly from sitting or lying positions to prevent a sudden drop in blood pressure. Commonly used calcium channel blockers are Calan or Isoptin (verapamil).

Box 8-11 Commonly Used Anticonvulsant Agents

Tegretol (carbamazepine), Depakene (valproic acid), Depakote (divalproex)

Stimulants

Stimulants (Fig. 8-5) are readily available over the counter as well as by prescription. They are found over the counter in diet preparations, pills to prevent sleep, cigarettes, and caffeinated beverages such as coffee, energy drinks, and soda. They are used medically to combat narcolepsy and attention-deficit/hyperactivity disorder in children.

Amphetamines are one type of stimulant. Amphetamines can be abused, and they have many "street names," including "uppers," "speed," and "bennies." The ease with which they are available should not diminish the power and potential danger of the drug (see Chapter 17).

Action: Stimulants provide direct stimulation of the central nervous system (CNS).

Uses: These drugs promote alertness, diminish appetite, and combat narcolepsy (sleep disorder related to abnormal rapid eye movement sleep). They are used in the treatment of attention-deficit/hyperactivity disorder (ADHD).

Side Effects: Increased or irregular heartbeat, hypertension, hyperactivity, dry mouth, hand tremor, rapid speech, diaphoresis, confusion, depression, seizures, suicidal ideation, and insomnia.

Contraindications: Patients with known hypersensitivity should not use these medications.

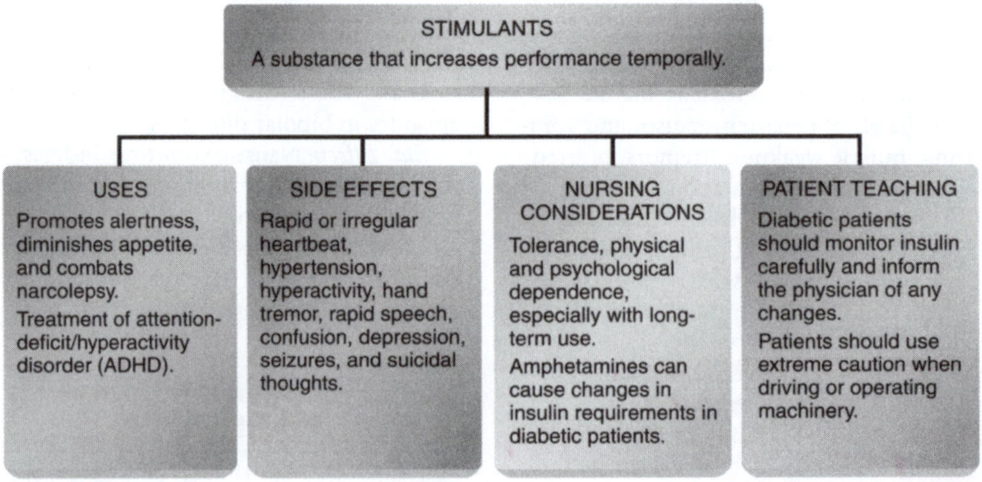

Figure 8-5 Stimulants.

Pregnant or lactating women should not use this classification of drugs. Because these are chemicals that increase stimulation of the CNS and respiratory systems, they should not be given to people who are alcoholic, manic, or who display suicidal or homicidal ideations. People who have heart disease or glaucoma also should not use these drugs because of the potential effect of the medications. Elderly people and patients who have diabetes, hypertension, or other cardiovascular conditions should use these drugs cautiously and with careful monitoring.

Nursing Considerations:

- Tolerance and physical and psychological dependence can occur with CNS stimulants, especially with long-term use.
- Do not discontinue medication abruptly.
- Monitor for suicide potential.
- Diabetic patients who take amphetamines should be informed that the amphetamines may cause changes in their insulin requirements.
- These medications can also cause changes in judgment; therefore, people should be counseled to use extreme caution when driving or operating equipment and should avoid these activities if possible.
- Encourage frequent rinsing of the mouth with water or use of hard, sugarless candy or saliva substitute to relieve dry mouth.

Box 8-12 provides some of the most commonly used stimulant agents.

Milieu

One of the areas that nurses have some control over is the therapeutic environment itself. In mental health terminology, this therapeutic environment is called the **milieu**, or therapeutic milieu. It is believed that the environment has an effect on behavior. Think about a person who goes to an event such as a concert or a ballgame that he does not feel excited about. That person might begin screaming or singing along and generally getting into the spirit of things shortly after arriving at the event.

Box 8-12 Commonly Used Stimulant Agents

Dexedrine (dextroamphetamine), Desoxyn (methamphetamine), Ritalin (methylphenidate), Adderal (dextroamphetamine/amphetamine)

Critical Thinking Question

You are to go on an assigned unit in a mental health floor to monitor a group discussing anger. You are feeling apprehensive and fearful about being on the same unit as these patients. Describe how you might feel after hearing how the patients' home life relates to this anger.

The milieu is the setting that will provide safety and help during the patient's stay. The milieu therapy is intended to combine the social and the therapeutic environments. In that way, every contact between nurse and patient gives the opportunity for a therapeutic interaction. The milieu must be comfortable and safe. Patients need to feel accepted as they learn new behaviors. It is best to have the milieu as appropriate to the situation as possible. Obviously, nurses cannot move walls and change decorating themes in the hospital, but they can allow the patient to choose the room for therapy or move to an area where the patient is more comfortable. If the patient is on a psychiatric unit rather than a medical or surgical unit, he or she is usually allowed to walk from area to area on the unit. A nurse can keep the area calm and quiet and arrange for roommate changes if needed. There are many things a nurse can and must do to maintain a milieu that is conducive to a patient's progress. As the patient progresses, the milieu will be changed to allow the patient to take on more responsibility.

Psychotherapies

Psychotherapy (Fig. 8-6) is the term used to describe the form of treatment chosen by the psychologist or psychiatrist or other mental health therapist to treat an individual. The goals of psychotherapy are to:

1. Decrease the patient's emotional discomfort.
2. Increase the patient's social functioning.

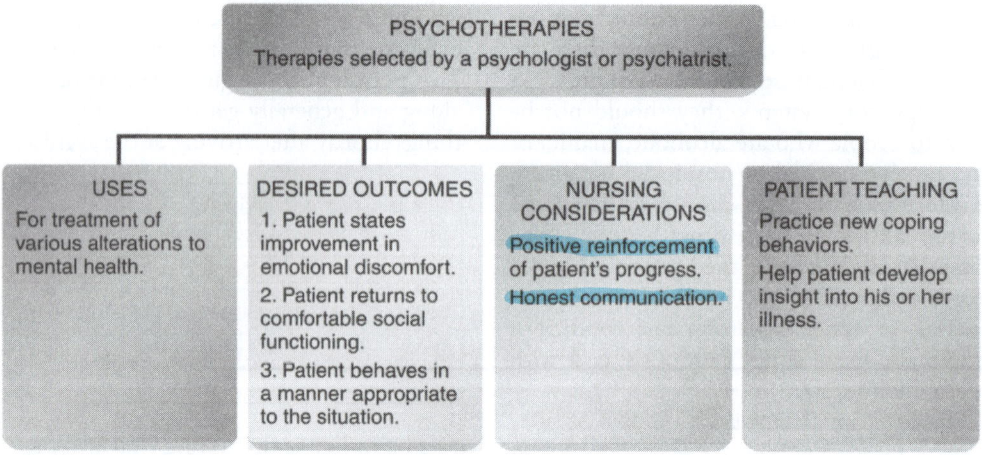

Figure 8-6 Psychotherapies.

3. Increase the patient's ability to behave or perform in a manner appropriate to the situation.

These goals are achieved in a variety of ways, including therapeutic relationships, open and honest venting of feelings and thoughts, allowing the patient to practice new coping skills, helping the patient to gain insight into the problem, and consistency in the team approach to the patient's care and treatment. Positive reinforcement of progress is encouraged. Some therapies may be focused on gaining insight into the reasons for current behavior and others are more focused on changing specific behaviors.

Several types of therapy are typically used. Nurses may or may not be actively involved in the therapy, but to provide continuity in the care of the patient, they must understand the basic ideas of the types of therapy.

Psychoanalysis

Psychoanalysis is the form of therapy that originated from the theories of Sigmund Freud. In psychoanalysis, the focus is on the cause of the problem, which is buried somewhere in the unconscious. The therapist tries to take the patient into the past in an effort to determine where the problem began. Chances are, according to Freud, that the problem is related to poor parent-child relationships and ineffective psychosexual development.

It is typical for the psychoanalyst to be positioned at the head of the patient and slightly behind, so that the patient cannot see the therapist. This decreases any kind of nonverbal communication between the two people. The patient is typically on the "couch," relaxed and ready to focus on the therapist's instructions.

Some of the techniques used in psycho analysis are as follows.

Free Association

In free association, the patient is allowed to say whatever comes to mind in response to a word that is given by the therapist. For example, the therapist might say "mother" or "blue," and the patient would give a response, also typically one word, to each of the words the therapist says.

The therapist then looks for a theme or pattern to the patient's responses. So, if the patient responds "evil" to the word "mother" or "dead" to the word "blue," the therapist might pick up one potential theme, but if the patient responds "kind" and "true" to the words "mother" and "blue," the therapist might hear a completely different theme. The theme may give the therapist an idea of the cause of the patient's emotional disturbance.

Dream Analysis

Because Freudians believe that behavior is rooted in the unconscious and that dreams are a manifestation of the troubles people repress, what better way to get an idea of the problem than to monitor and interpret dreams? The patient is asked to keep a "dream log." He/she is asked to awaken immediately after a dream and to write down the dream details right away in a notebook kept next to the bed. This is easier said than done, as many people remember only bits and pieces of a dream upon awakening. Psychoanalysts believe that dreams truly are the mirror to the unconscious and that it is possible to train the self to awaken long enough to record the dream. The dreams are then interpreted in much the same way as free association. Significant people or situations in the dreams are explored with the patient, and possible meanings are offered by the therapist.

Hypnosis

Many people are afraid of **hypnosis**. For many years, it was reputed to be quackery and presented in stage shows in which people did things such as cluck like chickens, which served as entertainment. Granted, this sort of thing can happen. Fraternity and sorority members love to invite stage performers to hypnotize pledgees during rush. Certainly, people like the entertainer David Copperfield have made comfortable livings with hypnosis.

Hypnotherapy, as professional therapists prefer to call it, is used for certain people in certain instances. It is not a magic solution to problems. It takes practice on the part of the patient. It can, however, be a very effective tool for unlocking the unconscious or for searching further into a technique called "past life regression."

Hypnosis is very deep relaxation. A person who has listened to a relaxation tape and felt the effects of it or who has driven a car and noticed that 20 minutes have passed that he or she cannot account for has been hypnotized.

In hypnotherapy, the relaxation is *guided* by the therapist, who has been trained in techniques of trance formation and who then asks certain questions of the patient or uses guided imagery to help picture the situation in an effort to find the cause of the problem (Fig. 8-7). At the end of the session, the therapist will leave some helpful hints for the patient. These are called posthypnotic

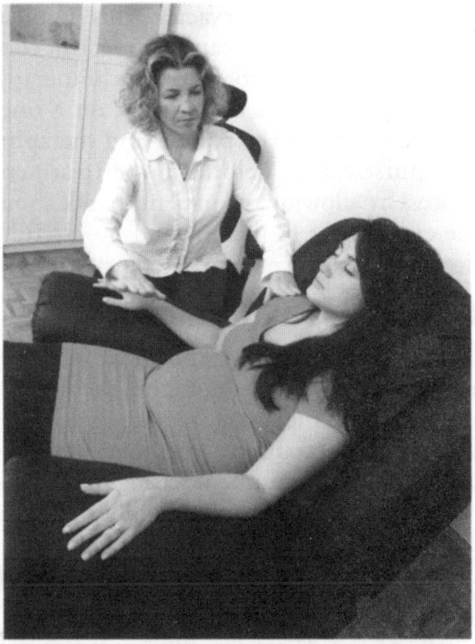

Figure 8-7 In hypnotherapy, a patient in a state of very deep relaxation is guided by the therapist.

suggestions and typically include positive, affirming statements for the patient to think about as well as instructions to help the person accomplish self-hypnosis.

Of course, just as there are unethical people in all walks of life, a small number of therapists may abuse this relationship, although it is very uncommon. People do not generally lose control when under hypnosis; they will, in most cases, still realize what is comfortable and acceptable to them personally, and they will not allow themselves to go deeper into hypnosis or to perform behaviors that they find objectionable.

Hypnosis and hypnotherapy are discussed in more depth in Chapter 9.

Catharsis

Catharsis is "the act of purging" or "elimination of a complex (problem) by bringing it to consciousness and affording it expression" (Merriam-Webster Online, 2013). In psychoanalysis, the therapist helps the patient see the root of the problem and then, by talking or expressing feelings, allows the patient to learn to evacuate this problem from the psyche. This can take place in conjunction with other forms of psychotherapy.

Psychoanalysis is undertaken on a one-on-one basis between patient and therapist. The nurse can be helpful in the treatment process by allowing the patient to talk about the experiences in therapy and by carefully documenting the patient's responses.

Behavior Modification

The treatment method known as **behavior modification** is based on the theories of the behavioral theorists (Skinner, Pavlov, and others). It is a common treatment modality used in multiple treatment settings (Fig. 8-8).

The purpose of behavior modification is to eliminate or greatly decrease the frequency of identified negative behaviors. One of the basic beliefs of behavior modification is that whenever a behavior is removed, it must be replaced by another behavior. Therefore, replacing the negative behaviors with ones that are more desirable is a major function of this type of psychotherapy.

As Skinner and Pavlov showed, behaviors can be learned and unlearned. The process of finding the appropriate stimuli and reinforcers determines the effectiveness of the change in behavior. According to some behaviorists, it takes approximately 20 repetitions of a behavior to make it a part of a person's lifestyle. However, anyone who has tried to lose weight or stop smoking might have a rebuttal to that theory.

Behavior can be changed, according to behavior modification theory, by either positive or negative reinforcement. Positive reinforcement is the act of rewarding the patient with something pleasant when the desired behavior has been performed. For instance, if Mrs. P has the habit of using foul language in an attempt to have a need met, it might be assumed that the desired behavior change would be for her to come to a staff member and ask quietly for what she needs. Mrs. P loves to be outside but is not allowed out except at supervised times. A suitable positive reinforcer might be to allow 15 additional minutes outdoors when she remembers to ask for her needs quietly. Generally, when the unacceptable behavior is exhibited by Mrs. P, the staff would either ignore it (because correcting it would in itself be a form of reinforcing the behavior) or quietly tell her that is not acceptable behavior and then acknowledge her only when the desired change has been demonstrated.

Classroom Activity

- Write out one behavior you personally would like to change. Include what a person could give you to create a change.

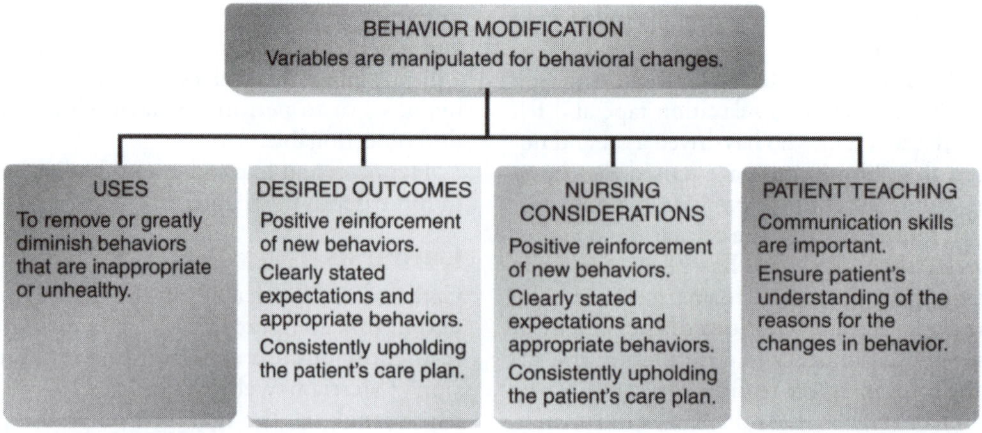

Figure 8-8 Behavior modification.

Negative reinforcement is interpreted by some as punishment. Great care must be taken when performing behavior modification with certain populations of people. It can look like an infraction of the Patient Bill of Rights and could be reported by someone who does not understand the situation.

Negative reinforcement is the act of responding to the undesired behavior by taking away a privilege or adding an unwanted responsibility. Critics of the legal system in this country sometimes cite imprisonment and capital punishment as forms of negative reinforcement. Parents who "ground" a child after the child behaves unacceptably are using negative reinforcement; requiring that child to perform extra household tasks for a stated period of time is reinforcing the fact that the negative behavior has consequences. The child may not repeat the negative behavior after either of these parental choices.

Whatever option is chosen, it is important to have the behaviors and consequences clearly stated. In a facility, this will be incorporated into the plan of care. At home, it can be stated in family meetings, agreed upon verbally by the family members, or made known by some other method of clear communication. The patient must have the ability to understand the ramifications of the behavior to be changed and the purpose for the type of consequence that is chosen. If the person is not capable of understanding the situation or is not able to remember due to some other problem, behavior modification could be considered a questionable alternative to other kinds of treatment.

Cognitive Therapies

Rational-Emotive Therapy (RET)

Dr. Albert Ellis, a "reformed" psychoanalyst, and other cognitive therapists have developed theories proposing that people teach themselves to be ill because of the way they think about their situations. Cognitive means "of, relating to, or being conscious of mental activity (as thinking, remembering, learning or using language)" (Merriam-Webster Online, 2013). Cognitive therapy emphasizes ways of rethinking situations. The therapist confronts the patient with certain behaviors and then works out ways of thinking about them differently.

Rational-emotive therapy (RET) is one of the best-known cognitive therapies (Fig. 8-9). Dr. Ellis's theory is based on an A-B-C format:

- A is the *activating* event, or the subject of the faulty thinking.
- B is the *belief* system a person has adopted about the activating event.
- C is the *consequence* to continuing the belief system.

Dr. Ellis has made up terminology that he uses with his therapy, such as "musturbation" (the act of insisting that something *must* go a certain way), "awfulizing" (the belief that something is not just inconvenient

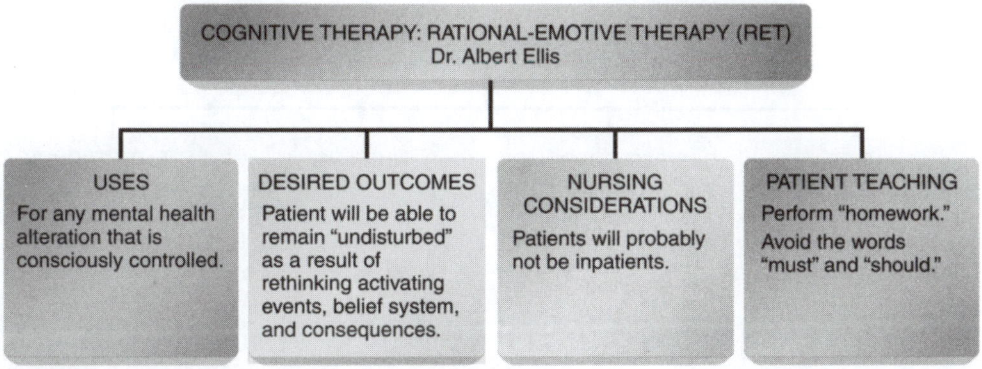

Figure 8-9 Cognitive therapy: rational-emotive therapy.

or unpleasant, but the extreme of "awful"), and "catastrophizing" (at which point, one has lost control of the situation). In RET, there are no "musts" or "shoulds." Feeling sad about an unpleasant experience (such as the death of a loved one) is acceptable and normal, but becoming depressed about the death is "awfulizing" and therefore considered by him to be unhealthy.

It is common for RET to be performed in groups. The patients are given homework to complete in the period between sessions. The expected outcome is that patients will no longer "disturb ourselves by the way we think" (Ellis, 1988).

> **Clinical Activity**
> Throughout your clinical experience, observe patients on the unit when they are instructed by the health-care provider that they "must or should" behave in a specific manner. During clinical post-conferences, discuss these episodes and whether the outcome was negative.

An offshoot of RET is known as cognitive behavior therapy (CBT). CBT is behavioral therapy that focuses on examining the relationships between thoughts, feelings, and behaviors. By exploring patterns of thinking that lead to self-destructive actions and the beliefs that direct these thoughts, people with mental illness can modify their patterns of thinking to improve coping. CBT is a type of psychotherapy that is different from traditional psychodynamic psychotherapy in that the therapist and the patient will actively work together to help the patient recover from the mental illness. People who seek CBT can expect their therapist to be problem-focused and goal-directed in addressing the challenging symptoms of mental illnesses. Because CBT is an active intervention, one can also expect to do homework or practice outside of sessions.

RET and other forms of cognitive therapies are gaining in popularity because usually they are significantly more short-term than psychoanalysis and therefore less costly to the patient.

Person-Centered/Humanistic Therapy

Theorists Abraham Maslow and Carl Rogers are most frequently credited with the concept of **person-centered**, or humanistic, therapy (Fig. 8-10). In this form of treatment, all caregivers are to focus on the whole person and to work in the "present." It is not important in humanistic treatment to understand the cause of the problem or what happened in the person's past; what is important is the here and now.

Unconditional Positive Regard

This is the phrase used by therapists who follow Rogerian theory. Unconditional positive regard means full, nonjudgmental acceptance of the patient as a person. It also means that the patient must work at accepting himself or herself. Being self-aware and having feelings

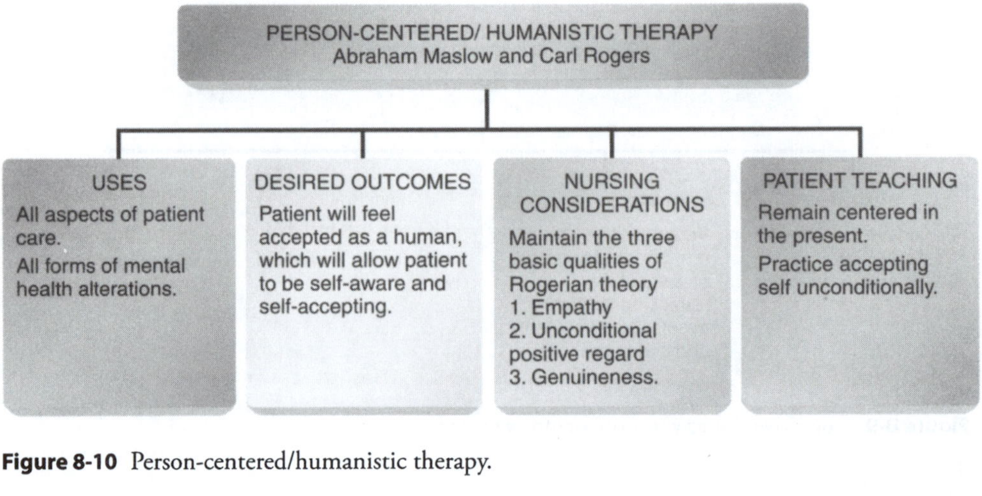

Figure 8-10 Person-centered/humanistic therapy.

that are congruent (equal) to that self-concept are some of the goals of humanistic therapy.

Rogers believed that people who care for other people must have three qualities. These qualities are:

- Empathy (the ability to identify with the patient's feelings without actually experiencing them with the patient)
- Unconditional positive regard
- Genuineness (honesty)

Although nurses may not be active participants in the actual therapy sessions with their patients, it is important for nurses to maintain these three qualities in *all* therapeutic relationships. When a patient feels betrayed, it usually results in deterioration of the nurse-patient relationship and loss of credibility for the nurse in that situation.

Counseling

Counseling is licensed and regulated differently not only state by state, but also sometimes municipality by municipality (Fig. 8-11). Some states require that a person be prepared at a PhD level to practice therapy independently; in some areas, only certain types of therapy are licensed. Nurses prepared at an LPN/LVN level or at an RN level can, in some localities, practice forms of treatment. It is up to nurses to do the appropriate research to determine their rights, responsibilities, and regulations in their locality, if counseling is a path they wish to pursue. Nurses may be asked or required to accompany their patients to counseling sessions at times. They may be asked to facilitate (lead) a group discussion sometimes. If nurses have the opportunity, they should take it. It is very interesting to see the dynamics of the group and the way the facilitator guides patients through issues.

Neeb's Tip These are confidential sessions, even if they are group oriented. Patients are there to work; others are there by invitation for special reasons.

Pastoral or Cultural Counseling

Some people prefer to obtain assistance or counseling from their church or spiritual leaders (Fig. 8-12). Sessions are often free, or on a "free-will" or "ability to pay" status. The person who provides therapy in this time or circumstance may or may not be trained in traditional mental health theories and modalities.

In some Christian faiths, nurses may have an opportunity to serve in ways they could not in a traditional setting. For example, "parish nurses" are licensed nurses who work through their church and perform tasks ranging from simply visiting a homebound church member to actually performing care and counseling or referrals for that individual. Depending on the particular church organization, nurses who serve as parish nurses may serve in a volunteer capacity or in a paid position. Training sessions are offered in some locales for nurses who wish to provide this service, although many churches do not yet require formal training for all their nurses.

Nurses may be in a position to counsel patients of their cultural or religious groups

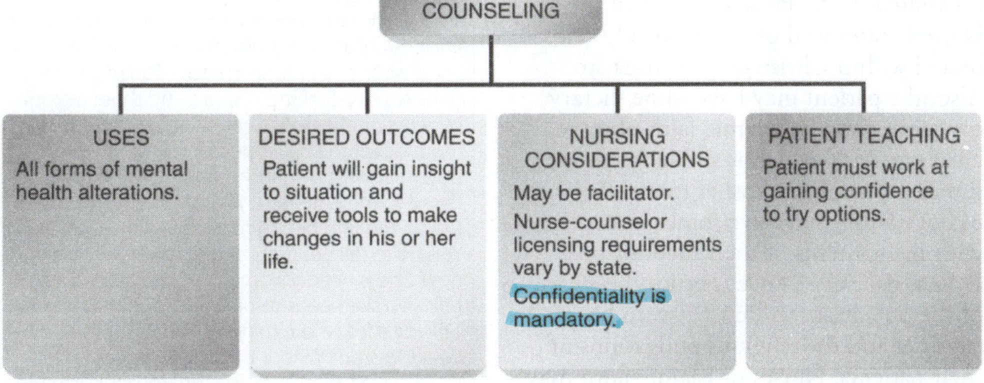

Figure 8-11 Counseling.

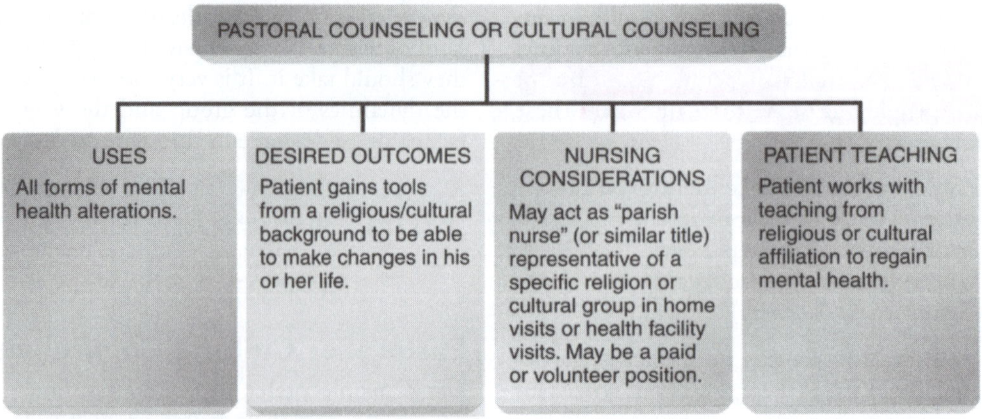

Figure 8-12 Pastoral or cultural counseling.

when the patient enters the health-care system. Here are some examples:

- Patients who profess Judaism, especially if those individuals observe kosher practices, may have concerns about dietary selections, may refuse to have certain procedures done between sundown Friday and sundown Saturday, and may insist on being admitted to a Jewish hospital if one is available.
- Patients of Islamic faith follow rituals that may conflict with schedules and routines within the hospital. Prayer times are proscribed by their faith and are strictly followed; therefore, medication times, treatment times, or attendance at therapy may meet with some conflict on the part of that patient. Prayers can be postponed in case of a conflict in schedules. Islamic belief follows holy times that are different from the traditional holidays or holy days celebrated in the social calendar in the United States or those traditionally celebrated within Christianity or Judaism. Also, the patient may have some dietary concerns; those of Islamic faith observe halal practices, which is similar to the Judaism practice of kosher foods. Patients of both faiths may have some concerns with the contents of their medications, such as gel caps. Nurses need to be aware of the potential conflicts between hospital routines and the religious obligations of their patients. Nurses of Islamic faith may find that one of their challenges working within their belief system is caring for patients of the opposite sex. Women of Islamic faith often wear a hijab (head covering) that completely covers the hair.

Neeb's Tip As a health-care provider, acknowledge and validate patients' beliefs regarding their religion or culture.

- Some Native American patients may have healing traditions that conflict with traditional Western medicine. Remember that it is not appropriate to label all Native Americans as one group; many tribes have their own unique beliefs and traditions. Shamans, healers, and medicine men are examples of people who may be present in the room with the Native American patient.

Critical Thinking Question

Maya is a new employee on your medical floor. Maya is Muslim. She has been given permission to wear her hijab. Maya "disappears" at odd times in addition to her assigned breaks. Today is exceptionally busy. Staffing is short, and there are new patients on the floor. The patient in the private room down the hall is deteriorating; she has the potential for stroke and is waiting to be transferred to the Emergency Department. Where is Maya? You find her on her knees deep in prayer. You try to tell her that things are very critical right now. She is needed; can't she pray later? Maya tells you she needs to pray now and that she will only be a few more minutes. What priorities must be addressed? Whose priorities are they? What potential problems could arise from this situation? What are some potential resolutions?

Table 8-1 examines a number of concepts that may affect certain cultural groups' willingness to seek and comply with mental health treatment.

Group Therapy

Group therapy is a very broad topic. Groups are formed for many reasons; they can be ongoing or short-term, depending on the needs of the patients or the type of disorder. Group therapy can include formal psychotherapy groups where patients meet with a therapist regularly as part of their treatment. Self-help programs are also a form of group therapy. For example, Alcoholics Anonymous (AA) and similar 12-step groups are well-established, ongoing groups. They are held not only in the treatment facility, but also in the community. Meeting times are established and published so that people know when and how to access them. As a rule, AA meetings are "closed" meetings; that is, only alcoholics are welcome. Sometimes, maybe once a month or once quarterly, a meeting is advertised as "open," so that other interested persons (and students) are welcome. Many people who have experienced alcoholism or other chemical dependencies have benefited from this 12-step approach to healing, and it is said that this type of peer group help is the

Table 8-1 Concepts That May Affect Certain Cultural Groups' Seeking or Complying With Mental Health Treatment

Caucasian	• Stigma remains attached to mental illness but is weakening somewhat. • Generally have more access to health insurance and to mental health professionals. • Tend to be more receptive to taking medications than other groups may be.
African American	• More likely than whites to receive initial treatment for mental health in emergency rooms (it is thought this may be because this population delays treatment). • Approximately 20% of African Americans do not have health insurance. • More likely to receive treatment from primary health-care provider rather than a mental health specialist. • If any treatment is rendered, it may be substandard. • Statistics may be skewed to show overrepresentation of African Americans having mental illness.
Hispanic	• Mental illness among Hispanics is about equal to that of Caucasians. • Currently the highest group not having health insurance. • Language barriers. • Young Hispanics tend to have higher rates of depression, anxiety disorders, and suicide. • Hispanics born in the United States tend to be diagnosed with a mental illness more frequently than those born in Mexico.
Native Americans	• Suicide rate approximately 50% higher than that of the general U.S. population. • Mental health treatment options very limited. • Lack of research into mental health issues for Native Americans. Also difficult to design and provide effective mental health care. • Cultural stigmas.
Asian Americans	• Cultural stigmas; depending on the group, the stigma is expressed differently. • Language barriers. • Tend to seek mental health services at lower rates than Caucasians. • Goal is to restore balance in life; often accomplished through exercise or diet rather than a mental health system.

Office of Minority Health. (2013). Accessed at http://minorityhealth.hhs.gov

most beneficial for this type of illness. Other types of support groups may have different formats.

Tool Box |▶ Alcohol Anonymous (AA)
www.aa.org

■ ■ ■ Clinical Activity
Attend an open AA meeting. Describe your views about AA prior to attending and write about your feelings after attending..

Group therapy also includes family therapy. Family counseling sessions are often set up with individual therapists with a specialty in the problem area for that family. It is expected that the whole family attend, but there may be times when only certain members are asked to attend or when the individuals will "break out" with another therapist and then return to the family group later.

Marriage counseling is set up either with an individual counselor or in a group with other couples. Many times, peer counselors are used. These are people who have experienced similar obstacles in their marriage and found creative, effective ways to manage their conflicts (Fig. 8-13). Sometimes, people choose to seek help from a spiritual leader. It is important for us to remember that the therapists and counselors are tools. They do not heal the patient; the patient heals himself or herself. Patients must take the suggestions given by the therapist, try them, and see what works for them. Nurses can help patients by reinforcing the good work they do in learning to keep themselves healthy. Nurses can also help by reminding patients gently that they do their own healing. Sometimes, when the road to healing gets rocky, patients may use the therapist as a scapegoat. Rather than agree or disagree with the patient, the nurse needs to remember the therapeutic communication skills, empathize with the hard work that is being done by the patient, and encourage the patient to discuss the frustration with the therapist.

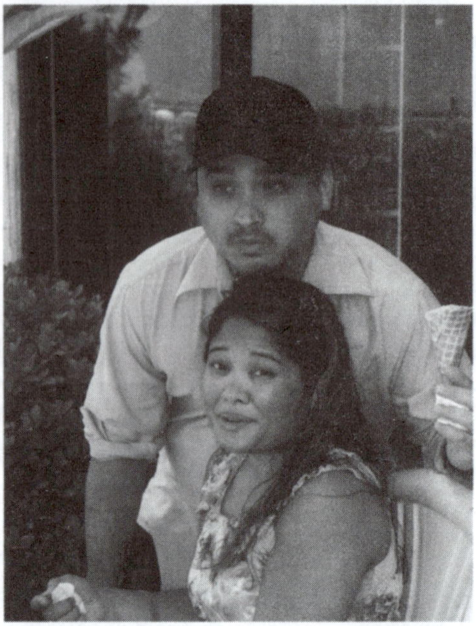

Figure 8-13 This obviously happy couple is a reminder that people can find creative, effective ways to manage conflicts within their relationships. A therapist may help them with suggestions, but they must try those suggestions themselves and find what works for them. *(Courtesy of Robynn Anwar.)*

Electroconvulsive Therapy

Electroconvulsive therapy (ECT), or electroshock therapy, as it is sometimes still called, is a form of treatment that is frightening to some patients. They envision the old movies in which the patient flopped relentlessly on the table. Fortunately, that is a no longer the case.

Because of these misperceptions, it is important for health-care providers to educate others (Fig. 8-14). Patients are generally given a sedative before the treatment. Nurses carefully monitor blood pressure and pulse before and after treatment. The amount of electricity used is individualized to the patient. A treatment usually lasts only a few minutes, and if one is slow to look, he or she might miss seeing a patient's so-called convulsion. Often, only a toe or a finger may twitch slightly; there are no more uncontrolled seizures on the treatment table.

ECT has a few side effects that can be fairly unpleasant. The patient may feel confused and forgetful immediately after the treatment. This can be from a combination of the ECT itself and the pretreatment medication. If there has been a stronger seizure, the

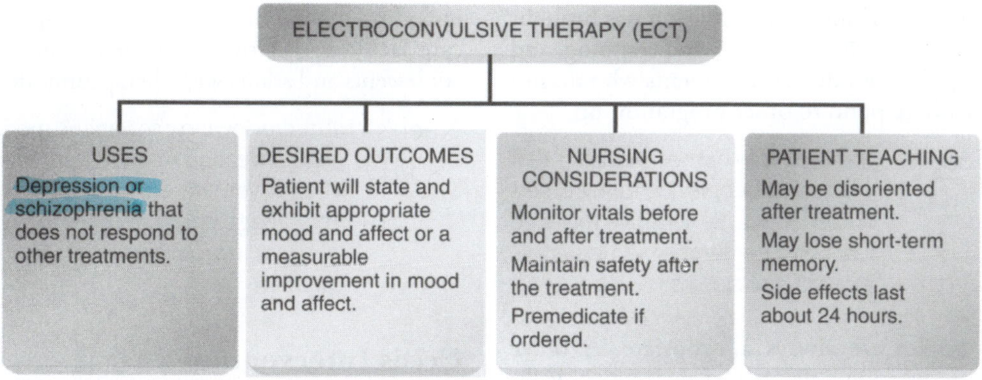

Figure 8-14 Electroconvulsive therapy.

patient may have some muscle soreness. Patients are secured with restraints during the treatment, however, so movement is minimal. Because of the possibility of confusion and forgetfulness, it is common to restrict the patient's activity for 24 hours after a treatment, and it is recommended that the nurse stay with the patient until the patient is oriented and able to care for himself or herself. ECT is not used indiscriminately as it once was. Today, it is used when other therapies have not been helpful, and it is usually reserved for severe or long-term depression and certain types of schizophrenia.

The nurse's responsibilities include careful monitoring of vital signs and accurate documentation relating to the patient's subjective and objective response to the treatment. The patient should have nothing by mouth (NPO) for at least 4 hours before a treatment. Reminding the patient to empty his or her bladder and to remove dentures, contact lenses, hairpins, and so on is also important. Ensuring that the patient is kept safe after therapy is also a major concern.

Humor Therapy

Many studies have been done over the years showing the effects of smiles, hugs, and laughter on mental health as well as physical conditions such as cancer (Fig. 8-15). The movie *Patch Adams,* based on a real-life doctor, portrayed the potential of humor therapy. Viewers saw breakthroughs take place in patients previously thought untreatable.

Humor therapy uses many modalities, from clowns to movies to just 10 good "belly laughs" daily. Whatever the medium, laughter alters outlooks and neurochemical production. Patients can show remarkable progress.

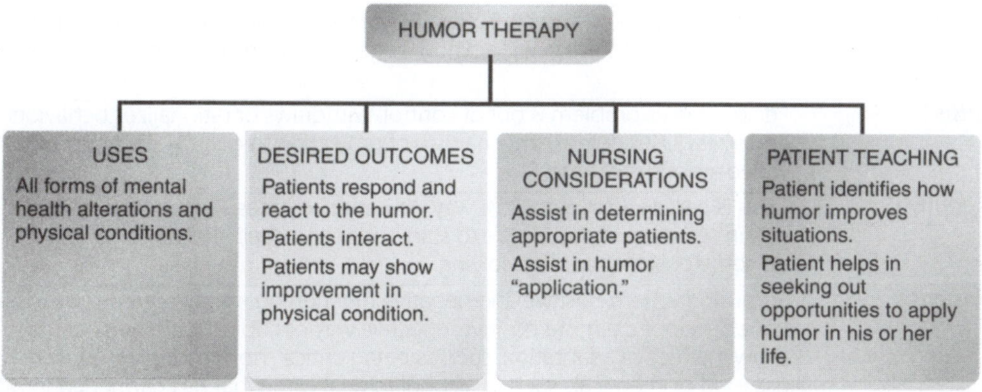

Figure 8-15 Humor therapy.

In fact, this kind of intervention has brought responses such as singing, hand clapping, and laughter from dementia patients who do not usually respond to other programming.

Neeb's Tip The danger in humor therapy is that what some people find funny, others find offensive. Be sensitive to varied reactions. Remember some people are fearful of clowns.

Smiles are always appropriate. A brave nurse wearing a red rubber nose when walking into the room of an appropriate patient might ease that person's pain—either mental or physical—even if only for a short while. Humor is important for nurses as well as for the patient, since caring for others on a daily basis can create unwarranted stresses.

Pet Therapy

Pet therapy has been found to reduce stress in patients. Unfortunately, not everyone can have a pet, due to finances, allergies, or living arrangements.

The well-renowned Dr. Oz sees pet therapy as a stress reliever, especially for lack of social interaction, such as the loss of a significant other. Pets are not judgmental. According to the National Institutes of Health (NIH), pet therapy can be used in several health-care settings, including mental health units and long-term care facilities. Pet therapy benefits children, adolescents and adults with therapeutic effects.

Neeb's Tip After reviewing the various modalities for treating mental health disorders: if you were using one of the modalities, could you discuss it as easily as if you were talking about a vitamin?

Crisis Intervention

Phases of Crisis

Although **crisis** is a highly individual situation, most experts agree that people experiencing a crisis pass through the five phases described in Table 8-2.

Crisis can happen at any time to anyone. It can involve one's child, next-door neighbor, or patient. Crisis is defined in several ways. In the health fields, a crisis is a sudden, unexpected event in a person's life that drastically changes his or her routine. Crisis has been defined as a state in which the body is out of homeostasis. It is thought of as a situation in which a person may "lose control of feelings and thoughts, thus experiencing an extreme state of emotional turmoil" (Shives and Isaacs, 2002).

A person in crisis is at risk for physical and emotional harm inflicted by self or by others.

Table 8-2 The Five Phases of Crises

Phase	Behaviors
Precrisis	Person feels "fine." Will often deny stress level and, in fact, state a feeling of well-being.
Impact	Person feels anxiety and confusion. May have trouble organizing personal life. High stress level. Person will acknowledge feeling stress but may minimize its severity.
Crisis	Person denies problem is out of control. Withdraws or rationalizes behaviors and stress. Uses defense mechanism of projection frequently. This may last varied amounts of time.
Adaptive	Crisis is perceived in a positive way. Anxiety decreases. Person attempts to regain self-esteem and is able to start socializing again. Person is able to do some positive problem solving.
Postcrisis	Surprisingly, both positive and negative functioning may be seen. Person may have developed a more positive, effective way of coping with stress *or* may show ineffective adaptation, such as being critical, hostile, depressed, or may use food or chemicals such as alcohol to deal with what has happened.

Examples of people who may be experiencing a crisis are those who have lost a job suddenly or were divorced recently, are in an abusive relationship, have experienced the death of a loved one, or are contemplating or attempting suicide. An important concept to remember is that each person has a different set of stressors and a different way of dealing with stress. What is a crisis for one person may be simply a minor nuisance for another person.

Many employers recognize the potential for crisis and offer some type of employee assistance program (EAP). The service is confidential, and usually the initial call is free to the employee. EAPs vary in what they are able to provide and may act as a referral service for the employee. Nurses should ask the patient if his or her employer provides this benefit.

Goals of Crisis Intervention

Nurses often have the unique opportunity of often being present for the first three phases of the crisis and not for the outcome (Fig. 8-16). In many agencies, nurses are not involved with longer term treatment, but they may very easily be the ones who walk into the room during a suicide attempt or who may take the call at the nursing station from a distraught parent who is about to hurt his or her child.

The goals of crisis intervention change according to the degree of treatment in which the nurse will be involved. Crisis intervention for the health-care provider is obviously provided at a different level than it would be from a law enforcement or emergency dispatch viewpoint. Since this text is meant to be an overview to prepare nurses at an entry level of practice, we will look at the goals of crisis intervention from a health-care perspective.

1. *Ensure safety:* Assess the situation. If the nurse or the patient is in physical danger, the nurse should signal for help. The nurse *should not* leave the patient unless danger to the nurse is imminent. It may sound harsh, but the nurse will be no good to anyone if he or she is hurt, or worse. The nurse must take care of his or her own safety, and then take care of the patient's safety.
2. *Diffuse the situation:* Nurses should do this verbally, when at all possible. A person in crisis is most likely not in control of his or her thoughts, feelings, or actions. Physical attempts at restraining or calming are best left until all verbal attempts have been made, and only when there is enough help to do it safely for the patient and the staff.
3. *Determine the problem:* The nurse should attempt to find out from the patient's viewpoint the cause of the crisis. It is very important that the nurse *not push* the patient for any reason and *remain calm* during the intervention. The last thing a patient in crisis needs is a nurse in panic. There is time for nurses to talk about their feelings when the patient is safe.

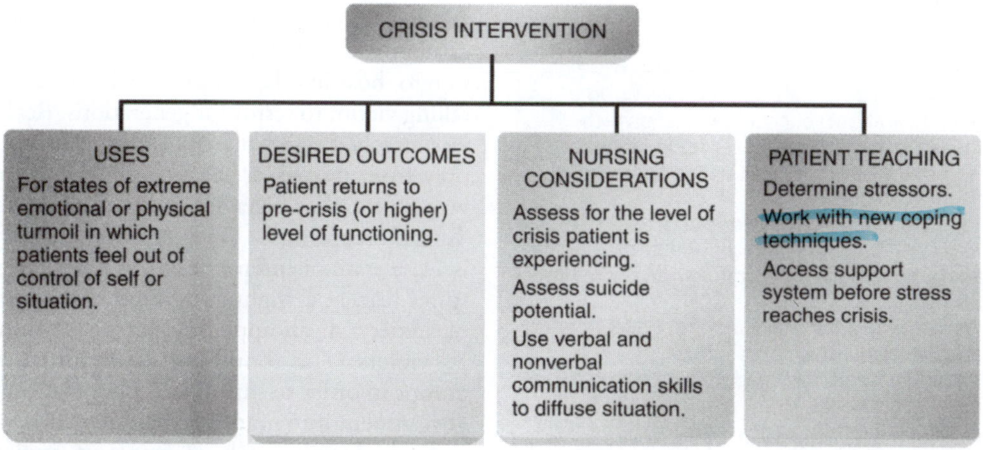

Figure 8-16 Crisis intervention.

4. *Decrease the anxiety level:* The nurse's adrenaline level will probably be at an all-time high, but it won't be even close to that of the person in crisis. The nurse should make every attempt to reassure the patient that he or she is in a safe place. The nurse should gently but firmly tell the patient that he or she is concerned, wants to help, and will do whatever is possible to make the situation more comfortable but that the patient's help and cooperation are needed. *Caution:* Nurses must be very careful with physical contact at this point. Touch as a nonverbal communication skill may be interpreted inaccurately as aggression or sexual innuendo by a patient whose thoughts and feelings are in turmoil.
5. *Return the patient to pre-crisis (or better) level of functioning:* A nurse may or may not be able to calm the patient to the point that he or she is able to understand what just happened. It might take a longer-term session of treatment to help the patient gain that kind of insight. No matter what level of intervention the patient requires, the ultimate goal is for him or her to learn the skills necessary to cope with stress in a more positive way than before the crisis. Much of that learning will come from the role modeling from the nurses. Quite often the most effective techniques are nonverbal where actions speak louder than words.

Critical Thinking Question

With a student partner, role-play one or more of the following potential crises (or think up your own). Think about your communication techniques. Do they change when dealing with crisis? If so, how? What about your nonverbal communication techniques?

- Parent whose child has been abducted at the mall
- Man who calls the clinic, stating he has just killed his wife
- Woman who is frantically seeking shelter from an abusive relationship
- You find a friend of your adolescent daughter slashing her wrists.
- Alcoholic, the main wage earner for the family, who has just been fired from his job

Classroom Activity

- Look in your city's telephone book for agencies that handle crisis intervention. Contact one in person. Inform the agency that this is a school project and you wish to ask them a few questions, such as: Whom does the agency service? What are its hours of operation? How is the agency funded? What does the emergency care cost the patient? Who is its staff? Write a short report of your findings. If possible, appoint someone to compile all the information so that each student nurse has a "starter set" to be able to help others.

Crisis, if treated in an appropriate and timely way, is usually temporary. Crisis intervention theories are changing to try to keep up with the current concepts of illness. Nevertheless, people will always be experiencing crisis. When crisis happens, it is important that the person who is there to help understand that this is a very frightening time for the person in turmoil. Nurses must understand that they are in a special position as they have some knowledge of crisis and communication skills and are able to help, yet they must always be aware of the legal ramifications of intervention.

Terrorism

September 11, 2001, changed life in the United States. Citizens of the United States became aware of a way of life experienced routinely by some of the country's global neighbors. Suicide bombers, anthrax, sarin gas, and tainted water and food sources—American citizens suddenly had a new kind of connection to those in other countries who have been falling victim to terror for generations. Reality was attached to what many Americans knew only from movies or the evening news. That way of life, that behavior, is called terrorism. Terror, according to Webster Online (2013), is "1: a state of intense fear; 2a: one that inspires fear, b: a frightening aspect, c: a cause of anxiety, d: an appalling person or thing; 3: violence (as bombing) committed by groups in order to intimidate a population or government into granting their demands."

Some words, such as fear and anxiety, which are used to define terrorism are also symptoms of many mental illnesses. Perhaps the most frightening part of this definition is that humans do not always know the source of the terror and thus are unable to defend themselves. They may feel a loss of personal control over their life and safety. It is difficult for adults to accept and deal with what has become an ever-present possibility in what Americans had always assumed was a safe place to live. How, then, do people help their children to process the potential dangers in the world at the same time they are moving through the normal stages of growth and development? How can people convey the message that while bad things happen, people are basically good and not to fear them? How do adults, parents, teachers, and health-care professionals prepare to help others who experience crisis, post-traumatic stress, depression, and other potential effects of terror? Suggestions will be offered in various chapters throughout this text; however, to borrow an idea from the sports world, the best defense is a good offense. Nurses need to be ready for the possibility of patients experiencing some effect of terrorism and must be willing to discuss the situation with that patient. As with so many other areas of nursing, it means nurses must take stock of their own thoughts and feelings about the topic.

Legal Considerations

The Nurse's Perspective: Today's society is a litigious one. It is easy to be tempted to stay uninvolved when people call out for help. In some states, nurses, physicians, and anyone else in the health fields are required by law to help. Some localities require health-care professionals to post identifying insignia on their vehicles. Most states do not require this yet, but many are considering it. This puts nurses in a sensitive position. Nurses want to help, but nursing curriculum at the entry level provides very little in the way of hands-on crisis intervention techniques. What if something goes wrong? Crisis intervention literature suggests that nurses risk a higher liability if they fail to try to help. In other words, it is safer legally for a nurse to do something to help than to do nothing.

Exactly what a nurse is able to do depends greatly on his or her locale, level of preparation, state's nurse practice act, and comfort level. Staying within the legal parameter of one's nursing licensure is of major importance; nurses should do only what they know and what is legal. The truth is that anyone can sue anyone for anything. The good news is that most states will find in favor of the medical professional who has, in good faith and in accordance with his or her licensure, made an effort to help a person in a crisis situation. The Good Samaritan law protects nurses as well. The Good Samaritan law *does not* generally cover nurses within the confines of their employment, however; only when acting to assist in a crisis or emergency situation are nurses protected.

Neeb's Tip

Remember: Crisis intervention has something in common cardiopulmonary resuscitation (CPR): Once a nurse starts and makes that commitment to help, he/she cannot quit until physically unable to continue. Starting to provide help and then changing one's mind can be interpreted as neglect or abandonment, and in such an instance, the nurse could be found at fault.

The Patient's Perspective: What happens to the patient experiencing the crisis? Because of the nature of crisis, the patient probably does not have a valid insight into the situation. The patient is very likely to be concerned about personal safety. On top of that, fear and inability to perceive the situation as it really is will interfere with communication. In most instances, the medical staff will encourage the patient to accept some form of treatment. The patient then has two choices: voluntary or involuntary commitment.

Voluntary treatment happens when the patient gives informed consent to be hospitalized or accept some formal treatment program. *Informed* consent means that the patient has been made aware of his or her behaviors, the implications of the behaviors, and expectations from the treatment. Informed consent can be verbal, nonverbal, or written. *Implied* consent allows people who are unconscious to be treated in such a way as to preserve life. If the patient is an adult of legal age who is considered to be competent in the eyes of the law (or an adolescent who has acquired legal emancipation), this patient can also sign himself or herself out at any time.

Involuntary commitment varies somewhat from state to state. Many states have the capability to place a "hold" on the patient, usually for 48 to 72 hours. During this time, the patient is confined to the treatment setting. Usually, a social worker is assigned to visit the patient and act as an advocate for him or her. The goal of the hold period is for the patient to see the need for help with his or her crisis and then consent to voluntary treatment. If, at the end of the hold period, the patient does not consent to treatment, he or she is free to leave the facility, as long as no other manifestation of crisis has surfaced during the hold.

In either instance, patients maintain all civil rights while in the treatment setting. The patient is covered under the Patient's Bill of Rights and most often the patient keeps a copy of the rights.

The Community Mental Health Centers Act made provisions for community-based treatment. Communities develop centers and provide treatment according to the needs of the area; not all centers provide all types of treatment or 24-hour service. However, the community is supposed to provide some method of emergency psychiatric treatment to help people in crisis as well as those who are chronically mentally ill. These centers can be in the form of freestanding crisis centers or walk-in clinics, and many are connected with the community hospital. In reality though, many communities may have minimal resources to provide these services, so nurses should know what is available in their communities

■ Summary

Table 8-3 summarizes treatment modalities that may be used alone or in conjunction with medications to treat a wide variety of mental health issues. The common uses and desired outcomes are covered.

Table 8-3 Summary of Commonly Used Treatment Modalities

Treatment Modality	Uses	Desired Outcomes
Psychotherapy	For treatment of various alterations to mental health.	**1.** Patient states improvement in emotional discomfort. **2.** Patient returns to comfortable social functioning. **3.** Patient behaves in a manner appropriate to the situation.
Behavior Modification	To remove or greatly diminish behaviors that are inappropriate or unhealthy.	Former undesirable behaviors have been replaced by new, healthy behaviors.
Rational-Emotive Therapy (RET)/ Cognitive Behavior Therapy(CBT)	Short-term, problem-focused therapy for any mental health alteration that is consciously controlled.	Patient will be able to remain "undisturbed" as a result of rethinking activating events, belief system, and consequences.
Person-Centered/ Humanistic	All aspects of patient care. All forms of mental health alterations.	Patient will feel accepted as a human, which will allow patient to be self-aware and self-accepting. Patient will gain insight into the situation and receive tools to make changes in his or her life.

Table 8-3 Summary of Commonly Used Treatment Modalities—cont'd

Treatment Modality	Uses	Desired Outcomes
Pastoral Counseling or Cultural Counseling	All forms of mental health alterations.	Patient gains tools from a religious/cultural background to be able to make changes in his or her life.
Group Therapy	Many uses, including family, couples, self-help.	Patient gains knowledge that there are others with similar problems. Patient learns from peers and helps others.
Electro-Convulsive Therapy (ECT)	Depression or schizophrenia that does not respond to other treatments.	Patient will state and exhibit appropriate mood and affect or a measurable improvement in mood and affect.
Humor Therapy	All forms of mental health alterations and physical conditions.	Patients respond and react to the humor. Patients interact. Patients may show improvement in physical condition.
Crisis Intervention	For states of extreme emotional or physical turmoil in which patients feel out of control of self or situation.	Patient returns to precrisis (or higher) level of functioning.

Key Concepts

1. The place in which treatment is given must be conducive to therapy. *Milieu* is the word used to describe the environment of the treatment area.
2. Psychopharmacology is very important to the effective treatment of the patient. There are many classifications of psychoactive medications and many individual medications within each classification. It is the nurse's responsibility to consult a drug reference regarding all the psychotropic medications they give their patients. It also is part of the nurse's role to reinforce teaching about the medications to the patient.
3. Psychotherapy, sometimes in conjunction with medications, is often used to treat patients. There are several methods of psychotherapy, including psychoanalysis, behavior modification, rational-emotive therapy, and humanistic, or person-centered, therapy.
4. Counseling is carried out in different ways, depending on the patient's needs and type of illness. Counselors may be licensed and the nurse's role in counseling regulated differently from state to state and municipality to municipality. Counseling is given individually or in group settings, according to the situation.
5. ECT is used for specific situations. Premedication is usually ordered. It is the role of the nurse to monitor vital signs, maintain safety, and document post-treatment observations.
6. Crisis intervention is very individualized. Crisis has five phases, and each person experiences them differently.
7. Employee support systems are becoming more accessible through employers. They are confidential and free or reasonably priced.
8. Pastoral or cultural counseling may be the treatment of choice for an individual. Nurses must do all they can to help the patient receive care that is personally meaningful.

CASE STUDY

Andrea, an emergency room nurse from San Diego, is on vacation with her friend. Andrea selected a road trip to a major theme park. There are two adults and two children in the vehicle. They are about minutes from the gate, Andrea sees smoke on the horizon. The radio in the vehicle alerts Andrea and her friend that the theme park has just experienced an explosion. Details are sketchy, but there are numerous injuries. The park has been closed. As Andrea and her friends approach what was the entrance to the park, they witness many individuals running, injured, and crying. People are on fire and rolling. There is a very unpleasant odor. Police, firefighters, and first responders are directing Andrea and her friend away from the site. Andrea tells them she is a nurse and offers to help. At this moment, her help is not wanted, but all are directed to a "holding" area. The children, whose ages are 4 and 13 (Olivia and Trinity), are crying and asking Andrea questions about the smoke. If you were Andrea, what would your emotional response be? How would you answer and calm the children? After a few minutes, the police accept Andrea's offer to help the wounded. The children become hysterical at Andrea's leaving the vehicle, yet Andrea feels responsible to help. What should Andrea do? What stages of crisis is she experiencing?

REFERENCES

CNN.com/Health. Report: *Minorities lack proper mental health care.* Dr. David Satcher, U.S. Surgeon General. August 27, 2001.

Deglin, J.F., Vallerand, A.H., and Sanoski, C.A. (2011). *Davis's Drug Guide for Nurses.* 12th ed. Philadelphia: F.A. Davis.

Ellis, A. (1988). *A Guide to Rational Living.* From the video series *Thinking Allowed.* Oakland, CA: InnerWork.

Meadows, M. (1997, September). Closing the Gap: Mental Health and Minorities. *Cultural Considerations in Treating Asians.* A Newsletter of the Office of Minority Health.

Office of Minority Health. (2013). Accessed at http://minorityhealth.hhs.gov

Oz, M.C., and Roizen, M.F. (2008). That Lovin' Feeling. In *You Being Beautiful: The Owner's Manual to Inner and Outer Beauty* (p. 292). New York: Free Press.

Sadock, B.J., and Sadock, V.A. (2008). *Kaplan and Sadock's Concise Handbook of Clinical Psychiatry.* Philadelphia. Lippincott Williams and Wilkins.

Sadock, B.J., Sadock, V.A. (2013). *Kaplan & Sadock's Pocket Handbook of Psychiatric Drug Treatment.* 6th ed. Philadelphia: Lippincott Williams and Wilkins

Shives, L.R., and Isaacs, A. (2002). *Basic Concepts of Psychiatric–Mental Health Nursing.* 5th ed. Philadelphia: JB Lippincott.

Townsend, M.C. (2012). *Essentials of Psychiatric and Mental Health Nursing.* 7th ed. Philadelphia: F.A. Davis.

Venes, D. (2013). *Taber's Cyclopedic Medical Dictionary.* 22nd ed. Philadelphia: F.A. Davis.

Webster Online. (2005). www.merriam-webster.com

Test Questions

Multiple Choice Questions

1. Which of the following is not a behavior noted in the crisis phase of crisis?
   a. Denial
   b. Feeling of well-being
   c. Use of projection
   d. Rationalization
2. One of the first statements a nurse might make to a person who has been abused might be:
   a. "Why didn't you leave the first time you were attacked?"
   b. "Do you want to prosecute or not?"
   c. "What do you think made that person hit you?"
   d. "You're safe here. I would like to help you."
3. A therapeutic environment (milieu) is *best* defined as:
   a. An environment in which a patient is under a 72-hour hold
   b. An environment that is locked and supervised
   c. An environment that is structured to decrease stress and encourage learning new behavior
   d. An environment that is designed to be homelike for persons who are hospitalized for life
4. Which of the following is *false* regarding ECT?
   a. It is used to treat depression and schizophrenia.
   b. It is used to stop convulsive seizures.
   c. Fatigue and disorientation are immediate side effects.
   d. Memory will gradually return.
5. Psychopharmacology (psychotropic drug therapy) is used:
   a. As a cure for mental illness
   b. Only to control violent behavior
   c. To alter the pain receptors in the brain
   d. To decrease symptoms and facilitate other therapies
6. Avoiding such foods as bananas, cheese, and yogurt should be emphasized to patients who are taking:
   a. Prozac
   b. Lithium
   c. MAOIs
   d. Tricyclic antidepressants
7. The goals of crisis intervention include all of the following *except:*
   a. Safety
   b. Increasing anxiety
   c. Taking care of the precipitating event
   d. Return to pre-crisis or better level of functioning
8. In order for psychotherapy to be effective, it is necessary to do all of the following *except:*
   a. Encourage the patient to repress feelings.
   b. Reinforce appropriate behavior.
   c. Establish a therapeutic patient-staff relationship.
   d. Assist patient to gain insight into problem.

Test Questions

9. Your patient, Mrs. L, is on your unit for bowel resection. She is exhibiting signs of nervousness and anxiety, which she attributes to the upcoming surgery. You note from her record that she has a history of ethyl alcohol (ETOH) abuse. Which of the following classifications of drugs would be potentially addictive for her?
a. Lithium salts
b. Antianxiety drugs
c. Antipsychotic drugs
d. Anticholinergics

10. James is a 13-year-old who has been transferred to your medical-surgical unit after being stabilized in the ED. He slit both wrists and took an overdose of his Wellbutrin. You know medications such as Wellbutrin:
a. Are antidepressants and should have stopped his suicidal impulse
b. Have no particular nursing considerations for children and adolescents
c. Are antidepressants and may have an increase in the suicidal ideation for children and adolescents
d. Are not effective as antidepressants for children or adolescents

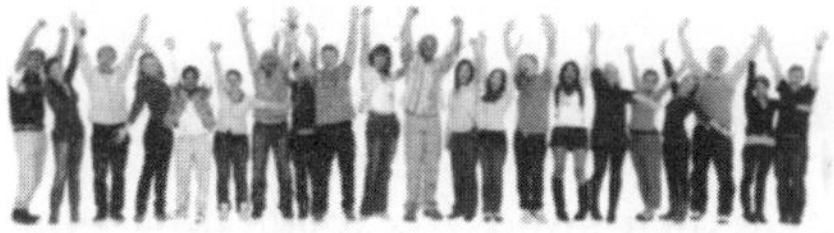

CHAPTER 9

Complementary and Alternative Treatment Modalities

Learning Objectives

1. Differentiate between alternative and complementary medicine.
2. Identify integrative medicine.
3. Identify the concept of the mind-body connection.
4. Identify support for patient beliefs and models.
5. Identify three alternative and complementary treatment modalities.
6. Identify three types of massage.
7. Differentiate between trance and sleep.
8. Identify the three primary channels of experience.
9. Define key terms.

Key Terms

- Alternative medicine
- Aromatherapy
- Beliefs
- Biofeedback
- Complementary medicine
- Holistic
- Hypnotherapy
- Integrative medicine
- Mind-body connection
- Models
- Placebo
- Presupposition
- Rapport
- Reflexology
- Reiki
- Trance

Medicine is a rapidly evolving field, and sometimes it is tempting for the nurse to assume that every patient is knowledgeable about the current state of the art. For some patients, conventional Western medicine is not the only course. Many factors affect a patient's choice of treatment modalities; education, experience, economic status, belief system, and culture are a few considerations.

There are many other means of treating illness and promoting good health in addition to traditional medicine. **Complementary** and **alternative medicine** (CAM) presents additional options. In general, alternative practices/medicines replace those of conventional medicine, and complementary methods are used together with traditional treatments. Many of these have been used for centuries. These present different choices to the pharmaceutical products dispensed at the local pharmacy. Often, these methods differ considerably from what is acceptable medical care in Western culture. Complementary or alternative methods may lack extensive scientific research to prove their effectiveness or even their safety according to the standards of conventional medicine. Those practices that do have at least some research validating that they are safe and do work comprise **integrative medicine,** which provides the best of both worlds.

An alternative practice, for example, would be to use an herbal preparation to combat depression instead of physician-ordered prescription medication. A complementary treatment might consist of using biofeedback to reduce the symptoms of anxiety associated with mental illness while the patient continues to participate in psychotherapy and take antianxiety medications. Both approaches address a key concept in alternative and complementary medicine: the **mind-body connection.**

Mind, Body, and Belief

The ways in which people's minds and bodies are interconnected stretch beyond the obvious physical world in which people live. First, there is the *brain,* an organ directly connected to the body by tissue such as nerves and blood vessels. The brain is contained within the bony cavity of the skull, which constitutes its protection and support. The *mind* represents the cognitive, emotional, and logical responses that make people individual human beings. The mind is clearly more than just the brain, the sum of its cells, chemicals, electrical activity, and connections.

It may seem strange to think that there was ever a question about the interconnectedness of the mind and the body. It has long been known that disease affects the mind, but conventional medicine has only recently started to accept that the reverse is also true, that the mind affects the disease. People's thoughts and emotions affect the way their bodies function, even on a cellular level. This **holistic** view makes complementary and alternative medicine increasingly popular choices for the treatment of all types of illness, including mental disorders.

Important to the effectiveness of any type of treatment are the patient's **beliefs.** Nursing requires respect for the beliefs and values of other people and cultures as fundamental to good practice. It is useful to remember that everyone has a different way of viewing the world. Everyone forms **models** of the world based on beliefs, values, education, and experience. Models are pictures or ideas that people form in their minds to explain how things work. Models help people understand and interact with others and their environment, and they help people to formulate beliefs.

To a large extent, a person's beliefs will determine the success of a given treatment. This can be plainly seen when a **placebo** medication is given and is effective in relieving symptoms like severe pain, even though the placebo is no more than a sugar pill. This illustrates that what the patient believes and expects the placebo to do can be more important than the actual composition of the tablet.

Even though the nurse might not be directly involved in the application of a complementary or alternative treatment, supporting the patient's cultural and belief systems is an important role in helping him or her move forward on a path to wellness. Each patient will have a different level of acceptance of various complementary and alternative approaches. How nonjudgmental, open, and accepting of different ideas for the success of the different methods is up to the patient. The nurse can ease that process by also remaining nonjudgmental, open, and accepting and at the same time being aware of any safety concerns for the patient.

As always, the boundaries of legal and acceptable nursing practice vary from state to state. Nurses need to check with their state's board of nursing or other regulating agencies to determine acceptable standards of practice in regard to using alternative, integrative, and complementary therapies.

Common Complementary and Alternative Treatments

Biofeedback

Stress-related anxiety is the common element of disorders relating to mental illness. It is known that the direct effects of sustained stress can be devastating (see Chapter 7, Coping and Defense Mechanisms). In a critical moment or progressively over time, the biological response to stress can impair the cognitive function of the mind and cloud a person's thinking. Prolonged stress can lead to emotional anguish that is experienced as fear, anxiety, anger, and depression. Prolonged stress can also lead to exhaustion and possible death. Anxiety contributes to physical symptoms—many of which can be reduced or controlled by biofeedback techniques. **Biofeedback** is a training program designed to develop one's ability to control the autonomic nervous system. While biofeedback only recently has become a complementary medical therapy, it has been widely accepted by traditionalists in the West because of its use of scientific measuring devices and proven techniques.

The primary purpose of biofeedback training is to teach patients to recognize tension within the body and to respond with relaxation (Fig. 9-1). Typically, training for patients takes place in a series of one-hour sessions, sometimes spaced a week apart. The patient is taught to obtain a deep level of relaxation as a means to control a light, buzzer, image, or a video game, to which he or she is attached by electrodes and cables. The machine is then gradually adjusted to greater sensitivity, and the patient learns improved control. When training is completed, all that is needed to obtain relaxation and symptom resolution at any time or place is recall of the particular thought and feeling that worked in the clinic.

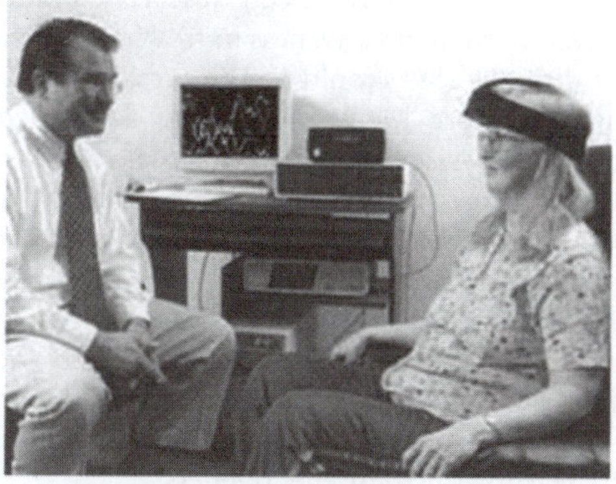

Figure 9-1 Biofeedback training teaches patients to recognize tension and respond with relaxation. *(Courtesy of Santé Rehabilitation Group, Euless, TX)*

Biofeedback is being used with good results for conditions including insomnia, some types of seizures, functional nausea and vomiting, tinnitus, and phantom limb pain. As with other forms of therapy, biofeedback practitioners must be aware of functional or even psychological symptoms that are actually caused by organic problems and require different treatment. It may not be appropriate to use biofeedback to treat extreme or acute states of mental illness, like severe depression, mania, agitation, schizophrenia, paranoia, obsessive-compulsive disorder (OCD), delirium, and identity or dissociative disorders. Critics have pointed out that the major effects from biofeedback can be more economical and easily obtained through relaxation training.

Patients with strong faith they can influence their own health are the most likely to be successful at mastering biofeedback. The experience of gaining control of one's physical reactions can have a tremendous effect on how the person will view stressful situations in the future. As an educational tool for more skeptical patients, learning biofeedback can demonstrate that they have a great deal more control over their responses and symptoms than they first expected.

Aromatherapy

Aromatherapy may well be one of the oldest methods used to treat illness in human beings. Related to herbal therapy, aromatherapy provides treatment by both the direct pharmacological effects of aromatic plant substances and the indirect effects of certain smells on mood and affect. Throughout human history and in many cultures, there are accounts of the use of aromatics to treat varying forms of illness. Applied in salves or ointments, used in incense, reduced to essential oils for topical application, or even ingested, these substances often appeal to patients who are seeking a "natural" approach to healing

People's response to the sense of smell has strong significance in their lives. People associate certain aromas with certain situations, conditions, and emotional states. Many individuals are able to relive particularly strong memories when exposed to an aroma that was present when the remembered event occurred.

For example, the fragrance of baking cookies or apple pie reminds some people of being at home and even experiencing some of the emotions connected to that memory. The ability for a particular smell to create positive alterations in mood makes aromatherapy attractive to many people and has created a large market in everyday products designed to evoke calm and well-being. Scented candles and personal care products like bath oils, shampoos, and body lotions are especially popular.

Treatment for anxiety-based mental illness and depression using aromatics like lavender, thyme, gardenia, and other botanicals is becoming a more acceptable adjunct to conventional methods. It is important to be aware that the oils and plant matter used in aromatherapy can be toxic if improperly administered and should be kept out of the reach of children and the cognitively impaired. Applied to skin, many plant oils are caustic or can trigger an allergic reaction. The nurse should observe and assess to determine if the products used are effective and if there are any side effects noted. As with all alternative treatment, it is advisable to find a competent and knowledgeable practitioner to benefit fully from the potential of aromatherapy.

Classroom Activity

- Bring several different aromatic herbs into class, pass them around, and have each student sniff the plant or a form of the plant. Students should discuss their immediate feelings after inhaling the aromas.

Herbal and Nutritional Therapy

Growing steadily in the United States today is the use of herbal compounds and nutritional supplements to treat illness. The popularity of self-treatment with herbs is in large part due to the desire of many people to return to a simpler lifestyle and as a means to avoid costly prescription medications. Most herbal products are considered nutritional supplements rather than medications, so these products avoid regulation by the Food and Drug Administration (FDA). They are also perceived by the public to be better, or safer, because they can be purchased over the counter and do not require a trip to the doctor's office. There are literally hundreds of products available to consumers seeking relief through herbal and nutritional means.

Neeb's Tip Belief plays a considerable role in the acceptance and use of these products.

With rapid changes in society since World War II has come people's awareness that their lives are no longer as pastoral, calm, and idyllic as they would like to remember them to be. This awareness became more evident after the events of September 11, 2001. In a world full of processed food, the quality of modern nutrition has come into question, and there is growing conviction that artificial additives lack the ability to provide the basics needed for good health.

Daily, people are assured in the popular press and the news media that the solution to many of their problems can be found in nutritional and herbal supplements. Lack of cortisol has been blamed for weight gain, and taking compounds rich in HGH (human growth hormone) has been credited with reversing aging. Infomercials tout the benefits of taking coral calcium and even improving sexual performance with herb-based preparations. The Internet is flooded with supplements that promise to improve people's lives by making them healthier and stronger.

Some herbs have been researched and proven in their effectiveness in treating disease conditions. This should not be surprising, for many modern medications were developed from herbal and other botanical origins. Native Americans knew the value of the inner bark of the willow tree, gathered and used for its ability to reduce fever and ease pain. They also used foxglove in their sweat lodges to energize the frail and restore vitality to the elderly. Little did they know that the salicylate in willow bark and digitalis in foxglove were the reasons for their effectiveness.

There is a tradition in Europe of using herbal medications and nutritional supplements to treat disease. For example, people in

Germany routinely plant and harvest herbs in their garden plots to create remedies for common ailments. Some herbal preparations are available there only by a doctor's prescription, and others can only be obtained through a licensed pharmacist. In the United States, the use of fresh or garden-grown herbs is discouraged because of the difficulty in determining the strength of the active compounds produced by plants under different growing conditions. Europeans are guided by generations of experience and practice to safely use available botanicals.

Unfortunately, the belief in the relative safety of herbs is a misunderstanding that has caused much concern among health-care providers. Deciding on an appropriate dose is difficult, because herbal preparations do not have to conform to any specific guidelines regulating strength or purity. People tend to think that if a small amount of the product is effective, more is better still. Some herbs are very toxic, particularly in pure form. Many herbs interact negatively with prescription medications. This point demonstrates the need for the nurse to include direct questions to the patient about the use of any CAMs. Nurses need to be able to teach their patients the importance of consulting with a physician before beginning any sort of herbal therapy. Table 9-1 describes the five most often used herbal medications and nutritional supplements in the treatment of mental illness in this country.

Neeb's Tip During the admission interview, ask the patient if he or she is taking any alternative or complementary products. Some of these may be contraindicated with medications ordered by the physician.

Tool Box | ▶ The National Institutes of Health division called the National Center for Complementary and Alternative Medicine (NCCAM) is an excellent resource for obtaining information on a specific CAM, including scientific data if available. This is available at www.nccam.nih.gov/

Massage, Energy, and Touch

Widespread among complementary and alternative treatment methods are modalities centered on manipulating the body's energy fields. Massage in one form or another has probably been known to man since before the dawn of history. Touch and movement are essential to life and well-being in both physical and psychological ways. Massage is the manipulation of the body using methodical pressure, friction, and kneading. People are shaped, almost literally, by their childhood experiences of touching. An infant has limited sensory discrimination but will react positively to being cuddled and held, and even to the feel of a snugly wrapped blanket.

Tool Box | ▶ Types of Massage Therapy www.massagetherapy.com/glossary/index.php

Massage has evolved into many variations as a result of its success (Fig. 9-2). Use of touch is common to many different treatment approaches, but there can be great variation in philosophical, theoretical, and practical ideas about how touch is applied. Western variations of massage include Swedish, which was developed in the early nineteenth century and is the type most people are familiar with. It is characterized by long, smooth strokes that go toward the direction of the heart.

The manipulation of specific body sites to relax muscle groups is known as trigger point massage. Conventional medical science has generated a similar trigger point therapy in which injections of steroids are applied at these key areas in place of massage to both relax the muscle group and reduce local inflammation.

Of course, there are also other means of massage available. Rolfing is a therapy designed to realign the body with gravity through fascial manipulation, a vigorous form of bodywork that is finding increasing acceptance. Eastern massage traditions have followed a different path. It is widely believed among Eastern practitioners that the body is governed by energy paths, called meridians. This energy is perceived as the life force, or

Table 9-1 Common Herbal and Dietary Therapies

Specific Therapy	Active Ingredients	Usual Dose	Uses	Side Effect	Contra-Indications	Drug/Food Interactions	Patient Teaching
Ginkgo Biloba	Ginkgentin, Ginkolic acid	120–140 mg PO daily, depending on what is treated; divide into 2–3 equal doses	Short-term memory loss though research is conflicting as to benefits	Bleeding, contact dermatitis, nausea, vomiting, diarrhea, headache; rarely, subdural hematoma, seizures (especially in children)	Pregnant or breast-feeding, children; use cautiously for patient taking anti-coagulants, MAOI medications because Ginkgo Biloba can act as an MAOI	May increase the effects of anticoagulant and antiplatelet drugs. Avoid foods containing large amounts of tyramine: aged meat and cheese, red wine, pickled herring, yogurt, raisins, sour cream, and other foods high in tyramine; also OTC cold and flu preparations.	Do not use if on Coumadin or aspirin. Works well for people over 50 as well as younger adults. May take 6–8 weeks to experience benefits. Use with some fruits and nuts can cause a poison ivy-like reaction.
Kava Kava	Kavapyrones, Piper methysticum, Kava pepper	10–110 mg PO dried kava extract three times daily, or freshly prepared kava beverages, 400–900 g *weekly*	Antidepressant, antianxiety, antipsychotic, to use as sleep aide	Drowsiness, changes in reflex and judgment, nausea, muscle weakness, burred vision, decreased platelet counts, decreased urea and bilirubin levels,	Pregnancy, breastfeeding Skin yellowing from accumulation of plant pigment can occur in chronic use. Liver disease	*Do not use with:* Alcohol: increases risk of kava toxicity. Alprazolam: risk for coma exists. CNS depressants: kava potentiates these. Levodopa: can increase Parkinson-like symptoms. Phenobarbital: can increase effects.	Symptom relief may occur in as little as 1 week. Potential for significant adverse reactions when using kava. Alcohol and CNS medications are enhanced with kava.

				dry skin, is a dopamine antagonist			
St. John's Wort	Hypericum perforatum	300 mg PO three times daily for 4–6 weeks	Antidepressant	Severe photosensitivity, dry mouth, constipation, GI upset, sleep disturbances, restlessness	Pregnant or breastfeeding, children; use cautiously for patient taking anticoagulants, MAOI medication	MAOIs, antidepressants, digoxin, birth control pills	Avoid prolonged exposure to sunlight. May increase the effects of MAOIs, OTC flu and cold medications, alcohol; do not use with these types of chemicals.
Omega 3 Fatty Acids (Dietary Supplement)	Alpha-linolenic acid (ALA), docosahexaenoic acid (DHA), and eicosapentaenoic acid (EPA) 3:2 EPA to DHA (fish oil)	1–2 g PO daily for health, cognitive enhancement	Depression, postpartum depression, bipolar disorder, anxiety, dementia	Loose stools with higher doses; "fishy" reflux	Use cautiously for patients taking anticoagulants	May increase effects of anticoagulants	If taking anticoagulant drugs or high doses of aspirin, practice good safety. The oils may increase clotting time.
Sam-E (Supplement for Naturally Produced Body Substance	s-adenosyl-L-methionine	See manufacturer's specifications and use as directed by a physician	Depression	Mild and transient anxiety, insomnia, heartburn, loose bowels	Can cause mania in patients with bipolar disorder; rule out before beginning treatment.		Patients with bipolar disorder should not use except under supervision of physician. Enteric coated preparations may reduce gastric upset.

Source: Spidle, R.A. (2006). Alternative and Complementary Treatment Modalities. In Neeb, K. (2006). Fundamentals of Mental Health Nursing. Philadelphia, F.A. Davis, pp. 164–166.
National Center for Complementary & Alternative Medicine at http://nccam.nih.gov

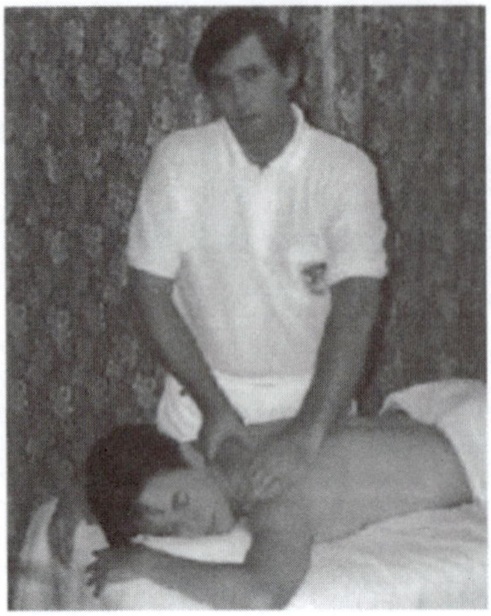

Figure 9-2 Massage can be an effective tool for relieving tension. *(Courtesy of everything-jersey.com)*

chi, *ki*, or *prana*. When the life force is obstructed, emotional and physical illnesses result. Various types of pressure, massage, and other techniques are employed along these meridians to release the flow of chi, restore balance, and improve health. Shiatsu is a Japanese form of acupressure that uses pressure from the fingers to free energy flow. **Reflexology** is also based upon the belief that energy pathways and zones cross the body, connecting vital organs and body parts (Fig. 9-3). Reflexologists use massage of the feet to act upon these pathways, unblocking and renewing the energy flow.

Therapeutic touch also deserves mention. **Reiki** is representative of methods of touch healing that are often associated with massage. Reiki is a term that means "universal life energy" and refers to the process whereby this energy is drawn along the body's meridians. Unlike methods that use physical movement, pressure, or massage to unblock these channels, Reiki uses the flow of life energy itself to accomplish the task. Practitioners are "attuned" to the energy channels and can manipulate them hands-on, hands just above the body, or even at a distance. Reiki techniques can even be employed as part of a more traditional massage session to enhance the physical benefits of the massage. Reiki has been demonstrated to increase warmth in the areas being treated and also to produce relaxation in the subject.

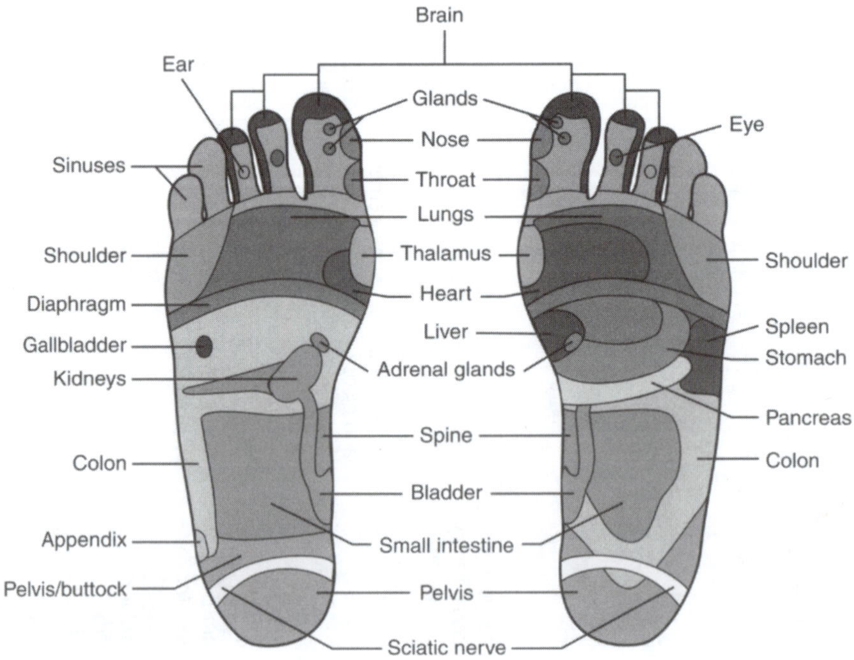

Figure 9-3 Reflexology foot diagram.

Hypnotherapy

Hypnotherapy is one of the most controversial complementary and alternative modalities. Hypnosis is a means for entering an altered state of consciousness, and in this state, using visualization and suggestion to bring about desired changes in behavior and thinking. Called **trance**, people enter this state of focused attention every day. The English language even contains references to this common experience of "zoning out." Trance is not sleep but rather describes a state of mind wherein a person is less aware of what is going on around him or her and instead is very focused on an internal experience, like a memory or an imagined event.

Everyone responds to suggestion to some extent. A person who is watching television and wants a snack after seeing commercials for a favorite fast-food restaurant has responded to suggestion. Fortunately, people's minds filter out suggestions that are unacceptably dangerous so they are not persuaded to imitate some of the more unsafe things seen on TV.

Neeb's Tip A hypnotherapist uses suggestion, both direct and indirect, to help the patient create change.

The general public has been subjected to an enormous amount of misinformation about hypnosis by stage hypnotists, movies, and books. As a result, hypnotherapy is widely misunderstood and wrongly feared by many people. Watching a stage hypnotist appear to make a volunteer cluck like a chicken or dance on a table certainly does not inspire confidence in hypnosis as a therapeutic tool. It is very hard for some people to overcome these fears, especially the stubborn belief in the myth that hypnosis is somehow "mind control" exercised for evil (or entertainment) purposes by the therapist.

Whereas some researchers and practitioners contend that hypnosis cannot stand on its own as a treatment modality, others are equally convinced that even lay practitioners can deliver effective therapy with a minimum of training and practice. No doubt this controversy will continue, as there are at present few regulations governing the use of hypnosis. In some states a therapist must be certified or licensed, but in others no one but a psychologist, psychiatrist, medical doctor, or other professional may practice the techniques.

Milton H. Erickson, M.D. (1901–1980), was one of the best-known figures in the development of hypnosis for modern therapeutic purposes. Dr. Erickson was a victim of polio, which left him partially paralyzed. He had little strength in his arms and upper body and was confined to a wheelchair. As if that were not enough, he was dyslexic, tone-deaf, color-blind, and had heart problems. Left alone during long periods of illness, Erickson became a master of observation and learned that subtle changes in facial expression, skin color, nuance of voice, and physical posture could tell him much about a person's inner state.

Dr. Erickson structured his therapeutic approach to patients in a new way. He refused to allow his own past disabilities ruin his living of life to its fullest and therefore refused to let old problems get in the way of his patients' enjoyment of living. Erickson ignored the past history of presenting patients, preferring instead to focus on present and future outcomes. In one classic case, Erickson gave the task of tending violets to a woman with depression. Combined with other therapeutic suggestions, she was kept too busy and involved in her community to remain depressed.

Traditional hypnotherapy and psychotherapy center on diagnosing problems and treating symptoms. Erickson promoted well-being, and study of his methods has challenged a whole new generation of hypnotherapists to do the same. Later, John Grinder and Richard Bandler would develop the field of neurolinguistic programming (NLP), based in large part upon their study of the extraordinary sensory acuity of Milton Erickson.

Neurolinguistic Programming

Investigating the techniques and methods of many successful therapists, Bandler and Grinder searched for ways to make psychotherapy more consistently effective. It was through these explorations that they realized that language cues could be used to understand how an individual experiences his or her world. Using those cues, a practitioner can help patients change their experiences and respond to problems in a different way. Unlike traditional hypnosis, neurolinguistic programming (NLP) does not use lengthy trance sessions and instead depends upon patients to take an active part in their treatment. When John Grinder and Richard Bandler began developing NLP, they based this extraordinary new type of therapy on a basic set of ideas, or **presuppositions.**

Presuppositions are the assumptions people make when forming communication. They are most often not spoken or written, but understood within the context of what is being communicated. For example, if the statement "I am so happy today!" is made, the presupposition, or unspoken assumption, is that the speaker is not normally happy. People's daily communications are filled with such assumptions, things that they take for granted. NLP differs from other therapies in that there is no presupposition that the patient is somehow "broken" and requires "fixing." Instead, practitioners are taught that patients are whole individuals who already possess the internal resources they need to recover from their illness. All that is required is to direct the patient to those resources and enable their use.

People observe their world through distinct channels of experience, tending to prefer one channel over another, but eventually using them all for important cues and sensory information about their environment and other people.

■ Primary Sensory Representation

The three primary methods of sensory representation are the visual, auditory, and kinesthetic channels (seeing, hearing, and touching). Of course, people also use taste and smell to gather information, but these paths are rarely the most important channel, and they are generally ignored.

Paying attention to speech patterns gives the practitioner a starting point for meaningful communication with the patient. The most obvious way to do this is to listen to the predicates a person uses while describing thoughts and ideas. The practitioner can then determine positive **rapport** if the person favors sight, hearing, or touch and match those predicates, using the same language patterns to create a starting point for meaningful communication. Recognizing these patterns can help improve a nurse's communication with patients. Table 9-2 illustrates types of word patterns people use.

Table 9-2 Representational System Predicates

Visual (Seeing)	Auditory (Hearing)	Kinesthetic (Touch)
an eyeful	clear as a bell	all washed up
appears to me	clearly expressed	boils down to
beyond the shadow of a doubt	call on	chip off the old block
bird's-eye view	describe in detail	come to grips with
catch a glimpse of	earful	control yourself
clear cut	express yourself	cool, calm, collected
dim view	give an account of	firm foundations
eye to eye	give me your ear	get a handle on
get a perspective on	grant an audience	get in touch with
scope out	heard voices	hand in hand
hazy idea	hidden message	hang in there
horse of a different color	hold your tongue	hold on

Table 9-2 Representational System Predicates—cont'd

Visual (Seeing)	Auditory (Hearing)	Kinesthetic (Touch)
in light of	idle talk	hold it
in view of	inquire into	keep your shirt on
make a scene	keynote speaker	know how
mental image	loud and clear	lightheaded
mind's eye	manner of speaking	moment of panic
naked eye	pay attention to	pain in the neck
paint a picture photographic	power of speech	pull some strings
memory	outspoken	sharp as a tack
plainly seen	rings a bell	slipped my mind
pretty as a picture	to tell the truth	start from scratch
sight for sore eyes	unheard of under pressure	underhanded

Of course, just about everyone uses all three forms of predicates at one time or another. The most important thing to remember is to match the dominant, or most used, form.

EXAMPLES

(Visual)

Mary: "I can't picture myself getting any better."

Nurse: "In light of your progress, see yourself going back to school. How does that look to you?"

(Auditory)

James: "I've heard that the doctor is tuned in to the newest treatments."

Nurse: "He can describe those in detail to you. I'll tell him you want to hear about them."

(Kinesthetic)

Diane: "I couldn't come to grips with the situation. I was under too much pressure all the time."

Nurse: "It is hard to get in touch with what's important when you feel that way."

These exchanges demonstrate communication on more than one level. By using the same language used by the patient, the nurse can establish that she or he is listening closely to the message that is being sent. This is a powerful tool in creating and maintaining rapport, the foundation to a therapeutic relationship.

Clinical Activity
Interact with a patient to determine if the person favors sight, hearing, or touch. Afterward, communicate with patient on his or her level. In post-conference, share with fellow students if this enhanced your rapport with the patient.

Summary

Nursing practice is evolving and is incorporating "alternative" or "complementary" therapies into traditional care delivery systems (Table 9-3). State boards of nursing can determine at what level and scope of practice nurses should provide the alternative therapy.

Tool Box In 2003, the Minnesota Board of Nursing adopted guidelines and statements for appropriate use of complementary therapy in Minnesota. Those guidelines can be found at http://mn.gov/health-licensing-boards/nursing/licensees/practice/integrative-therapies.

Table 9-3 Alternative Therapies

Disorder	Mind-Body Experience	Herbal	Nutritional Therapy and Lifestyle	Hands -on Therapy	Alternative Therapy
Anxiety	√	√	√	√	√
Arthritis	√	√	√	√	√
Asthma	√	√	√	√	√
Cancer Prevention and Treatment	√	√	√	√	
Congestive Heart Failure	√	√	√	√	√
Coronary Heart Disease	√	√	√		√
Depression	√	√	√	√	√
Diabetes	√	√	√	√	√
GERD	√	√	√	√	√
Gastrointestinal Problems	√	√	√	√	√
Migraine Headache	√	√	√	√	√
Tension Headache	√	√	√	√	√
Hepatitis	√	√	√	√	√
Hypercholes-terolemia	√	√	√	√	√
Hypertension	√	√	√	√	√
Irritable Bowel Syndrome	√	√	√	√	√
Musculoskeletal Problems	√	√	√	√	√
Upper Respiratory Infection	√	√	√	√	√
Urinary Tract Infection	√	√	√	√	√

Source: Adapted from Complementary and alternative medicine. (2009). In D. Venes (Ed.), *Taber's cyclopedic medical dictionary* (21st ed., pp. 2540–2552). Philadelphia, F.A. Davis.

Key Concepts

1. Alternative and complementary treatments provide options for patients other than those offered by conventional (Western) medicine. Alternative modalities are used instead of, and complementary are used in addition to, conventional practices.
2. The mind-body connection is an important concept in all types of medical treatment. Disease and wellness affect the whole person. Holistic treatments address both the illness and the person.
3. An individual has beliefs, based upon his or her model of the world. These beliefs must be respected by the nurse.
4. Anxiety is common to disorders relating to mental illness. Prolonged stress and anxiety lead to physical as well as mental and emotional afflictions.
5. Biofeedback is a technique that teaches the patient to recognize and control stress responses in the body. It is widely accepted because of its use of scientific measuring devices to demonstrate the effectiveness of the treatment.
6. Aromatherapy uses a person's emotional response to smell as well as the pharmacological effects of various fragrant botanical and other substances to treat illness.
7. Herbal and nutritional therapies are becoming more prevalent as the public embraces "natural" healing. Many modern medications have evolved from uncultivated botanical products. Relative safety and effectiveness is still in question, as the industry is largely unregulated, with no set standards for these products.
8. Other types of alternative and complementary therapy focus on manipulation, strengthening, and removing blockage from the free flow of energy in the human body. Massage and therapeutic touch modalities are successful groups of both stand-alone and adjunctive treatment for disease.
9. Hypnotherapy and neurolinguistic programming are two prominent modalities that address mental and bodily illness by empowering change in the patient's thought patterns. Both tightly focus on communication patterns and the patient-therapist relationship.

REFERENCES

Complementary and alternative medicine. (2009). In D. Venes (Ed.), *Taber's Cyclopedic Medical Dictionary.* 21st ed., pp. 2540–2552. Philadelphia: F.A. Davis.

F.Y.I.—A Publication of the Minnesota Board of Nursing (2003). *Complementary therapies.* Spring/Summer 2003, *19*(1), 7.

National Center for Complementary and Alternative Medicine. Available at http://nccam.nih.gov

Skidmore-Roth, L. (2010). *Mosby's Handbook of Herbs and National Supplements.* 4th ed. St. Louis: Mosby-Elsevier.

Test Questions

Multiple Choice Questions

1. Alternative therapy modalities are used:
a. Infrequently, as they have no value to patients today
b. In combination with conventional therapies
c. In place of conventional therapies
d. Only when there is no hope for recovery

2. A treatment modality used with conventional medical therapies is:
a. A medical approach
b. A model approach
c. A holistic approach
d. A complementary approach

3. When traditional medicine is combined with less traditional methods, it is:
a. Integrative medicine
b. Exclusive medicine
c. Based on the physician's opinions
d. Biofeedback

4. The mechanism that describes thought and expectation affecting health is:
a. A complementary therapy
b. A misconception that is dangerous to the patient
c. An integrated therapy
d. The mind-body connection

5. Mrs. Lucas is telling you about her ideas for curing her depression by taking herbal medication. She is convinced that because St. John's wort is a natural product, it is better for her than her prescription therapy. You should:
a. Quickly get the drug handbook and show her she is wrong.
b. Remain open and supportive.
c. Point out to her that herbal therapy is contraindicated.
d. Suggest some available brands for her to use.

6. Of the following, which are either complementary or alternative modalities?
a. ECT, Reiki, rolfing
b. Hypnotherapy, shiatsu, antianxiety medications
c. NLP, psychotherapy, SAM-e
d. Aromatherapy, biofeedback, massage

7. Mr. Douglas wants to know more about massage therapy. Which one of the following is *not* a massage modality?
a. Reiki
b. Trigger point
c. Rolfing
d. Swedish

8. Which of the following is *false* about trance?
a. It is an altered state of consciousness, just like sleep.
b. Humans move in and out of trance states during the day.
c. It is a state of relaxed awareness.
d. Trance is a common experience even if you are not aware of it.

9. Which of the following statements indicates a visual channel preference for information?
a. "That really feels good! My gut feeling is that it will work!"
b. "It sounds good to me; this idea is worth paying attention to."
c. "I can see the solution, and clearly it will work."
d. "I smell a rat. I think the whole thing stinks."

10. Which of the following should be *avoided* when communicating with a mentally ill patient?
a. Having an expectation that the patient will get better
b. Making the presupposition that the patient will not improve
c. Taking the time to convey respect for the patient
d. Demonstrating through your expression and posture that you are listening

UNIT 2

Threats to Mental Health

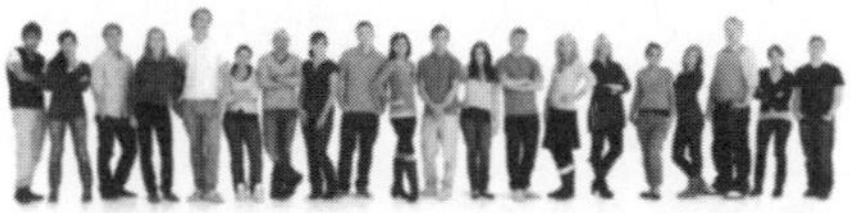

CHAPTER 10

Anxiety, Anxiety-Related, and Somatic Symptom Disorders

Learning Objectives

1. Define anxiety disorders.
2. Identify the changes in DSM-5 and how they relate to current anxiety disorders
3. Identify the new classified anxiety disorders.
4. State physical and behavioral symptoms of anxiety disorders.
5. Identify treatment modalities for anxiety disorders.
6. Identify nursing interventions in anxiety disorders.
7. Define the difference in diagnosing somatic symptom disorder and diagnosing somatic symptoms
8. Identify medical treatments for people with somatic symptoms and related disorders.
9. Identify nursing interventions for people with somatic symptoms and related disorders.

Key Terms

- Anxiety
- Compulsion
- Conversion
- Dysmorphophobia
- Eustress
- Free-floating anxiety
- Generalized anxiety disorders
- Hypochondriasis
- "La belle indifference"
- Malingering
- Obsession
- Obsessive-compulsive disorder (OCD)
- Panic disorder
- Phobia
- Post-traumatic stress disorder
- Primary gain
- Secondary gain
- Signal anxiety
- Somatization
- Somatoform disorder
- Somatoform pain disorder
- Stress
- Stressor
- Survivor guilt

Anxiety Disorders

Stress produces **anxiety.** Stress is everywhere in today's society. Most often, stress is associated with negative situations, but the good things that happen to people, such as weddings and job promotions, also produce stress. This stress from positive experiences, such as becoming newly married, promoted at work, or something similar, is called **eustress.** It can produce just as much anxiety as the negative stressors. A **stressor** is any person or situation that produces anxiety responses. Stress and stressors are different for each person; therefore, it is important that the nurse ask what the stress producers are for that patient. What is extremely stressful for one person (driving in rush hour traffic, for example) might be relaxing to someone else (go with the traffic flow and relax after a busy day).

Anxiety can be described as an uncomfortable feeling of dread that is a response to extreme or prolonged periods of stress. According to Gorman and Sultan (2008), anxiety is an unpleasant feeling of tension, apprehension, and uneasiness or a diffuse feeling of dread or unexplained discomfort.

The four commonly accepted levels of anxiety are:

- Mild
- Moderate
- Severe
- Panic

Hildegard Peplau teaches that a mild amount of anxiety is a normal part of being human and that it is necessary to change and develop new ways of coping with stress (Fig. 10-1).

Anxiety may also be influenced by one's culture. It may be acceptable for some people to acknowledge and discuss stress, but others may believe that one should keep personal problems to oneself. This can be a challenge to the nurse during an assessment.

Anxiety is usually referred to in one of two ways: **free-floating anxiety** and **signal anxiety.** Free-floating anxiety is described as a feeling of impending doom. The person might say something like "I just know something bad is going to happen if I go on vacation," without knowing when or where the event might occur. Signal anxiety, on the other hand, is an uncomfortable response to a known stressor (e.g., "Finals are only a week away and I've got that nagging nausea again."). Both types of anxiety are involved in the various anxiety disorders.

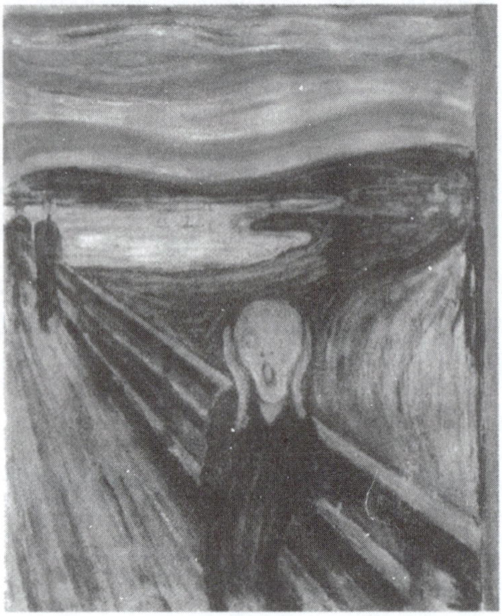

Figure 10-1 Anxiety ranges in severity from mild through panic. "The Scream," a famous painting by Norwegian artist Edvard Munch, depicts a person in a very high state of anxiety.

Nurses working with children and teenagers must be aware that they also experience anxiety and stress. They may not be able to verbalize their feelings, and they may display symptoms differently than adults do. Some indicators of stress and anxiety in these age groups include decline in school performance, changes in eating habits and sleeping patterns, and withdrawal from friends and usual activities. Nurses can be instrumental in screening children and adolescents for signs of anxiety.

The Diagnostic & Statistical Manual, 5th edition (DSM-5, 2013) has made a number of revisions to anxiety disorders from the 4th edition known as DSM-IV-TR (2000). These will be noted in this chapter. In DSM-5, some disorders that were previously listed as anxiety disorders, including **post-traumatic stress disorder** and obsessive compulsive disorder, have now been listed under new categories. In this text these will be discussed in the section "Types of Anxiety and Anxiety-Related Disorders" in this chapter.

■ Etiology of Anxiety and Stress

Psychoanalytic theory says that there is a conflict between the id and the superego, which causes anxiety. At some time in the individual's development, this conflict was repressed but emerged again in adulthood. When conflict emerges, patients realize they have "failed," and the manifestations of anxiety are once again felt.

Biologically the basic stress response is called the fight-or-flight response and contributes to feelings of anxiety. In this response to stress the blood vessels constrict because epinephrine and norepinephrine have been released. Blood pressure rises. If the body adapts to the stress, hormone levels adjust to compensate for the epinephrine-norepinephrine release, and the body functions return to homeostasis. If the body does not adapt to the stress, there are many long-term health problems that can be created including lowered immunity, heart disease, and many other conditions (Fig. 10-2).

Studies are continually being conducted trying to correlate the condition of stress to physical illness. In 2002, researchers at Carnegie Mellon University in Pittsburgh (Cohen, 2003) studied 334 paid individuals. They introduced a rhinovirus into the participants' noses. Then they placed the participants into individual, private hotel rooms. Several days later, they tested the individuals for symptoms. People who had described themselves as happier, contented types of personalities demonstrated cold/flu symptoms only one third as often as the individuals who did not use those kinds of words to describe themselves and their stress level. This is one study. Experts do not know all of the variables, but it does make a fairly strong argument for a positive correlation between emotional stress and physical illness.

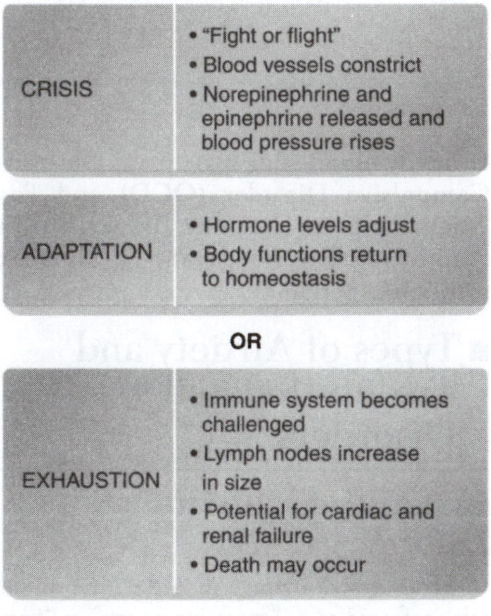

Figure 10-2 General Adaptation Syndrome (GAS) model of stress.

The LPN/LVN will frequently encounter stress in medical-surgical patients. Physical and emotional symptoms can interrelate. It is important for nurses to recognize the relationship between physical and emotional responses to stress. Nurses can be instrumental in gaining accurate planning and interventions for their patients by providing accurate assessment and documentation of the patient's symptoms as his or her body adapts to stress. Table 10-1 gives examples of medical conditions and the effects of the body's adaptation response to stress.

■ Differential Diagnosis

Differentiating normal anxiety from an anxiety disorder can be challenging. Because so many symptoms are associated with anxiety disorders, it is important for people to have a complete physical workup before being checked for these disorders. The symptoms of anxiety disorders are listed with each of the specific disorders (see section "Types of Anxiety Disorders"). Symptoms of anxiety disorders can mimic those seen in diabetes, cardiac problems, medication side effects, electrolyte imbalances, or physical trauma. The physician must rule out a systemic infection or an allergy that might be related to chills or swallowing difficulty. Hot flashes, which can occur in some anxiety states, could be related to a fever or to menopause. The physician must always consider the possibility of drug or alcohol abuse as partial causes for the symptoms. Certainly, more than one condition can occur simultaneously. A psychiatric evaluation is often needed to confirm a diagnosis of an anxiety disorder.

Common symptoms of anxiety can be present in many other conditions. It is easy to see how mistakes in diagnosing can happen.

Table 10-1 Adaptation Responses to Stress and the Outcome of Stress on the Body

Stress-Related Medical Condition	Body's Adaptation to the Stress	Outcome of Stress on the Body
Lowered Immunity	Interferes with effectiveness of the body's antibodies; possibly related to interactions among the hypothalamus, pituitary gland, adrenal glands, and the immune system.	Increased susceptibility to colds, viruses, and other illnesses
Burnout	Associated with stress-related depression.	Emotional detachment
Migraine, Cluster, and Tension Headaches	Tightening skeletal muscles, dilating of cranial artery.	Nausea, vomiting, tight feeling in or around head and shoulders, tinnitus, inability to tolerate light, weakness of a limb
Hypertension	Role of stress is not positively known but is thought to contribute to hypertension by negatively interacting with the kidneys and endocrine system.	Resistance to blood flow through the cardiovascular system, causing pressure on the arteries; can lead to stroke, heart attack, and kidney failure.
Coronary Artery Disease	Stressor increases the amount of epinephrine and norepinephrine.	Constricted coronary vessels, increased pulse and respirations
Cancer	Same mechanisms that lower immunity.	Lowered immunity may allow for overcolonization of opportunistic cancer cells.
Asthma	Automatic nervous system stimulates mucus, increases blood flow, and constricts bronchial tubes; may be associated with other stress-related conditions such as allergy and viral infection.	Wheezing, coughing, dyspnea, apprehension; may lead to respiratory infections, respiratory failure, and/or pneumothorax.

Symptoms of anxiety may include:

- Muscle aches
- Shakes
- Palpitations
- Dry mouth
- Nausea
- Vomiting
- Diarrhea
- Hot flashes
- Chills
- Polyuria
- Insomnia
- Difficulty swallowing

DSM-5 has made changes in some disorders that were once categorized under anxiety. Formerly found with anxiety was **Obsessive-Compulsive Disorder (OCD)** and Post-Traumatic Stress Disorder (PTSD). In this chapter, revisions from DSM-IV-TR will be mentioned periodically as a comparison.

Types of Anxiety and Anxiety-Related Disorders

Generalized Anxiety Disorder (GAD)

In **generalized anxiety disorder**, the anxiety (also referred to as "excessive worry" or "severe stress") itself is the expressed symptom. It is diagnosed when excessive worry is related to two or more things and lasts 6 months or longer.

Patients who have GAD may display any number of symptoms. The DSM-IV-TR lists 18 symptoms of anxiety, and the patient must show six or more in order to be considered to have GAD. DSM-5 has reduced the symptoms to include at least 3 of the following:

- Restlessness
- Easily fatigued
- Difficulty concentrating or mind going blank
- Irritability
- Muscle tension
- Sleep disturbances

These symptoms become pervasive as the person is unable to control the worry and other symptoms. All aspects of life become involved. This disorder can be debilitating.

Neeb's Tip Generalized anxiety disorder can be paralyzing and impact all areas of a person's life.

Panic Disorder

Panic disorder is a recurrent condition that is a state of extreme fear that cannot be controlled. It is an abrupt surge of intense fear or discomfort that reaches a peak in a short period of time. It can lead to intense fear and worry about it happening again. It is also referred to as "panic attack," and people may not consider it to be a serious disorder initially. In the past, panic disorder was linked to agoraphobia. DSM-5 now has them as two separate disorders.

Some traits of panic disorder include:

- Fear (usually of dying, losing control of oneself, or of "going crazy")
- Dissociation (a feeling that it is happening to someone else or not happening at all)
- Nausea
- Diaphoresis
- Chest pain
- Increased pulse
- Shaking
- Unsteadiness
- Feelings of being suffocated or unable to catch one's breath

Neeb's Tip Panic symptoms can develop suddenly and unexpectedly in the susceptible person. People with history of panic disorder need to be prepared to identify early signs in the hope that they can gain some control before the symptoms are out of control.

Phobia

This is the most common of the anxiety disorders. **Phobia is defined as an "irrational fear."** The person is very aware of the fear and even of the fact that it is irrational, but the fear continues. People develop phobias to many different things—approximately 700 different things, in fact (Box 10-1). Snakes, spiders, enclosed spaces, and the number 13 are some of the more common phobias (Fig. 10-3). People also develop phobias of things such as caring for their children (because they might hurt them) and eating in places other than their own home.

The psychoanalytic view of phobias that the fear is not necessarily from the object itself but rather a displaced, unconscious fear that is displaced on the object/event such as a snake or height. Learning theory views phobias as learned responses. When the person avoids the phobic object, fears is escaped and that is a powerful reward. Most phobias start in childhood but people can develop them later in life. In older people it is common is see fear of falling or choking.

Box 10-1 Some Common Specific Phobias

Acrophobia: Fear of height
Ailurophobia: Fear of cats
Carcinomatophobia: Fear of cancer
Decidophobia: Fear of making decisions
Nyctophobia: Fear of darkness
Odontophobia: Fear of teeth or dental surgery
Scoleciphobia: Fear of worms
Thanatophobia: Fear of death

Source: Adapted from Townsend (2012). Essentials of Psychiatric Mental Health Nursing, 7th ed. Philadelphia: F.A. Davis Company, with permission.

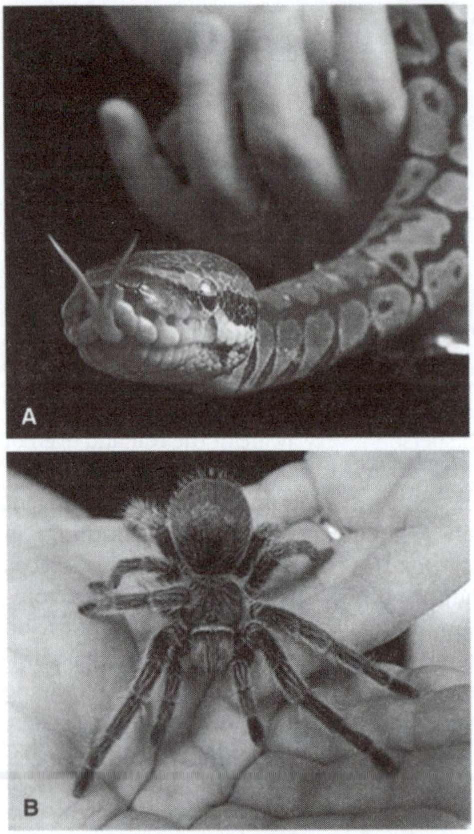

Figure 10-3 A, Fear of snakes (ophidiophobia), and B, fear of spiders (arachnophobia), are two of the most common phobias. *(Courtesy of the University of Texas Libraries, The University of Texas at Austin.)*

It is not uncommon for more than one phobia to develop in a person. They most often begin in childhood, perhaps repeated into a traumatic event.

Phobias have three subcategories: agoraphobia, social phobia, and specific phobias.

Agoraphobia is the irrational fear of being in open spaces and being unable to leave or being very embarrassed if leaving is required.

EXAMPLE

Agoraphobia: People who fear shopping in large malls or who fear going to sporting events may actually fear the possibility of being unable to escape in the event of an accident.

Social phobias are those in which people avoid social situations as a result of fear of humiliation or being judged negatively. This reaction is out of proportion to the situation. There are correlations between people with this type of phobia and self-medicating with alcohol and/or drugs.

EXAMPLE

Social phobias: The fear of speaking in public and the fear of using public facilities such as bathrooms or laundromats are examples of social phobias.

Specific phobias include having an irrational fear of a specific object or situation. These are the classic phobias that most people are familiar with.

EXAMPLE

Specific phobias: Claustrophobia (fear of enclosed places), hematophobia (fear of blood), and acrophobia (fear of heights).

Tool Box |▶ For a comprehensive list of phobias go to http://phobialist.com/#A-

■ ■ ■ Clinical Activity

When your hospitalized patient has a phobia such as agoraphobia, anticipation of the patient's reaction to leaving his/her room for testing must be addressed with the patient to prevent distress.

Obsessive-Compulsive Disorder

Obsessive-compulsive disorder (OCD) is reoccurring thoughts, ideas, and actions that interfere with a person's daily ability to function. DSM-5 no longer categorizes OCD as an anxiety disorder but puts it in its own category. This disorder is now believed to be a neurological short circuit that causes repetitive behaviors. A genetic link among families who display OCD has also been suggested. OCD is different than obsessive compulsive personality disorder. See Chapter 14.

OCD has two components: the **obsession** (repetitive thought, urge, or emotion) and the **compulsion** (repetitive act that may appear purposeful). It is not uncommon for people to be double and triple checking that doors are locked before one is able to sleep or leave the house. When these obsessive thoughts and compulsive actions begin to prevent a person from sleeping or leaving the house, it becomes OCD. The person with this kind of disorder is unable to stop the thought or the action. Behaviors become very ritualistic (Fig. 10-4).

Behaviors in patients with OCD vary. Some people wash their hands unceasingly. Others have a strict ritual that, if interrupted, requires starting over from the beginning. Some people have to check something or clean something over and over. People with this disorder tend to be perfectionistic and very rule-oriented.

Physical symptoms also vary. If the person is prevented from performing the obsession or compulsion, the anxiety converts itself into somatic (body-related) symptoms.

A related disorder to OCD is hoarding disorder. This is a new disorder in DSM-5. Hoarding disorder is severe distress caused by persistent difficulties discarding or parting with possessions.

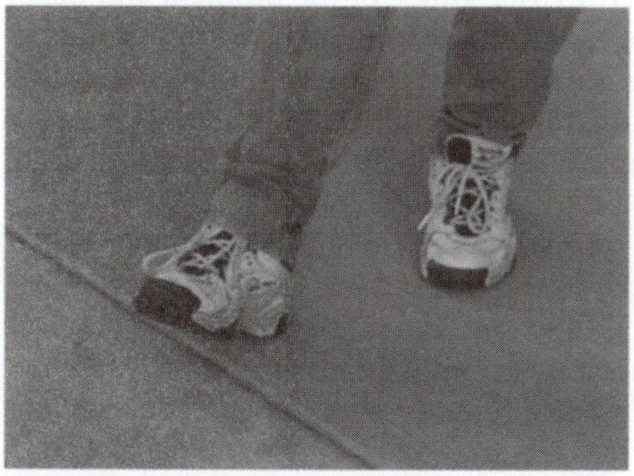

Figure 10-4 Compulsive behaviors include refusing to step on a crack in the sidewalk. The behavior is very ritualistic, and performing the action reduces the person's anxiety. *(Courtesy of the National Institute of Mental Health, Bethesda, MD.)*

Critical Thinking Question

Tommy has come to your clinic with numerous cracks on his hands, which are bleeding and very sore. Tommy tells you that he just has to wash his hands all the time. His mother says he will wash for 2 to 3 hours at a time, and he will not stop when she tells him to. The physician has diagnosed Tommy with OCD and has explained the illness to Tommy and his mother. When the physician leaves the room, Tommy's mother begins to cry: "What did he just say? What am I supposed to do? What did I do wrong that Tommy got this illness?" What will you tell her? What areas will you explore with her?

Classroom Activity

- See the movie *As Good as It Gets* for a depiction of OCD.

Clinical Activity

When caring for a patient with OCD, identify what the staff has been doing to accommodate the patient's obsessions and compulsions.

Post-Traumatic Stress Disorder

Post-traumatic stress disorder (PTSD) is developed in response to an unexpected emotional or physical trauma that could not be controlled. A victim of PTSD will probably have reoccurring, intrusive, disturbing memories of the incident that may last over a period of time. This disorder was once viewed as an anxiety problem in DSM-IV-TR, but the current view is that it belongs in a new category—Trauma and Stress or Related Disorders (DSM-5, 2013). So now it is viewed less as an anxiety problem and more related to the physical and emotional responses to a trauma. One reason for this change is the increasing recognition that people suffering from PTSD often are more troubled with pervasive sadness, aggressive behaviors, and dissociative symptoms such as flashbacks than anxiety symptoms. Young children can also suffer from PTSD.

People who have fought in wars, who have been raped, or who have survived violent storms or other actual or threatened traumatic events are examples of those who are susceptible to suffering from this disorder. Police, fire, and rescue personnel are at risk for PTSD when they see victims of violence and destruction whom they cannot help. The assault on the United States during the attacks on the World Trade Center towers, the Pentagon, and the passengers and crew on the ill-fated flight in Pennsylvania on September 11, 2001, has brought new attention to the condition of post-traumatic stress disorder. The horror of witnessing tragedy such as this now reaches anyone with a television or Internet; such a person can also suffer from PTSD. People in countries far away are able to experience tragedy in "real time." Certainly those citizens who were on the scene and attempting to save lives, saw destruction the likes of which most of us, hopefully, will never experience directly. They and their families will deal with the post-traumatic effects of that day for some time to come.

Critical Thinking Question

Think for a moment where you and your family members were on September 11, 2001. Think about the things you felt and shared with each other at that time. Do you feel as though you might have experienced a mild, moderate, or severe PTSD from 911?

Magnify that as you think, "what if I were the one standing on that sidewalk watching people die or jump from those buildings, wanting to help and knowing I couldn't?" Dramatic? Maybe. Realistic? Yes. And just a very slight taste of the intensity of the fears and flashbacks people with PTSD experience.

A term associated with PTSD is "**survivor guilt.**" This is the feeling of guilt expressed by survivors of a traumatic event. A Vietnam veteran may say, "Why me? Why did that lady and her kids get blown away and I lived? They didn't deserve that." Another concern associated with PTSD is the suicide rate among military who served in the wars. Since the Afghanistan war began, there has been a rise in suicide among military, suggesting that PTSD is a factor. This population continues to be in need for more mental health services (Drummond, 2012).

PTSD symptoms may appear immediately or be repressed until years later. Symptoms of PTSD can include:

- "Flashbacks," in which the person may relive and act out the traumatic event
- Social withdrawal
- Nightmares
- Insomnia
- Feelings of low self-esteem as a result of the event
- Changes in the relationship with a significant other and difficulty forming new relationships
- Irritability and outbursts of anger toward another person or situation, apparently for no obvious reason
- Depression
- Distress when thinking about the event
- Making efforts to avoid reminders of the event

Self-medicating with alcohol and other substances to treat the discomfort is a concern with many patients. The evaluation process should include a substance abuse assessment and treatment if needed.

Trust and communication and listening skills are very important tools for nurses who have patients with PTSD. Encouraging expression of thoughts and feelings surrounding the experience and the survivor guilt is an important first step in the patient's ability to identify the source of the problem and begin the process of healing (Fig. 10-5). It is important to validate the patient's feelings regarding the situation. Honesty and genuineness in communicating with these patients will help to build a working rapport.

Family members and significant others such as spouses can suffer from the effects of PTSD as well. Often, these people experience the same trauma, even though they were not present for the original event. The term "vicarious trauma" may apply in this situation.

Classroom Activity

- Watch the movies "Coming Home" and "The Best Years of Our Lives" to get a perspective of the return to civilian life after war.
- Watch the movie "Nuts" about trauma after rape and incest.

Critical Thinking Question

Jeanne is a 21-year-old single woman admitted for pneumonia. Her social history indicates that she survived a house fire when she was 10 years old and that her twin sister died in that fire. Today is the day for the monthly fire drill at the hospital. You note that Jeanne is not in her bed. You are unable to find her during the drill. After the drill, you search her room and find her sitting on the floor of the closet. She is wrapped in a blanket and is crying. She does not respond to your verbal cues. What do you think is happening to her? What illness might she have? How will you get her out of the closet? What can you do to help her?

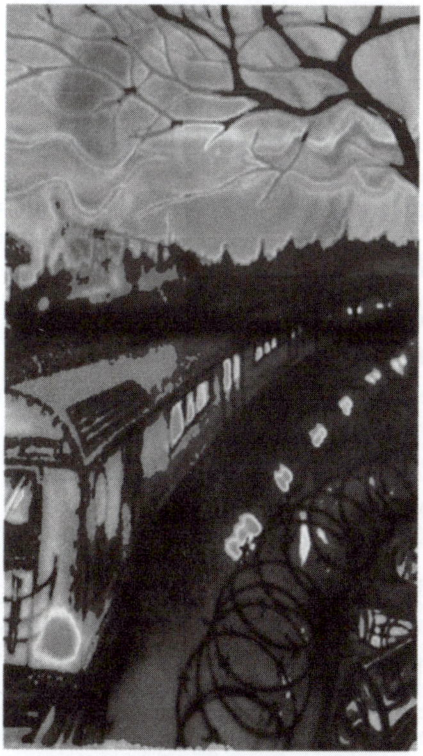

Figure 10-5 Encouraging the patient's expression of thoughts and feelings about the traumatic experience, as in this painting, is an important first step in identifying the problem and beginning the healing process. *(Courtesy of the National Institute of Mental Health, Bethesda, MD.)*

Medical Treatment of People With Anxiety and Anxiety-Related Disorders

Treatment is individualized to the patient and may include one or more of the following: psychopharmacology, individual psychotherapy, group therapy, systematic desensitization, hypnosis, imagery, relaxation exercises, and biofeedback.

Psychotherapy includes individual treatment, group therapy, and systematic desensitization

Pharmacology Corner

Medications are being used effectively to control chronic anxiety. The most common are anti-anxiety medications, which include benzodiazepines. See Table 10-2 for a list of common anti-anxiety medications. The benzodiazepines are commonly used and are effective in most cases. Use of the anti-anxiety drugs is short-term whenever possible because of the strong potential for dependency. Individuals with anxiety disorders who are chemically dependent are managed with other medications having calming qualities but not the same high potential for addiction as the anti-anxiety drugs. Hydroxyzine hydrochloride (Atarax) and clonidine (Catapres) are examples.

The antidepressant class of selective serotonin reuptake inhibitors (SSRIs) is being used as primary treatment in many cases of GAD, panic disorders, social phobias, OCD, and PTSD. For example, the FDA has approved fluoxetine, paroxetine, and fluvoxamine for treatment of OCD. Sometimes higher doses of the drugs than are used with depression are needed, so close monitoring of side effects is important. For PTSD, paroxetine and sertraline have been approved by the FDA. Panic disorders have been successfully treated with paroxetine, fluoxetine, and sertraline. Dosing increases must be done slowly as these patients are especially sensitive to overstimulation from these medications. More research in under way to identify more effective medications for these conditions.

Table 10-2 Commonly Used Anti-Anxiety Medications

Alprazolam (Xanax)
Buspirone (BuSpar)
Chlordiazepoxide (Librium)
Clonazepam (Klonopin)
Clonidine (Catapres)
Diazepam (Valium)
Hydroxyzine (Atarax)
Lorazepam (Ativan)
Oxazepam (Serax)
Prazepam (Centrax)
Zolpidem (Ambien)

techniques to help the patient experience the anxiety-producing situation in a controlled environment and integrate the painful feelings associated with the anxiety. Patients concentrate on esteem needs and reality.

■ Alternative Interventions for People With Anxiety and Anxiety-Related Disorders

Aromatherapy

Essential oils, such as peppermint or eucalyptus, are popular aids in relaxation. Methods of application include using diffusers (machines that turn the oil into droplets that diffuse into the air), placing a drop on a piece of clothing, or applying directly to the skin, such as the temple area. Patients can purchase these essential oils and equipment at specialty stores, some bath oil supply stores, or even in some pharmacies. There are online resources as well. Prescriptions are not needed, but patients should be cautioned to use essential oils in very small amounts (drops at a time) and that some individuals may experience allergic responses, especially if the oils are applied directly to the skin.

Biofeedback

Biofeedback is a form of behavior modification. It is a system of progressive relaxation. There are many tapes and products on the market to assist patients in this "do-it-yourself" method of relaxation. Biofeedback done effectively alters the brain to a slower wave frequency and can actually increase the immune response for humans. The patient should discuss with the doctor if biofeedback is appropriate. The nurse may assist with providing information and resources.

Hypnotherapy

Hypnosis, done by a qualified, licensed therapist, may be helpful. It will assist the patient in relaxation. Some people joke about "going to my happy place," but there is validity in finding pleasure or a lighthearted memory. Patients need to continue to take time to do the relaxation as directed by the therapist. Hypnosis is not a "one-time" therapy. It, like biofeedback, needs to be done routinely to be effective. The nurse's role may be as simple as to remind the patient to find quiet time for this, or if the patient is being seen as an outpatient, the nurse may ask the patient how frequently she or he has been able to do the self-hypnosis and what kind of results the patient has experienced thus far.

Additional Alternative Interventions

The following may provide additional relief:

- Stress and relaxation techniques
- Yoga
- Acupuncture
- Kava

■ Nursing Care for People With Anxiety and Anxiety-Related Disorders

Common nursing diagnoses for people with anxiety and anxiety-related disorders:

- Anxiety, coping, ineffective
- Fear
- Thought process, disturbed
- Violence, risk for

General Interventions

1. *Maintain a calm milieu:* Patients who have anxiety disorders need to have a calm and safe treatment area. Minimizing the stimuli helps the patient to keep centered and focused.

2. *Maintain open communication:* Encourage the patient to verbalize all thoughts and feelings. Honesty in dealing with patients helps them learn to trust others and increases their self-esteem. Patients will feel the value that nurses have in that relationship. Observe the patient's nonverbal communication. As previously stated, affect and body language often reveal more about a patient's thoughts and feelings than the words that are spoken.
3. *Observe for signs of suicidal thoughts:* Patients with anxiety disorders, especially those suffering with PTSD, are at risk for suicide as a result of feelings of low self-esteem or decreased self-worth. Nurses must be alert to this possibility and should observe and confront the patient and document any suspicions or statements the patient expresses.
4. *Document any changes in behavior:* Any change, no matter how small, can be significant to the patient's care. Positive or negative alterations in the way a patient responds to the nurse, to the treatment plan, or to other people and situations should be documented. The data collected and documented will allow the nurse to provide accurate feedback.
5. *Encourage activities:* Activities that are enjoyable and nonstressful help the patient in several ways. Activities provide a diversion, give the patient time to concentrate on something other than the anxiety-producing situation, and give an opportunity to provide positive feedback to the patient about the progress he or she is making. These activities should be purposeful, not just "busy work." The patient should not be put in a situation of competition as a result of activities. Competition could increase the anxiety and be counterproductive to treatment.

Table 10-3 summarizes the types of anxiety and related disorders, the general symptoms, and common nursing actions for them, and Table 10-4 outlines a Nursing Care Plan for

Table 10-3 Nursing Care for Patients With Anxiety and Related Disorders

Disorders	Symptoms	Nursing Actions
Generalized Anxiety Disorder	Muscle aches, shakes, palpitations, dry mouth, nausea, chills, vomiting, hot flashes, polyuria, difficulty swallowing, feeling of dread	• Provide calm milieu • Open communication done calmly and clearly • Focus on brief messages • Teach early signs of escalating anxiety • Suicide precautions if the person indicates any self-destructive thoughts • Document behavior changes • Encourage activities • Promote deep breathing and other relaxation methods • Reassurance
Panic Disorder	Fear, dissociation, nausea, diaphoresis, chest pain, increased pulse, shaking, unsteadiness, paralysis	Same as above • Stay with patient during attack
Phobia	Irrational fear of a particular object or situation	Same as above • Focus on nonthreatening topics • Reassure about patient's safety

Continued

Table 10-3 Nursing Care for Patients With Anxiety and Related Disorders—cont'd

Disorders	Symptoms	Nursing Actions
Obsessive-Compulsive Disorder	Repeated thoughts and/or repeated actions	Same as above • Allow patient to express the anxiety • Recognize and accept need for obsessions and compulsions • Allow time for rituals • Provide structured schedule and give patient some control • Explore alternative methods of anxiety reduction
Post-Traumatic Stress Disorder	"Flashbacks," social withdrawal, low self-esteem, relationships that may change or be difficult to form, irritability, anger seemingly for no reason, depression, chemical dependency	Same as above • Keep patient oriented to the present • Encourage patient and significant others to attend groups for patients with PTSD • Encourage patient to talk about traumatic events if he/she is able

Table 10-4 Nursing Care Plan for Patient With Anxiety

Assessment/ Data Collection	Nursing Diagnosis	Plan/Goal	Interventions/ Nursing Actions	Evaluation
Patient is: • Restless • Irritable • Pacing • Hyperventilating • Verbalizing negative thoughts and expecting a calamity	Anxiety	Demonstrates a sense of increased comfort	• Calm environment • Promote relaxation techniques including deep breaths • Soothing music • Verbalize reassurance about current situation resolving	Patient appears more relaxed and verbalizes more positive outcomes

a patient with anxiety. See Figure 10-6 concept map care plan for panic disorder and GAD.

■ Somatic Symptom and Related Disorders

Somatic Symptom Disorder (SSD)

Somatic refers to the body. The new term somatic symptom disorders (SSD) replaces the old term **somatoform disorders** in DSM-5.

SSD is characterized by somatic symptoms that are either very distressing or result in significant disruption of functioning, as well as excessive and disproportionate thoughts, feelings, and behaviors regarding those symptoms. To be diagnosed with SSD, the individual must be persistently symptomatic (typically at least for 6 months). It is a category of disorders in DSM-5 as well as a specific diagnosis.

In the past the term somatoform disorders was more associated with physical symptoms with no organic cause. This still may be

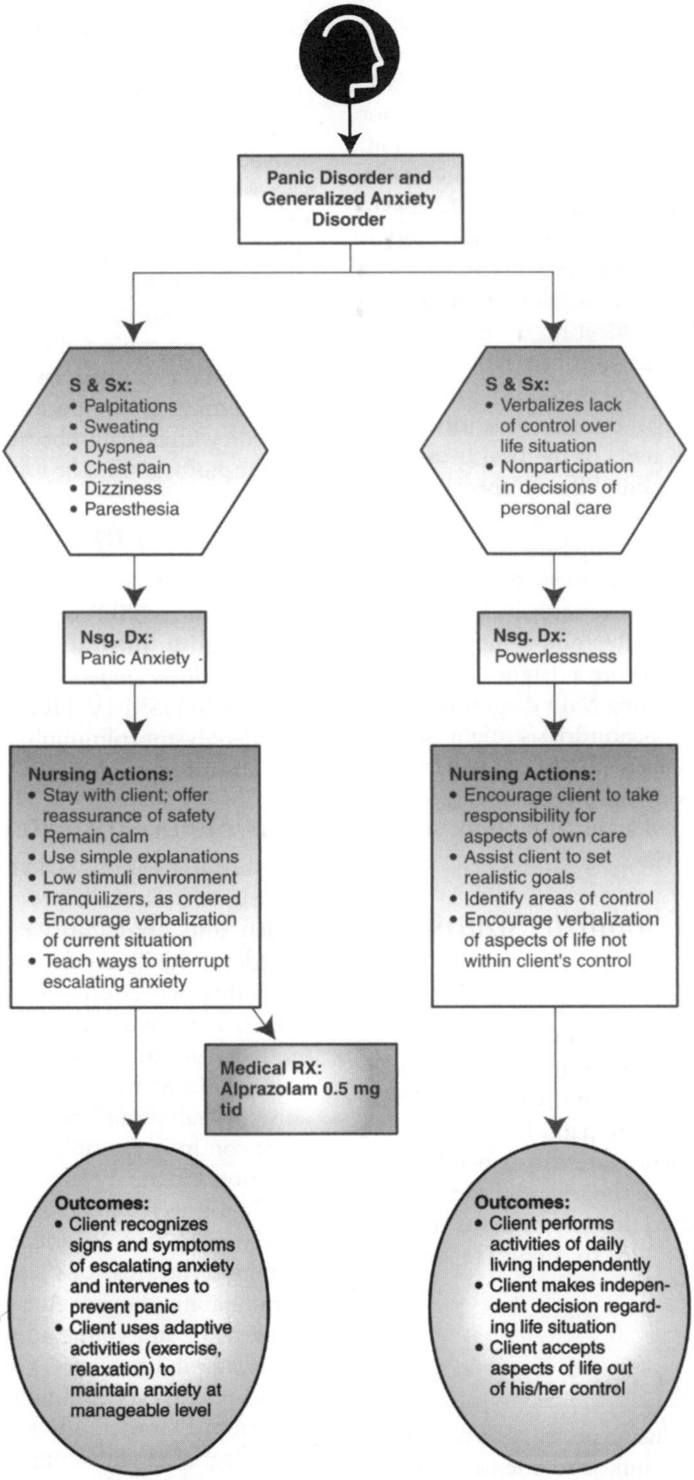

Figure 10-6 Concept map care plan for panic disorder and generalized anxiety disorder. *(From Townsend (2011): Essentials of Psychiatric Mental Health Nursing, 5th ed. Philadelphia: F.A. Davis Company, with permission.)*

the case in SSD but is not required. A prominent feature is excessive focus on one's physical symptoms, that interferes with one's daily functioning. These symptoms may or may not be associated with an actual medical condition. For example, a patient with a small sore seeks multiple opinions out of fear of skin cancer. Despite negative biopsies, the patient keeps checking it, talking about it, and seeking other possible providers who might offer other tests despite great financial burden. In SSD high levels of worry about one's health becomes the central focus in the person's life even to the point of becoming the person's identity. These patients are high users of the health-care system, often seeking out different specialists and testing. So nurses will encounter these patients more often in nonpsychiatric settings. There is a definite anxiety component to this disorder as the individual worries excessively. Although distress is normal with a new symptom, exaggerated responses before a diagnosis would be a factor in considering SSD diagnosis. In the past the term **hypochondriasis** might be used to describe someone with SSD. A patient who focuses extensively on physical symptoms is sometimes referred as suffering from **somatization** or somatizing.

Etiology of Somatic Symptom Disorder

Biologically, research has been conducted concerning the possibility of a genetic or biological predisposition to somatic difficulties. For example some individuals may have increased sensitivity to pain. Early childhood traumatic experiences are also associated with SSD. Psychological theories include physical symptoms rooted in unconscious mechanisms that develop to deny, repress, or displace anxiety.

❃ Cultural Cons

How an individual experiences a bodily sensation can be linked to one's cultural perspective. Some symptoms may be more or less acceptable to acknowledge in different cultures.

Differential Diagnosis

People with somatic disorders present many challenges in obtaining an accurate diagnosis. Nurses must be alert to physical illness that may actually be causing the symptoms. Multiple sclerosis, for example, can present with many and varied symptoms that may be as yet undiagnosed. Discuss with the patient's medical doctor all possibilities for physical illness rather than a somatoform disorder. These patients can end up being subjected to many tests, procedures, and even surgeries with no improvement in symptoms. It is important to avoid labeling a person with SSD just because a physical basis for symptoms cannot be found.

Somatic Symptom Related Disorders

In addition to SSD, several related disorders are covered in this text including conversion disorder, illness anxiety disorder, and factitious disorder. In DSM-IV-TR additional diagnoses included **dysmorphophobia** and **somatoform pain disorder**.

Conversion Disorder

Conversion reaction, as defined in the defense mechanisms (see Chapter 7), is converting anxiety into a physical symptom. Conversion disorder is the illness that emerges from overuse of this mechanism. In conversion disorder, there is a loss or decrease in physical functioning that cannot be explained by any known medical disorder or pathophysiological mechanism. Paralysis and blindness are two of the more common examples of this disorder. It is common for the dysfunction to somehow be deeply connected to denial and to a prior negatively perceived experience (e.g., someone who loses the sense of vision after watching a pornographic movie). Age of onset is usually adolescence and young adulthood, but it can occur later in life as well. Conversion disorder is also referred to as Functional Neurological Symptom Disorder. The rationale is that persons diagnosed with Functional Neurological Symptom Disorder will likely be seen by a neurologist.

The symptoms, although not supportive of organic disease, are very real to the patient.

The nurse should not convey to a patient that he or she thinks the patient is "faking" the illness; it is real to the patient. The patient is truly experiencing the symptoms. Even though the patient is concerned enough about the symptoms to consult a physician, he or she may give the impression of really not caring about the problem. **"La belle indifference"** is the clinical term used to describe this condition.

The belief about this disorder is that the symptom, e.g., the paralysis or blindness, is allowing the patient to avoid a situation that is unacceptable to him or her. This unacceptable situation is the source of extreme anxiety, which is converted into the dysfunction. The dysfunction, then, is relieving the anxiety. This is called **primary gain** and is believed to be the function of the paralysis or blindness. **Secondary gain** is the extra benefits one may acquire as a result of staying ill. Secondary gain includes extra emotional support such as sympathy and love or financial benefits. Much of this is occurring at the unconscious level.

Malingering is a situation for achieving personal gain that differs from the others mentioned. Malingering is a conscious effort to avoid unpleasant situations. The patient "fakes" or pretends to have the symptoms.

> **Critical Thinking Question**
> Will the DSM-5 change reduce the social negativity associated with the word *hypochondriasis*?

Illness Anxiety Disorder

In this disorder somatic symptoms are not present or if present, are only mild in intensity. The person's distress is not from the physical complaint itself but rather from his/her anxiety about the meaning, significance, or cause of the complaint. Historically these patients are often referred to popularly as hypochondriacs. These people are sometimes referred to as "professional patients." Hypochondriasis has been a recognized, official diagnosis according to DSM-IV-TR. In DSM-5 hypochondriasis was changed to *Illness* Anxiety Disorder.

A major difference between illness anxiety disorder and conversion disorder is that the person with conversion disorder focuses on the symptoms of the illness, while the person with illness anxiety disorder is afraid he or she will *get* a serious disease.

Factitious Disorder

Falsification of medical or psychological signs and symptoms in oneself or others is called a factitious disorder. The diagnosis requires demonstrating that the individual is taking secretive actions to misrepresent, simulate or cause signs or symptoms of illness or injury in the absence of obvious external rewards. When the individual falsifies information for another as in a child or pet, the diagnosis is factitious disorder imposed on another or by proxy.

> **Critical Thinking Question**
> Penny is a 35-year-old married mother of three children, ages 2 years, 3 years, and 4 months. She works as a clerk in a large office. She has been visiting the clinic regularly since her last pregnancy. She is experiencing severe, intermittent pain in her right arm and left foot. The pain does not interfere with her life as a wife and mother, and she is not able to detect any kind of pattern to the pain. She tells you that she is not especially concerned about the pain. "When it gets too bad for me, my husband cooks and cleans the kitchen."
>
> Penny says that she thinks the source of her pain is related to "the day I banged my right hip real hard on the door of the copy machine." She also has begun expressing concern that things are going so well for her that she "just has the feeling that something terrible is about to happen." What is your preliminary impression of Penny's illness? What other information might you want to obtain from Penny?

Medical Treatment of Patients With Somatic Symptom and Related Disorders

Patients with these disorders are usually admitted to a medical unit rather than a psychiatric unit. Treatment focuses on the symptoms, which more than likely are medical in nature. The patient does not generally display unusual or unmanageable behavior that indicates the need for mental health unit admission.

Treatment is, of course, individualized for each patient. Once a somatic disorder is diagnosed, the ongoing involvement of a psychiatrist is helpful to give insight to managing this patient. Some approaches that may be used to treat these disorders include individual and group psychotherapy, hypnosis and relaxation techniques. It is beneficial for the therapist to help the patient express the underlying cause of the anxiety. Hypnosis can be very effective in making this determination. Behavior modification can be effective if the patient is prone to secondary gains from the somatic symptoms. Methods of stress management are also taught as the person learns new ways to handle anxiety. Patients may resist accepting that their problem has a strong psychological or emotional component and therefore cannot understand how a paralyzed limb or pain has anything to do with anxiety. People who have a somatic symptom disorder may feel insulted, become resistive to treatment, and search for other ways to explain the physical problem.

Alternative Interventions for Patients With Somatic Symptom and Related Disorders

Alternative treatment of choice is related to the particular condition or symptom set. Choices may include the following treatments in addition to biofeedback, hypnosis, relaxation, and imagery.

Massage

Massage therapies are believed to not only relieve tensions and discomforts in the musculoskeletal system, but also may assist with blood and lymph flow. Massage may be effective, especially with medication, to assist the patient to overcome physical symptoms. Caution should be used, however, not to actually emphasize the body complaint and reinforce the illness.

Herbal/Nutritional Supplements

It is possible that a patient is experiencing a nutritional deficiency or possibly a condition such as arthritis along with the somatoform disorder. Herbs or supplements geared to the specific pain issue may help the patient to experience less pain, either physically or psychologically.

Nursing Care of the Patient With Somatic Symptom and Related Disorders

Common nursing diagnoses include the following:

- Anxiety
- Coping, ineffective
- Sensory perception, disturbed
- Thought processes, disturbed

Pharmacology Corner

Medications are used sparingly because these patients typically have a history of being overprescribed. When medications are ordered for a patient, the classifications of choice are usually selective serotonin reuptake inhibitors (SSRIs) (e.g., fluoxetine); other antidepressants, particularly the tricyclics, such as imipramine; anti-anxiety drugs; or combinations of these medications. At this time, if medications are considered, SSRIs are greatly preferred over the other classes of antidepressants and probably should be first-line agents. See Table 10-5 for medications commonly used to treat somatic symptom and related disorders.

Table 10-5 Commonly Used Medications for Somatic Symptom and Related Disorders

Medications are ordered judiciously for these disorders. When a medication is used, it is generally an antidepressant or an anti-anxiety agent.

Amitriptyline (Elavil)
Bupropion (Wellbutrin)
Doxepin (Sinequan)
Fluoxetine (Prozac)
Paroxetine (Paxil)
Sertraline (Zoloft)
Trazodone (Oleptro)

Table 10-6 summarizes the symptoms and nursing interventions for the somatic symptom disorders discussed previously. Figure 10-7 is a concept map of somatoform disorders.

Communication Skills

Honesty in dealing with the patient is very important. Gaining trust that will encourage the patient to verbalize thoughts and feelings about the physical and emotional aspects of this type of disorder is crucial. Do not discount the patient's disorder. An example of a way to be honest about the situation follows.

EXAMPLE

Nurse: "Ms. P, your physician can find no physical or life-threatening conditions at this time. We will continue to observe and examine you. We will make every attempt to help you improve."

In this way, the patient understands that nothing is showing up in the tests that have been made to this point. The person hears that nothing life-threatening is causing the symptoms. The nurse has said that the staff is attempting to help the patient but has stopped short of promising improvement or of "curing" the patient.

Socialization and Group Activities

Keeping the patient focused on other topics may help in the recovery. Nurses will involve the patient in the goal setting and interventions of the care plan. Aiding the patient in learning assertive communication skills can be helpful. Working with other health-care staff in occupational therapy, recreational therapy, and social activities can also act to divert the patient's focus from the dysfunction.

Support

It is important for the nurse caring for patients with somatoform disorders to remember to pay attention to the patient but not to

Table 10-6 Nursing Care for Patients With Somatic Symptom and Related Disorders

Type	Symptoms	Nursing Interventions
Somatic Symptom Disorder	• High level of anxiety about health • Excessive time and energy devoted to symptoms • May or may not have an organic disorder	• Listen to patient's concerns but then focus on other issues • Promote trust • Encourage patient to express self about other issues than the symptoms
Conversion Disorder	• Loss or decrease in physical functioning that seems to have a neurological connection (paralysis, blindness) • Indifference to the loss of function • Primary and secondary gain	• Use therapeutic communication skills. • Encourage therapy (occupational therapy, physical therapy, etc.). • Provide emotional support. • Respond to the patient's symptoms as real.
Illness Anxiety Disorder	• "Professional patient" • Intense fear of becoming seriously ill • Preoccupation with the idea of being seriously ill and not being helped—may be concerned about not being taken seriously or evaluated properly	• Do not reinforce the symptom. • Be nonjudgmental. • Continue to focus on trusting relationship.

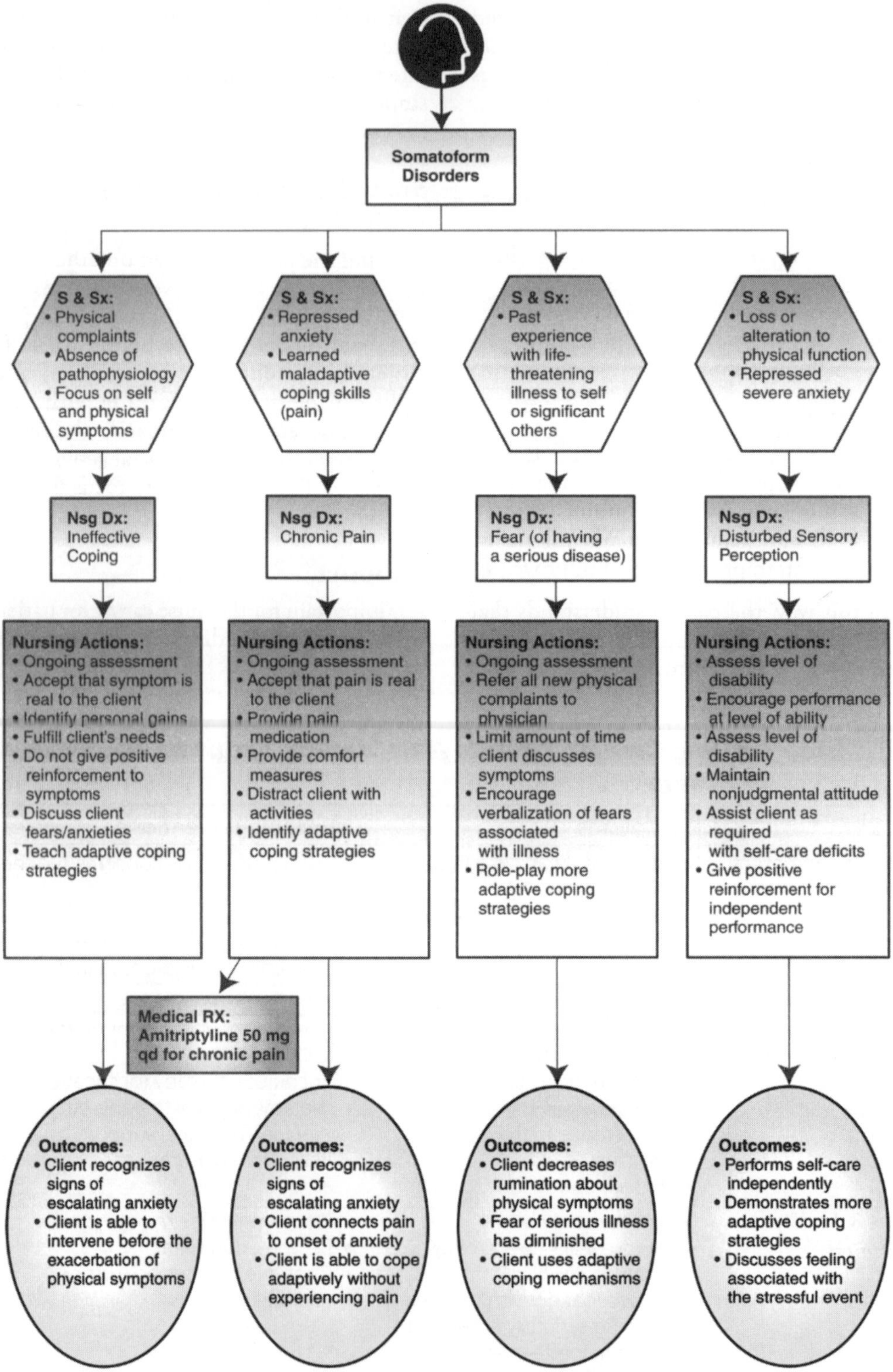

Figure 10-7 Concept map care plan for somatoform disorder. *(From Townsend (2011): Essentials of Psychiatric Mental Health Nursing, 5th ed. Philadelphia: F.A. Davis Company, with permission.)*

reinforce the symptom. The nurse should always make a thorough head-to-toe assessment. This shows the patient that the nurse is concerned for the patient's health but will not be focusing on the area of dysfunction or reinforcing the problem. Nurses should document all findings in a matter-of-fact way. Patients need to know that they are being taken seriously, even though they may not agree with the medical findings of their illness.

Key Concepts

1. Anxiety disorders have many common characteristics. Psychoanalytic theories propose that it is important to find the underlying cause of the anxiety. Biological theories postulate that the causes are not the primary concern, but rather the physical reasons may result in the anxiety.
2. Medications and therapies should be individualized for the patient.
3. Trust and communication techniques are important tools for the nurse caring for a patient with an anxiety disorder. Maintaining a calm milieu is also essential.
4. Somatic symptom disorder is characterized by somatic symptoms that are either very distressing or result in significant disruption of functioning, as well as excessive and disproportionate thoughts, feelings, and behaviors regarding those symptoms. The symptoms may or may not have an organic cause.
5. Treatment and nursing care for patients with somatoform disorders may be difficult and long-term, as these are chronic disorders. Patients may use the defense mechanisms of denial and conversion reaction.
6. DSM-5 (2013) is the current major for psychiatry.

CASE STUDY

A patient comes for his scheduled appointment with Dr. Sneeze. The patient is a well-known politician. He has been the subject of negative press in recent months. His main symptoms are general malaise, sneezing, chronic headache, and "feeling like I have a constant cold." Dr. Sneeze orders blood work and a chest x-ray and does a complete physical exam of the patient. You have collected vital signs and the health history when you roomed the patient. The patient does not have a young family at home but is on the road campaigning and meeting his constituents almost daily. He believes he has become infected with something serious, since his symptoms do not seem to subside. Dr. Sneeze delivers the news to the patient that he is "healthy." His examination and lab work do not show any physical illness, and the doctor suggests perhaps the symptoms are "most likely viral in nature and probably stress and anxiety related." Dr. Sneeze suggests the patient take over-the-counter medications for his symptoms and find methods to reduce his stress. Dr. Sneeze leaves the room. The patient expresses his extreme disappointment at not being given "something to take" and asks you to explain to him how stress can give one a cold.

1. How will you respond to the patient's request for medication?
2. What are your thoughts about the patient's expectation for receiving medications? How will you discuss that with him?
3. What alternatives (for example, dietary, herbal, etc.) can you discuss with him or ask the doctor to discuss with him?

REFERENCES

American Psychiatric Association. (2000). *Diagnostic and Statistical Manual of Mental Disorders IV-Text Revision.* Washington DC, Author. (Known as DSM-IV-TR.)

American Psychiatric Association. (2013). *Diagnostic and Statistical Manual of Mental Disorders 5.* Washington, DC, Author. (Known as DSM-5.)

Anderson, R.A. (2001). *Clinician's Guide to Holistic Medicine.* New York: McGraw-Hill.

Braiker, H. (2002). *September 11 Syndrome.* New York: McGraw-Hill.

Cohen, S. (2003). *Sociability and Susceptibility to the Common Cold.* Washington, DC: Carnegie Mellon University (copyright American Psychological Society), *14*(5) September 2003.

David, J., and Kupfer, M. (n.d.). Retrieved from http://www.dsm5.org/Pages/Default.aspx

Drummond, K. (2012). Army suicides: July deaths set a magic new record. *Forbes.* Retrieved from www.forbes.com/sites/katiedrummond/2012/08/16/army-suicide-rate/

Gorman, L.M. and Sultan, D.F. (2008). *Psychosocial Nursing for General Patient Care.* Philadelphia: F.A. Davis.

Nicholson, R.A. (2003). *Chill Out: Anger Can Give You a Headache.* St. Louis, MO: Saint Louis University.

Shives, L., and Isaacs, A. (2002). *Basic Concepts of Psychiatric-Mental Health Nursing.* 5th ed. Philadelphia: JB Lippincott.

Sierpina, V.S. (2001). *Integrative Health Care—Complementary and Alternative Therapies for the Whole Person.* Philadelphia: F.A. Davis.

Somatic symptom disorders. (2012). In *American Psychiatric Association DSM-5 Development.* Retrieved from www.dsm5.org/proposedrevision/Pages/SomaticSymptomDisorders.aspx

Townsend, M. (2008). *Essentials of Psychiatric and Mental Health Nursing.* 4th ed., p. 389. Philadelphia: F.A. Davis.

Townsend, M. (2012). *Essentials of Psychiatric and Mental Health Nursing: Concepts of Care in Evidence-Based Practice.* 7th ed. Philadelphia: F.A. Davis.

Test Questions

Multiple Choice Questions

1. Your significant other is a veteran of the war in Iraq. It is very difficult for him or her to drive through a parking ramp because "There are people hiding behind the pillars! They have guns! Be careful!" This person is most likely experiencing:
a. Auditory hallucinations
b. Flashbacks
c. Delusions of grandeur
d. Free-floating anxiety

2. Ms. T cannot leave her home without checking the coffee pot numerous times. This makes her late to many functions, and she misses engagements on occasion because of it. Ms. T probably is suffering from what kind of disorder?
a. Generalized anxiety disorder
b. Phobia
c. Post-traumatic stress disorder
d. Obsessive-compulsive disorder

3. Mr. L has a severe fear of needles. He is hospitalized on your medical unit. The lab technician enters to draw blood for the routine CBC, and Mr. L begins to cry out, "Get away from me! I can't breathe! I'm having a heart attack!" Your first response to Mr. L would be:
a. "I'll take your vital signs and call my supervisor."
b. "Why do you think you're having a heart attack, Mr. L?"
c. "Don't worry. She's done this many times before."
d. "Mr. L, relax. Take a few deep breaths. I'll stay with you."

4. Which of the following is *not* an anxiety disorder? *(select all that apply)*
a. Panic disorder
b. Obsessive-compulsive disorder
c. Multiple personality disorder
d. Agoraphobia

5. A patient with an obsessive-compulsive disorder is:
a. Suspicious and hostile
b. Flexible and adaptable to change
c. Extremely frightened of something
d. Rigid in thought and inflexible with routines and rituals

6. Which of the following is *true* regarding a phobic disorder?
a. It involves repetitive actions.
b. It involves a loss of identity.
c. It results in sociopathic behavior.
d. It is an irrational fear that is not changed by logic.

7. In obsessive-compulsive disorder, a compulsion is:
a. A repetitive thought
b. A repetitive action
c. A repetitive fear
d. A repetitive illusion

8. The medication(s) of choice for the treatment of OCD is (are): *(select all that apply)*
a. Paxil (paroxetine)
b. Prozac (fluoxetine)
c. Luvox (fluvoxamine)
d. Effexor (venlafaxine)

9. The three subcategories of phobia include all *EXCEPT:*
a. Agoraphobia
b. Social phobia
c. Acrophobia
d. Specific phobia

10. Which of the following are NOT nursing intervention(s) for people with anxiety disorders? *(select all that apply)*
a. Maximize stimuli to create diversion from the anxiety.
b. Encourage the patient to verbalize all thoughts and feelings.
c. Observe the patient's nonverbal communication for data on a patient's thoughts and feelings.
d. Observe for signs of suicidal thoughts.
e. Document only positive changes in behavior.
f. Discourage activities; activities might only increase a patient's anxiety level.

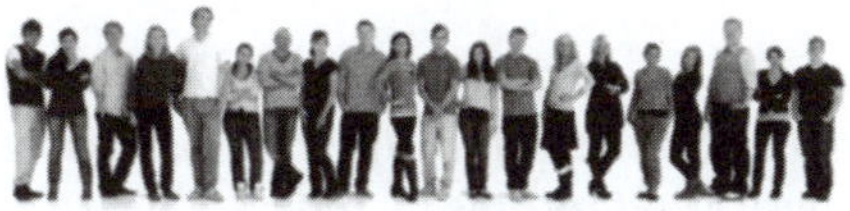

CHAPTER 11

Depressive Disorders

Learning Objectives
1. Define depressive disorders.
2. Identify three types of depressive disorders.
3. Describe common physical and behavioral symptoms of major depressive disorder.
4. Identify treatment modalities for depressive disorders.
5. Describe key nursing care interventions for depressive disorders.

Key Terms
- Depression
- Dysthymic disorder
- Major depressive disorder
- Mood

Feeling down, discouraged, and depressed is something all people experience at some time in their lives. Periods of emotional highs and lows are normal. Depressive disorders are very different from a transient bout of the "blues" or depressed **mood. Depression** is a painful and debilitating illness that affects all areas of one's life. There are several types of depression that are collectively called depressive disorders. These can change or distort the way a person sees himself, his life, and those around him. People who suffer from depression usually see everything with a more negative attitude. They cannot imagine that any problem or situation can be solved in a positive way. Depression can take a variety of forms and affect all age groups. Depressive disorders all have similar symptoms that vary by duration, timing and presumed etiology. It is more common in women, but men with depression may be underdiagnosed (Figure 11-1). See Box 11-1 for list of general facts about depressive disorders.

> **Cultural Considerations**
>
> Depression crosses all cultures and socioeconomic groups. However, depressive disorders may be misdiagnosed or underdiagnosed in some cultures due to language barriers and lack of access to mental health services. This is particularly true in cultures that are more fearful of being "labeled" with a psychiatric diagnosis. Some cultures may express depressive symptoms as physical symptoms, such as fatigue and headache, while others may be more prone to speak in psychological terms of sadness and guilt.

Types of Depressive Disorders

Major Depressive Disorder

Major depressive disorder, or major depression, is characterized by a combination of symptoms that severely interfere with a person's ability to work, sleep, study, eat, and enjoy once-pleasurable activities. These symptoms must last at least 2 weeks and very often last much longer to receive this diagnosis. Major depression is disabling and prevents a person from functioning normally. Some people may experience only a single episode of depression within their lifetime, but more often a person has multiple episodes. Major depressive disorder affects approximately 5% to 8% of the U.S. population age 18 and older annually. A person has a 16.6% chance of developing a major depressive disorder in one's lifetime (Kessler, 2005).

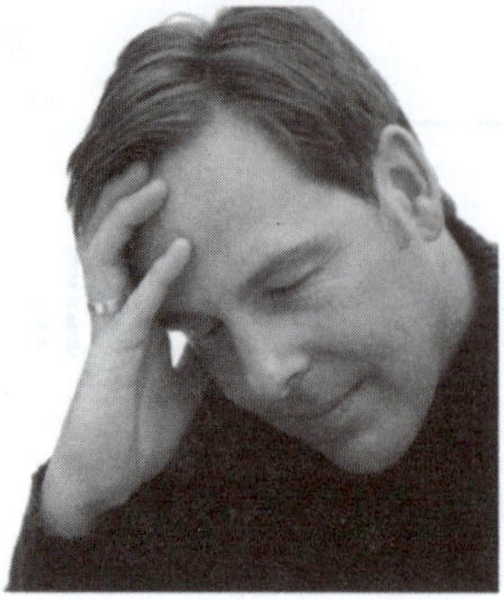

Figure 11-1 Depression is less reported in the male population, but this may be caused by male tendency to mask emotional disorders with behaviors such as alcohol abuse.

Box 11-1 General Information About Depressive Disorders

- Common not only in the United States but also internationally.
- Most common reason for seeking out mental health professional.
- Nearly twice as many women as men are affected by a depressive disorder annually. However, men frequently suffer from depression that may be masked.
- The elderly are prone to depression often related to multiple losses and decline of health, among other variables.
- Depressive disorders are being diagnosed earlier in life than they were in previous generations, including in children and adolescents.
- Because symptoms can be hidden and vague, the primary physician is often the first to identify depression.
- Symptoms often go unrecognized and can be a factor in poor work performance, family conflict, and substance abuse.
- Once one is diagnosed with a depressive disorder, there is a high probability of recurrence.

Source: Adapted from Kessler et al. (2005): "Major Depressive Disorders Among Adults—National Institute of Mental Health."

Major depressive disorder is characterized by a classic cluster of symptoms. Behavioral and physical symptoms include:

Five or more of the following for at least a 2-week period that represent a change in functioning:

- Sad mood
- Sleep pattern disturbances
- Increased fatigue
- Increased agitation
- Feelings of guilt or worthlessness
- Weight loss or gain
- Decreased interest in pleasurable activities (anhedonia)
- Decreased ability to think, remember, or concentrate
- Recurrent thoughts of death or suicide

These symptoms are often the same behaviors someone experiences in a low period of his or her life, but the duration and intensity are increased (Figures 11-2 and 11-3).

Tool Box Clinicians use a number of depression scales to follow the severity of the patient's symptoms over time. These include:

1. Beck Depression Inventory, www.ibogaine.desk.nl/graphics/3639b1c_23.pdf_
2. Hamilton Depression Rating Scale, www.psy-world.com/online_hamd.htm

Differentiating a grief response to a major life loss from major depressive disorder can be difficult as some of the symptoms, such as sadness, insomnia, and poor appetite, may resemble a depressive episode. See Table 11-1 for tips to differentiate grief from depression.

Neeb's Tip A period of depression following the death of a loved one is normal. When this response goes on longer than expected and interferes with a person's self-esteem, it may indicate a depressive disorder.

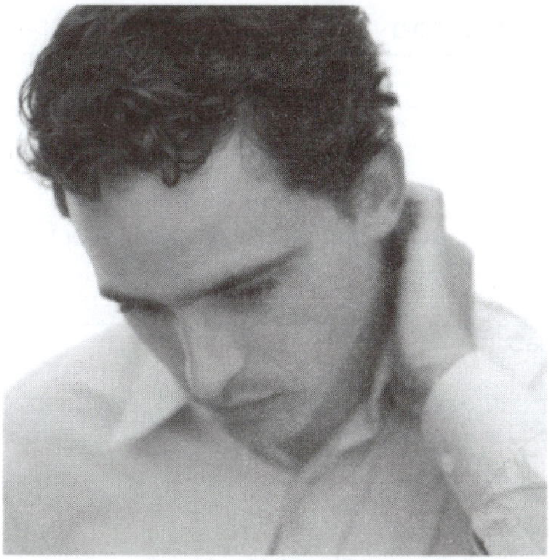

Figure 11-2 Sadness becomes depression when it lasts a long time and interferes with day-to-day functioning.

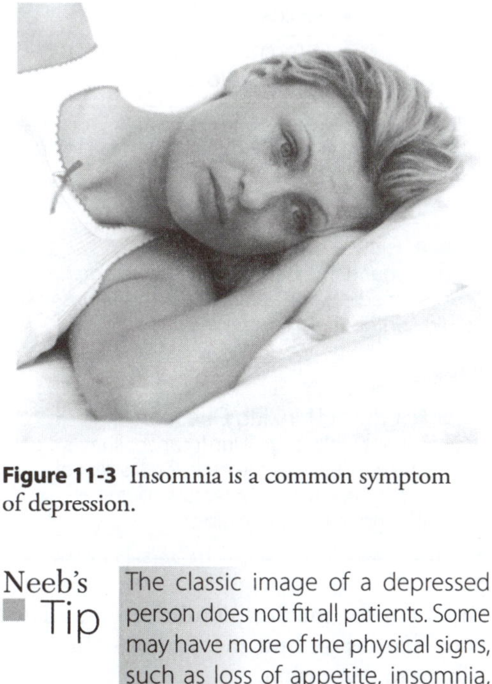

Figure 11-3 Insomnia is a common symptom of depression.

Neeb's Tip

The classic image of a depressed person does not fit all patients. Some may have more of the physical signs, such as loss of appetite, insomnia, and early morning wakening, and not display the outward sadness that is usually associated with depression.

Dysthymic Disorder

Dysthymic disorder is a less severe form of depression that is characterized by its chronic nature. It is sometimes called persistent depressive disorder. It affects approximately 5% to 6% of the U.S. population age 18 and older at some point in their lifetimes (Kessler, 2005). It often begins in childhood, adolescence, or early adulthood. About 40% of adults with dysthymic disorder also meet criteria for major depressive disorder or bipolar disorder.

Dysthymic disorder is characterized by a depressed mood for most of the day, for more days than not, as indicated by either subjective account or observation by others, for at least 2 years and 1 year in children. These symptoms are less severe than those of major depressive disorder but have gone on for long periods.

Symptoms often include:

- Poor appetite or overeating
- Insomnia or hypersomnia
- Low energy or fatigue
- Low self-esteem
- Poor concentration or difficulty making decisions
- Feelings of hopelessness

Critical Thinking Question
Describe the behaviors that would differentiate dysthymic disorder from major depressive disorder.

Postpartum Depression

Postpartum "blues" is a common response a few days after giving birth and may be related to fatigue, hormone changes, and anxiety. It resolves in a short time with rest and support. Postpartum depression, also called postpartum onset depression, occurs up to 6 months after childbirth and is a much more serious condition. Postpartum onset depression is classified as a major depressive disorder with the same classic cluster of symptoms as above with the addition of lack of interest in the baby, which can progress to rejection of the baby and lead to a psychotic state. A patient suffering from this disorder needs intensive treatment with medications and psychotherapy. See Chapter 20 for more information.

Major Depressive Disorder With Seasonal Pattern

Previously called seasonal affective disorder (SAD), this is a depression associated with seasonal patterns. Symptoms generally are exacerbated during the winter months and

Table 11-1 Differentiating Grief From Depression

	Uncomplicated Grief	Major Depression
Reaction	• Labile • Heightened when thinking of loss	• Mood consistently low • Prolonged, severe symptoms lasting more than 2 months
Behavior	• Variable, shifts from sharing pain to being alone • Variable restriction of pleasure	• Completely withdrawn or fear of being alone • Persistent restriction of pleasure
Sleep Patterns	• Periodic episodes of inability to sleep	• Wakes early morning
Anger	• Often expressed	• Turned inward
Sadness	• Varying periods	• Consistently sad
Cognition	• Preoccupied with loss • Self-esteem not as affected	• Focused on self • Feels worthless; has negative self-image
History	• Generally no history of depression	• History of depression or other psychiatric illness
Responsiveness	• Responds to warmth and support	• Hopelessness • Limited response to support • Avoids socializing
Loss	• Recognizable, current	• Often not related to an identified loss

Source: Adapted from Ferszt (2006): How to distinguish between grief and depression? *Nursing, 36*(9), 60–61; Brown-Saltzman (2006). Transforming the Grief Experience. In Johnson, Gorman, Bush (eds.). Psychosocial Nursing along the Cancer Continuum, 2nd ed., pp. 293–314, Oncology Nursing Press: Pittsburgh, PA.

subside during the spring and summer. This type of depression is thought to be related to the hormone melatonin. During months of longer darkness, there is increased production of melatonin that seems to trigger depressive symptoms in some people.

Substance-Induced Depressive Disorder

Substance-induced depressive disorder is depressed mood from the physiological effects of withdrawal, intoxication, or after exposure to a substance. This can include drugs of abuse such as alcohol, opioids, sedatives, and anti-anxiety medications as well as exposure to toxins.

Depressive Disorder Associated With Another Medical Condition

This condition is characterized by a prominent and persistent depression that is judged to be the result of direct physiological effects of a general medical condition. See Boxes 11-2 and 11-3 for medical conditions associated with depression and medications that contribute to depression.

Clinical Activity

Review your depressed patient's risk factors, including medications and medical conditions that could contribute to the depression.

Critical Thinking Question

Your patient with Stage II lung cancer shows signs of depression. Besides the emotional stress of having cancer, what other factors could be contributing to the depression?

Premenstrual Dysphoric Disorder

This form of depressive disorder was added to the Diagnostic and Statistical Manual 5th edition in 2013. The features include a consistent pattern of markedly depressed mood, excessive anxiety, and mood swings during the week prior to menses, which start to

Box 11-2 Medical Conditions Associated With Depression

- Stroke (especially frontal lesions)
- Myocardial infarction
- Adrenal disorders
- Dementia
- Diabetes
- Cancer
- Hypothyroidism
- Brain tumors
- Parkinson's disease
- Multiple sclerosis
- Chronic pain
- Chronic kidney disease

Source: From Gorman and Sultan (2008): Psychosocial Nursing for General Patient Care, 3rd ed. Philadelphia: F.A. Davis Company, with permission.

Box 11-3 Drugs That Can Cause Depression

Antihypertensive agents including:
- Reserpine
- Beta blockers
- Methyldopa

Oral contraceptives
Steroids
Psychoactive agents
Benzodiazepines
Anabolic steroids
Amphotericin-B

Cancer chemotherapeutic agents including:
- Vincristine
- Vinblastine
- Interferon
- Procarbazine
- L-asparaginase

Alcohol
Amphetamine or cocaine withdrawal
Opioids

Source: From Gorman and Sultan (2008): Psychosocial Nursing for General Patient Care, 3rd ed. Philadelphia: F.A. Davis Company, with permission.

improve after the onset of menses and then become minimal or absent after menses.

Etiology of Depressive Disorders

Depressive disorders are complex and may have multiple etiologies. Biochemical theories have become more important with the identification of insufficiency of neurotransmitters, especially norepinephrine and serotonin. These insufficiencies may be the result of inherited or environmental factors. The effectiveness of antidepressants seems to result from enhancing levels of these neurotransmitters, giving strong credibility to these theories. Family history remains an important risk factor indicating genetic links. Psychological theories have focused on personal history of deprivation, trauma, and significant loss. Classic psychoanalytic theory views depression as the reaction to the loss of a significant person who has been both hated and loved. An individual can also be prone to low self-esteem and a sense of helplessness due to environmental factors and have a tendency toward depression. Physical illness and medications are also frequent contributors to depressive symptoms.

Treatment of Depressive Disorders

Treatment involves a combination of pharmacological and psychotherapeutic approaches. This approach has the best outcomes. The advent of so many new antidepressants has provided many more opportunities for successful treatment (see Pharmacology Corner). Individual psychotherapy to address past losses and stressors, short-term cognitive behavioral therapy to develop new strategies to alter negative thinking, and group therapy to address socialization and poor self-esteem can all be helpful. For the patient with severe depression who does not respond to drugs or psychotherapeutic approaches, electroconvulsive therapy is sometimes suggested. It can be used in conjunction with other modalities such as medication. People may have a therapeutic session of 6–10 treatments over 4–8 weeks. Patients are given sedation prior to the treatment. The side effect of memory loss is frequently seen.

Alternative Treatments

Light Therapy

Light therapy is being prescribed and used successfully in the treatment of depression with seasonal pattern. It consists of special lights to be

Classroom Activity
- Arrange for a psychiatrist to talk to the class about psychotherapy and pharmacotherapy in depressive disorders.
- Arrange for a hospital social worker to discuss depression with physical illness.

used for certain amounts of time during the day. Also, exposure to natural light has been shown to reduce depression and increase alertness.

Herbal and Nutritional Therapy

General dietary changes such as avoiding caffeine, sugar, and alcohol or adding servings of whole grains and vegetables may help a person with mild depression. Herbs such as St. John's wort, kava, gingko, fish oil, and SAMe have been shown to provide antidepressant effects in some patients with mild depression. St. John's wort probably should not be used with selective serotonin reuptake inhibitors (SSRIs) or monoamine oxide inhibitors (MAOIs) (Skidmore-Roth, 2010).

> **Pharmacology Corner**
>
> Antidepressants are the medications of choice in treating depressive disorders. See Table 11-2 for the categories of antidepressants. They are also used to treat depression associated with bipolar disorders, schizophrenia, and dementia. Selected agents may be used to treat anxiety disorders and bulimia as well. Some of the target symptoms that antidepressants may treat include sadness, inability to experience pleasure, change in appetite, insomnia, restlessness, poor concentration, and negative thoughts. These medications work to increase concentration of neurotransmitters such as serotonin and norepinephrine. The early antidepressants were called tricyclics and MAOIs. The newer antidepressants, including SSRIs, SNRIs, and heterocyclics, also called tetracyclics, have much better side-effect profiles. The anticholinergic actions of tricyclics and the rigid dietary restrictions needed for MAOIs often limit the use of these medications, but they can still be effective for some patients who are resistant to the other categories. These medications all require several weeks of use before some improvement in depression can be expected; they should not be stopped abruptly. These medications are all oral preparations. Sometimes combinations of antidepressants may be prescribed. See Chapter 8 for more information on these medications.
>
> When severely depressed patients are started on antidepressants, they need close monitoring. As the drugs take effect, the person's mood begins to lift and he or she may have the increased energy to implement a suicide plan.

Nursing Care of the Patient With Depressive Disorders

Common nursing diagnoses with this population include the following:

- Hopelessness
- Self-care deficit
- Self-esteem, disturbed, deficit
- Social interaction, impaired

General Nursing Interventions

- Identify small, achievable goals the patient can meet. Provide support and encouragement. Break down tasks into small parts for the severely depressed patient. For example, rather than encouraging the patient to get dressed, have the patient focus on putting on a t-shirt.
- Encourage the patient to speak about his or her concerns without judgment. Use open-ended questions, such as "Tell me what concerns you today." Avoid blanket reassurance like "you are doing fine" or minimizing the patient's feelings as in "you're lucky you have a job." This might alienate a patient who is not feeling fine. Help a patient who verbalizes hopelessness to focus on describing his feelings and concerns. Then discuss one concern at a time to prevent it from being overwhelming for the patient.
- Encourage independence.
- Avoid activities that might tax memory or concentration if the patient is struggling with these.
- Monitor patient compliance with antidepressants. Include education about potential side effects and not to expect results for several weeks.
- Encourage participation in activities to reduce time spent ruminating on negative thoughts.
- Promote a trusting relationship.

Table 11-2 Antidepressants

Drug Category	Examples	Important Considerations
Tricyclics	amitriptyline (Elavil), nortriptyline (Pamelor), desipramine (Norpramine)	Major side effects are anticholinergic symptoms requiring close monitoring. Symptoms include: dry mouth, urinary retention, constipation, blurred vision, sedation. Use with extreme caution in the elderly.
SSRIs (selective serotonin reuptake inhibitors)	paroxetine (Paxil), sertraline (Zoloft), fluoxetine (Prozac)	SSRI withdrawal syndrome can occur with sudden discontinuation; includes dizziness, nausea, cholinergic rebound (salivation, loose stool)
SNRIs (serotonin norepinephrine reuptake inhibitors)	duloxetine (Cymbalta), venlafaxine (Effexor)	Monitor for insomnia, restlessness
Heterocyclics	bupropion (Wellbutrin), mirtazapine (Remeron), trazodone (Oleptro)	Monitor for dizziness, headache, tachycardia
MAOIs (monoamine oxidase inhibitors)	phenelzine (Nardil), tranylcypromine (Parnate), isocarboxazid (Marplan)	Serious, potentially fatal hypertensive crisis may occur in presence of foods high in tyramine (aged cheeses, red wine, smoked and processed meats). Special diet must be followed.

Source: Adapted from Townsend (2012), Gorman & Sultan (2008), and Pederson & Leahy (2010).

- Encourage the patient to challenge negative thoughts. For example, identify an alternative solution to one problem, and encourage one example such as why the patient is a good parent.
- Promote physical activity where possible, for example, ambulating in the hall twice a day. Focusing on physical activity can promote the patient's sense of well-being.
- Promote the patient's self-esteem by identifying improvements or recent successes. The depressed patient may tend to focus only on negatives.
- If a patient gives any clues of contemplating suicide, notify other team members and the physician immediately. See Chapter 13 for more interventions for suicidal patients.

Neeb's Tip

Depressive disorders can contribute to confusion and social withdrawal in the elderly and can lead to misdiagnosis of dementia (sometimes called pseudodementia). These patients need multidisciplinary assessment to obtain the correct diagnosis and treatment.

Table 11-3 provides the nursing care plan for depressed patients.

Clinical Activity

- Review effective interventions used by the nursing team to approach the depressed patient.
- Identify small goals that the depressed patient has achieved.

Neeb's Tip

As antidepressant drugs take effect, the patient may initially feel more energized before the mood lifts. A suicidal patient can be at increased risk during this period because he or she has more energy to initiate a suicide plan while still feeling hopeless. Any patient who is suicidal should be closely monitored during the first few weeks on antidepressants. All antidepressants carry a black box warning from the FDA about increased risk of suicidality in children and adolescents.

Table 11-3 Nursing Care Plan for the Depressed Patient

Data Collection	Nursing Diagnosis	Plan/Goal	Interventions	Evaluation
Withdrawn, refusing to leave his room	Impaired social interaction	To participate in conversation with nurse once a day. Establish a trusting relationship.	Spend time with patient each day without pressure or demands. Ask questions that do not require demanding answers. Accept periods of silence. Encourage participation in structured activities if possible to reduce pressure on patient to "perform."	Track frequency of patient talking with others. Verbalizes concerns to nurse.

Clinical Activity

Review the side-effect profile of your patient's antidepressants and incorporate teaching as appropriate to promote patient compliance.

Critical Thinking Question

A patient is complaining of nausea and dizziness. In reviewing the medications from home, the patient has been taking paroxetine for 5 years. The patient is now NPO due to surgery. What do you need to know about this medication that could be a factor in the patient's postoperative recovery?

Critical Thinking Question

Identify some of the differences in side-effect profiles from tricyclic antidepressants and from SSRIs.

Key Concepts

1. Depressive disorders are treatable, and most people respond positively to the appropriate medications.
2. Major depressive disorder is a debilitating illness that often recurs in one's lifetime.
3. Depression is the most common reason for seeking out a mental health professional
4. Mood disorder due to a general medical condition is frequently seen in physically ill patients in the hospital.
5. Nursing care of the depressed patient should include promotion of self-esteem and socialization.
6. Antidepressants are very effective in treating depression, but side-effect profiles may require a change in drug as needed.

CASE STUDY

Marge is a 55-year-old single woman who works as a librarian. Over the past few months she has had increasing difficulty in sleeping, poor concentration, and an overwhelming sense of sadness. Her mother died 1 year earlier, and Marge attributed these changes to a grief reaction. However, as time has gone on, the symptoms have become more distressing. She has stopped exercising, has turned down social invitations, and spends most of her time alone at home. She has begun missing work because of oversleeping, and her supervisor has approached her with concern. Marge has agreed to see her physician for a checkup. Marge presents to the doctor with a depressed appearance. On specific questioning she reports feeling that she no longer feels competent in her job despite advanced degrees and certification and over 20 years' experience. These feelings have increased over the past 3 months and occur daily.

The physician considers major depressive disorder as a diagnosis and prescribes paroxetine.

1. What teaching would you provide to the patient about the antidepressant?
2. What other forms of treatments might be proposed?
3. What other concerns would you have for this patient?

REFERENCES

American Psychiatric Association. (2000). *Diagnostic and Statistical Manual of Mental Disorders IV-Text Revision*. Washington DC, Author. (Known as DSM-IV-TR)

American Psychiatric Association. (2013). *Diagnostic and Statistical Manual of Mental Disorders 5*. Washington, DC, Author. (Known as DSM-5)

Brown-Saltzman, K. (2006). Transforming the Grief Experience. In R.C. Johnson, L.M. Gorman, and N.J. Bush (Eds.). *Psychosocial Nursing Along the Cancer Continuum*. 2nd ed., pp. 293–314. Pittsburgh, PA: Oncology Nursing Press.

Ferszt, G. G. (2006). How to distinguish between grief and depression? *Nursing, 36*(9), 60–61.

Gelenberg, A. J. (2010). *Practice Guideline for the Treatment of Patients With Major Depressive Disorder*. 3rd ed. American Psychiatric Association. Retrieved from http://psychiatryonline.org/content.aspx?bookid=28&sectionid=1667485#654166

Gorman, L., and Sultan, D. (2008). *Psychosocial Nursing for General Patient Care*. 3rd ed. Philadelphia: F.A. Davis.

Kessler, R.C., Berglund, P., and Demler, O. (2005). Lifetime prevalence and age-of-onset distributions of DSM-IV disorders in the National Comorbidity Survey Replication. *Archives of general psychiatry, 62*(6), 593–602.

National Institute of Mental Health. *Major Depressive Disorders Among Adults*. Retrieved from http://mentalhealth.gov/statistics/1MDD_ADULT.shtml

Pederson, D.D., and Leahy, L.G. (2010). *Pocket Psych Drugs*. Philadelphia: F.A. Davis.

Sadock, B.J., and Sadock, V.A. (2007). *Synopsis of Psychiatric/Behavioral Sciences/Clinical Psychiatry*. Philadelphia: Lippincott Williams & Wilkins.

Skidmore-Roth, L. (2010). *Mosby's Handbook of Herbs and Natural Supplements*. 4th ed. St. Louis: Mosby-Elsevier.

Townsend, M.C. (2012). *Psychiatric Mental Health Nursing*. 7th ed. Philadelphia: F.A. Davis.

Test Questions

Multiple Choice Questions

1. Ms. S is admitted to your medical unit with a diagnosis of dehydration and a history of depression. She tells you, "I just can't eat. I'm not hungry." Your best therapeutic response would be:
a. "You aren't hungry?"
b. "If you can't eat, what is that candy bar wrapper doing in your bed?"
c. "Why aren't you hungry?"
d. "You really should try to eat some real food."

2. Your patient has a diagnosis of major depressive disorder and has been started on sertraline (Zoloft) 50 mg bid. After taking the medications for three days, the patient says, "I don't think this medicine is working. I don't want to take it any longer." What would be your best response?
a. I'll let your doctor know and he may order a different medication.
b. These medications usually take a few weeks to bring about an improvement to your symptoms.
c. The important thing now is getting you more involved in patient activities.
d. It is important to eat a more balanced diet to help this medication work.

3. Your patient appears withdrawn and depressed. Which of the following would not be an effective intervention?
a. Develop a trust.
b. Show acceptance.
c. Be judgmental.
d. Be honest.

4. The nurse who is assessing a patient with major depression would expect to observe which of the following symptoms?
a. Euphoria
b. Extreme fear
c. Extreme sadness
d. Positive thinking

5. The nursing interventions for a patient with major depression would include all of the following *except:*
a. Active listening skills
b. Maintaining safe milieu
c. Encouraging adequate nutrition
d. Reassuring the patient everything will be "just fine"

6. Your new patient is taking an MAOI for severe depression. What would you tell the Dietary Department about her upcoming meals?
a. No caffeine
b. No processed lunch meat
c. No extra salt
d. Gluten-free diet

7. Your patient with major depressive disorder isolates herself in her room for the whole day. You find her sitting and staring out the window. What is the best therapeutic response when you walk in the room?
a. "Come with me. It's time for group therapy."
b. "I'd like to introduce you to other patients."
c. "What are you thinking about?"
d. Make frequent short visits to her room and just sit there.

8. Your patient, Mr. A, had a recent myocardial infarction and open heart surgery with an uncomplicated recovery. His wife tells you that Mr. A has changed and is now uncommunicative, sad, and discouraged about the future. How would you respond to Mrs. A?
a. I'll let the doctor know.
b. This is normal. I would just ignore it for now.
c. Tell me more about the changes in his behavior.
d. We should get a psychiatric consult.

Test Questions

cont.

9. Mrs. J has been diagnosed with dysthymic disorder and has been taking paroxetine for 3 years. On arrival in your mental health clinic, she presents very differently than on her last visit. She is cheerful, energetic, and talkative. Previously she had been fatigued and negative. What should you do?

a. Encourage the patient to no longer take her antidepressant.
b. Get more information from the patient about how she is feeling.
c. Recommend that she not be seen in the clinic today.
d. Talk with the patient's husband to confirm these behavior changes.

10. Which of the following is not true about depression?

a. It is more common in men than in women.
b. It is common after myocardial infarction.
c. Grief after a major loss can mimic depression.
d. Children and adolescents can suffer from depression.

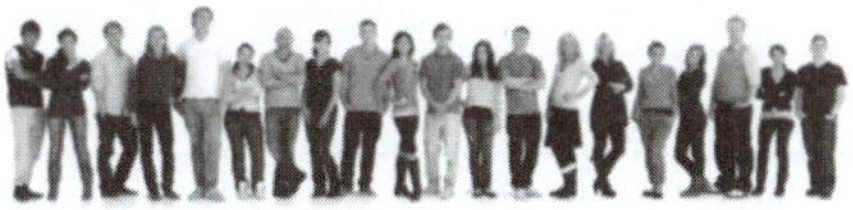

CHAPTER 12

Bipolar Disorders

Learning Objectives

1. Describe three different types of bipolar disorders.
2. Describe factors that make bipolar disorder difficult to diagnose.
3. Describe nursing interventions for behaviors associated with mania.
4. List three medications useful in treatment of bipolar disorders and the potential side effects of each.
5. Describe two teaching points for bipolar patients on mood stabilizers.

Key Terms

- Bipolar disorder
- Cyclothymic
- Hypomania
- Mania

■ Characteristics of Bipolar Disorders

Bipolar disorder (previously known as manic depression) is characterized by marked shifts in mood, energy, and ability to function, often with profound depressions to periods of hyperactivity or **mania** with periods of normalcy. The common forms of bipolar disorders include bipolar I, bipolar II, and cyclothymic, as well as several others. These are listed in Table 12-1. Bipolar disorders are often hard to diagnose until the behavior becomes exaggerated, such as grandiosity, high-risk behaviors, violence. During **hypomania** phases (less severe hyperactivity), a person may be highly productive, so this disorder might not get diagnosed. Some highly creative people, such as Ernest Hemingway and Jackson Pollock, had this disorder. **Cyclothymic** disorder is a chronic disorder marked by multiple episodes of hypomania and depression.

Mania episodes (also known as manic) are characterized by a distinct period of abnormality and persistently elevated, expansive, or irritable mood. Extreme mania can include psychotic behaviors such as hallucinations and delusions. There is a high risk of suicide with bipolar disorder. Patients may also abuse alcohol or other substances in an effort to self-medicate to feel better. Bipolar disorder can be confused with depression, personality disorders, schizophrenia, substance abuse, and anxiety disorders. Clues that the illness is bipolar disorder include early onset, family history of bipolar disorder, recurrent depressions, repeated loss of efficacy of antidepressants, and hyperactivity during depressive episodes (Akiskai, 2009).

See Box 12-1 for general information about bipolar disorders.

Manic Phase

The manic phase may last from days to months and cause marked disruption of occupational and social functioning. It can include the following symptoms:

- Easily distracted
- Little need for sleep (may feel rested after 3 hours of sleep)
- Poor temper control, easily agitated and irritable
- Reckless behavior and lack of self-control, including:
  - Drinking, and/or drug use, binge eating
  - Poor judgment

Table 12-1 Forms of Bipolar Disorders

Type	Description
Bipolar I	The classic image of bipolar disorder—a full syndrome of manic symptoms and most likely depression episodes
Bipolar II	At least one bout of major depression with episodic occurrence of hypomania. This patient may never have experienced a full episode of mania.
Cyclothymic	A chronic mood disturbance of at least 2 years (one year in children) duration involving numerous episodes of hypomania and depressed mood but of less intensity.
Bipolar disorder due to another medical condition	Prominent and persistent disturbance in mood characterized by mania that is a direct result of physiological effects of a general medical condition
Substance/medication - induced bipolar disorder	Disturbance characterized by elevated, expansive mood with or without depression that is the direct result of the physiological effects of a substance, e.g., alcohol, amphetamines, cocaine, heavy metals

Source: Adapted from Diagnostic and Statistical Manual of Mental Disorders, 5th ed. (2013), American Psychiatric Association; and Townsend (2012), Psychiatric Mental Health Nursing: Concepts of Care in Evidence-Based Practice, 7th ed. Philadelphia: F.A. Davis Company, with permission.

Box 12-1 General Facts About Bipolar Disorders

- 3.9% of the American population will suffer from this disorder in their lifetime.
- Affects males and females at approximately the same rate.
- Episodes may or may not be associated with periods of depression
- It is usually initially diagnosed between ages 15 and 24.
- After the first episode, there is a high risk of recurrence.
- Some have periodic episodes separated by years, and others have much more frequent cycles.
- There is strong evidence for a genetic/inherited link, but a specific genetic defect has not yet been identified.
- Occurs in children but is difficult to diagnose. Symptoms can be confused with attention-deficit/hyperactivity disorder or substance abuse.

Sources: NIMH: www.nimh.nih.gov/health/publications/bipolar-disorder/complete-index.shtml . Kessler RC, Chiu WT, Demler O, Walters EE. Prevalence, severity, and comorbidity of twelve-month DSM-IV disorders in the National Comorbidity Survey Replication (NCS-R). Archives of General Psychiatry, 2005 Jun;62(6):617–27.

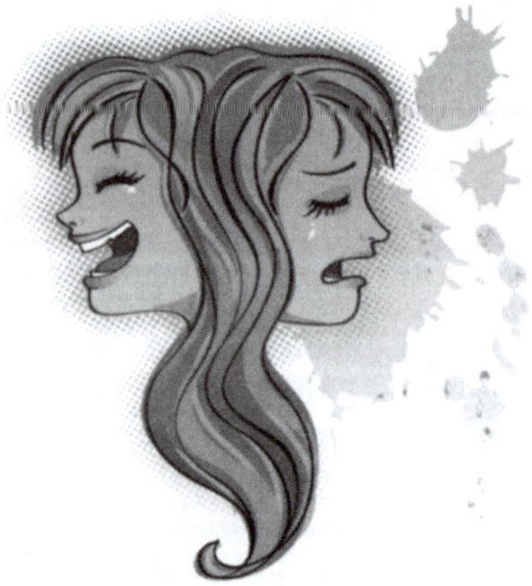

Figure 12-1 Depiction of bipolar disorder.

  - Sex with many partners (promiscuity)
  - Spending sprees
- Very elevated mood
  - Excess activity (hyperactivity)
  - Increased energy
  - Racing thoughts, flight of ideas
  - Talking a lot
  - Very high self-esteem (false beliefs about self or abilities)
- Very involved in activities

In the early phase of a manic episode, an individual can become more engaging and outgoing with high achievement, energy, and success. As a manic phase accelerates, this individual can become frenzied and out of control, leading to impaired decision making and even altered appearance. For example, females experiencing a manic episode may apply their make-up in a distorted manner, especially lipstick. The person may be more reckless in other areas such as business decisions and potentially hazardous actions. The individual in a manic phase may be prone to abuse substances such as tranquilizers and/or alcohol to sleep and control some aspects of this behavior. Substance abuse may also trigger bipolar disorders. The presence of substance abuse with bipolar disorder increases the negative outcomes and can confuse the illness presentation.

Neeb's Tip Patients in a manic phase can go for days without sleep and not feel tired.

Classroom Activity

- Watch films depicting people with bipolar disorder, including *Pollack* and *Lust for Life*.

Depressed Phase

The depressed phase of bipolar disorder is similar to those described for major depressive disorders in Chapter 11. The following symptoms may be seen:

- Low mood or sadness
- Difficulty concentrating, remembering, or making decisions
- Eating problems
  - Loss of appetite and weight loss
  - Overeating and weight gain
- Fatigue or lack of energy
- Feeling worthless, hopeless, or guilty
- Loss of pleasure in activities once enjoyed
- Loss of self-esteem
- Thoughts of death and suicide
- Trouble getting to sleep or sleeping too much
- Pulling away from friends or activities that were once enjoyed

The conversion to manic phase from the depressed phase may appear quickly. Sometimes the two phases of manic and depression overlap. They may occur together or quickly one after the other in what is called a mixed state.

Cultural Considerations

- Bipolar disorder is more common in higher socioeconomic groups.
- As with other psychiatric disorders, misdiagnosis can occur due to misunderstood practices and language barriers. Bipolar disorder can be misdiagnosed as schizophrenia when culturally accepted behaviors are misunderstood.

Tool Box General Behavior Inventory, which has been useful as a self-report monitoring tool in bipolar disorder, is found in Depue, R. A., Slater, J. F., Wolfstetter-Kausch, H., Klein, D., Goplerud, E., & Farr, D. (1981). A behavioral paradigm for identifying persons at risk for bipolar depressive disorder: A conceptual framework and five validation studies. *Journal of Abnormal Psychology, 90,* 381–437.

Mood Disorder Questionnaire: Five-question screening tool: www1.nmha.org/bipolar/questionnaire.cfm

Critical Thinking Question

Your patient on the surgical unit has a diagnosis of cyclothymic disorder. Describe what behaviors you might expect postoperatively.

Etiology of Bipolar Disorders

Biological theories predominate as the cause of bipolar disorder. Studies indicate this disorder is caused by an imbalance in neurotransmitters, particularly norepinephrine, dopamine, and serotonin. Increased levels are believed to be present in manic episodes and decreased in depressive ones. A genetic link has also been demonstrated through family studies. A combination of genetics and biochemical factors, along with environmental triggers such as stressful life events, may present the most comprehensive picture. Medical conditions and medications can trigger an episode in susceptible people. See Box 12-2 for drugs and medical conditions that can precipitate a manic state.

> **Critical Thinking Question**
> Your new patient on the substance abuse unit has a diagnosis of bipolar disorder I as well as alcohol use disorder. How would alcohol use contribute to symptoms in bipolar I?

Treatment of Bipolar Disorders

Treatment for bipolar disorder often starts emergently when family members realize the patient is in a mania state. People are more likely to seek treatment for themselves during depressive phases than during manic phases. When someone is in a state of euphoria, he or she is less prone to accepting treatment and less likely to think there is a need for it (Hirschfeld, 2008). Medications, the most common being mood stabilizers, are the primary treatment. These can be used during an exacerbation as well as for control of frequency and intensity of future episodes (see the Pharmacology Corner).

Treatment should include psychotherapy in combination with medications to reduce the severity of relapse and promote medication compliance. Early diagnosis is also consistent with improved outcomes. Patients are sometimes resistant to taking these medications when they have stabilized due to potential side effects. Therefore, education on medication compliance is an essential part of the treatment plan. After a manic phase, psychotherapy and family therapy may help patients and families cope with the shame and long-term effects of the manic phase. During a manic phase, the patient may have hurt loved ones emotionally with words and actions. As life becomes flatter and less exciting without mania, the patient may need support to cope with life with less highs and more stability. It is common for patients to use alcohol and sedative drugs to try to sleep during manic episodes as well as stimulants during

Box 12-2 Drugs and Physical Illnesses That Can Cause Manic States

Drug Related	Infections
Steroids	Influenza
Levodopa	Q fever
Amphetamines	St. Louis encephalitis
Tricyclic antidepressants	**Red-like infections**
Monoamine oxidase inhibitors	Hyperthyroidism
Methylphenidate	Multiple sclerosis
Cocaine	Systemic lupus erythematosus
Thyroid hormone	Brain tumors
	Stroke

Source: Adapted from Gorman and Sultan (2008), Psychosocial Nursing for General Patient Care, 3rd ed. Philadelphia: F.A. Davis Company, with permission.

Pharmacology Corner

Mood stabilizers are the cornerstone treatment of bipolar disorders. See Table 12-2 for a listing of mood stabilizer medications. These include lithium and a number of anticonvulsants including carbamazepine, valproic acid, and lamotrigine. These medications often are a lifelong regimen. People with bipolar disorder may also continue on antidepressants and may require anti-anxiety and/or antipsychotic drugs such as olanzapine during the acute manic phase. The antipsychotic aripiprazole is also used to treat bipolar disorder. Many patients will continue on more than one medication to remain in remission. Patients must be counseled to report side effects rather than stop medications abruptly. If side effects are too distressing, alternative medication combinations can be prescribed. See Chapter 8 for additional information on mood stabilizers.

Table 12-2 Mood Stabilizers

Drug Category	Drug Examples	Important Considerations
Lithium Carbonate	Lithium, Eskalith, Lithobid	Toxic symptoms can occur even at normal blood levels, so monitoring of adverse effects must be ongoing. May take several weeks to achieve full therapeutic effect. Used with caution in the frail elderly who are at risk for dehydration. Rapid discontinuation can increase risk of relapse. Patient needs to report all other medications to avoid drug interactions.
Anticonvulsants	carbamazepine (Tegretol), gabapentin (Neurontin), valproic acid (Depakene), lamotrigine (Lamictal)	Monitor CBC for possible blood dyscrasias. Increased risk for suicide. May take several weeks to take effect.

Source: Adapted from Townsend (2012), Psychiatric Mental Health Nursing: Concepts of Care in Evidence-Based Practice, 7th ed. Philadelphia: F.A. Davis Company, with permission.

depressive phases, so substance abuse counseling may be part of the treatment plan.

Treatment should also include monitoring adequate fluid and food intake, as these can become compromised during all phases of this disorder.

In the early phases of a manic episode, alternative treatment that includes herbs such as chamomile and valerian can help with mild anxiety and insomnia.

Lithium requires close monitoring, including regular blood levels. Therapeutic levels are between 0.5 and 1.2 mEq/L for most patients (1.0 and 1.5 in acute mania). There is a narrow range between therapeutic and toxic levels, so close monitoring is needed. The blood levels can become elevated in dehydration, profuse sweating, and chronic diarrhea leading to toxicity. Toxicity can cause tremors, confusion, seizures, coma, and even death. Early warning signs of toxicity include nausea, vomiting, and sedation. See Table 12-3 for signs of lithium toxicity. Lithium takes about 7–10 days to reach the desired effect and is only available orally.

A variety of anticonvulsants are used as mood stabilizers. Regular CBCs to monitor for anemia and blood dyscrasias are an important part of the follow-up and patient teaching. Each anticonvulsant has a specific side-effect profile, so this should be incorporated in patient teaching.

Compliance with medication regimen is an ongoing issue with bipolar patients. If

Neeb's Tip

Lithium has a FDA black box warning that toxicity can occur at doses close to therapeutic levels. It should be prescribed when there are resources to provide ongoing blood tests.

Neeb's Tip

Lithium toxicity can develop quickly, especially in dehydration. Patient education must be an ongoing process so patients are reminded to monitor themselves.

Table 12-3 Signs of Lithium Toxicity

Serum Levels	Symptoms
1.5–2.0 mEq/L	Blurred vision, ataxia, tinnitus, nausea, vomiting, diarrhea
2.0–3.5 mEq/L	Excessive output of dilute urine, increased tremors, muscle irritability, confusion
↑3.5 mEq/L	Seizures, coma, oliguria, arrhythmias, cardiovascular collapse

Source: Adapted from Townsend (2012), Psychiatric Mental Health Nursing: Concepts of Care in Evidence-Based Practice, 7th ed. Philadelphia: F.A. Davis Company, with permission.

they are in a euphoric state, they may believe they don't need medications. When they are in remission, they may be more concerned about side effects and stop their medications. Patient teaching and follow-up counseling continue as part of the nursing care of these patients.

See Table 12-4 for the side effects of mood stabilizers.

Neeb's Tip

Bipolar patients on medications should be counseled to use birth control as many of these medications are not safe to use in pregnancy. Patients need to be counseled to speak with their physicians about associated risks.

Neeb's Tip

Anticonvulsant drugs have an adverse effect of increased risk of suicidality. Patients taking such drugs must be monitored closely for worsening depression and suicidal thoughts or behaviors.

Cultural Consideration

Ethnically diverse populations may metabolize medications differently.

Critical Thinking Question

A 29-year-old patient with a history of bipolar I disorder is NPO for surgery. He is routinely taking lithium and lamotrigine. Since he is unable to take these medications, what concerns would you have and what would you monitor?

Nursing Care of the Patient With Bipolar Disorders

Common nursing diagnoses for patients with bipolar disorder include the following:

- Anxiety
- Coping, ineffective
- Nutrition, imbalanced: less than body requirements
- Self-care deficit
- Sleep pattern, disturbed
- Thought process, disturbed

General Nursing Interventions

- Provide clear, firm limits. Clearly define what is expected and what is not allowed. For example, if the patient needs to pace, set a specific area where that can be done; if he is talking too loudly, point

Table 12-4 Side Effects of Mood Stabilizing Agents

Side Effects	Medication	Nursing Implications
Drowsiness, dizziness,	Lithium, anticonvulsants	Educate patient on safety, driving. Determine if dosing schedule allows evening dose.
Dry mouth	Lithium	Sugarless candies, saliva substitute
GI upset	Lithium, anticonvulsants	Administer meds with meals.
Fine hand tremors	Lithium	Report to MD, dosage adjustment may be needed, avoid caffeine.
Polyuria, dehydration	Lithium	Monitor I&O and weight.
Weight gain	Lithium	Need to maintain adequate sodium even if reducing calories.
Increased suicide risk	Anticonvulsants	Monitor for worsening depression, suicide risk.

Source: Adapted from Townsend (2012), Psychiatric Mental Health Nursing: Concepts of Care in Evidence-Based Practice, 7th ed., pp. 622–623. Philadelphia: F.A. Davis Company, with permission.

this out and encourage the need to lower his voice.

- Focus on reality, especially when the patient describes grandiose ideas. Present reality without arguing with patient.
- Remove hazardous objects from the patient's room. Promote safety for all involved in the patient's care by identifying signs of increasing potential for violence.
- Reduce external stimulation such as extraneous noise.
- Provide an outlet for excess energy by letting the patient pace or exercise.
- Encourage activities that don't require a lot of concentration
- Encourage patient compliance with medication regimens and lab testing.
- Take the time to establish a relationship with the patient to promote a sense of safety.
- Identify ways to ensure the patient is eating and drinking adequately; for example, provide food that is easy to eat on the move.
- Encourage the patient to complete thoughts or actions rather than jumping from item to item.
- If the patient is depressed, see the nursing interventions in Chapter 11.

Neeb's Tip

Patients can move quickly from social, affable, highly energetic, fun behavior to angry, violent behavior.

Neeb's Tip

Patients in a manic phase exhibit poor insight and judgment, so this provides a challenge to nurses to manage inappropriate behavior.

Clinical Activity

- Monitor lithium levels.
- Review potential medication side effects that can contribute to the patient's symptoms as well as compliance with mood stabilizers.

Critical Thinking Question

A 45-year-old patient with a long history of bipolar II disorder has been in remission for 5 years. She tells you she has stopped taking her valproic acid because she feels so good and the medication prevented her from losing weight. How should you respond?

Clinical Activity

Identify the family support network for the bipolar patient and ensure that they are knowledgeable on monitoring signs of manic episodes.

Table 12-5 provides the nursing care plan for patients with bipolar disorders.

Classroom Activity

- Review the drug categories for treatment of bipolar disorder and develop patient teaching materials for each.

Key Concepts

1. Bipolar disorders can include severe depressions with periods of extreme mania, as well as severe depressions with minor bouts of mania.
2. The manic phase can last for days, weeks, or months and cause severe disruption in all areas of functioning.
3. Lithium remains a recognized treatment for bipolar disorder and requires monitoring of blood levels to ensure safety.
4. A number of new medications to treat bipolar disorder are now used as well, including many anticonvulsants.
5. Ongoing medication management is challenging as the euphoric patient will often deny the need for these medications.
6. Primary nursing interventions for a patient in mania include maintenance of safety, promotion of health, and medication compliance.

Table 12-5 Nursing Care Plan for Patients With Bipolar Disorders

Data Collection	Nursing Diagnosis	Plan/Goal	Interventions	Evaluation
Inappropriate behavior including loud conversation, swearing, domineering	Ineffective coping	Patient will display more socially acceptable behaviors	Calmly point out to patient what behavior is not appropriate, e.g., "you're talking too loud again." Avoid sounding angry or judgmental. Set limits on swearing. Do not argue, bargain, or threaten patient. Explore how the patient can vent his frustration/energy in more socially acceptable ways. Provide alternative ways to express self.	Patient is able to control one behavior for a set period of time.

CASE STUDY

Jonathan is a 30-year-old single attorney living in New York City. He recently joined a prestigious law firm and is anxious to make a strong impression with the partners. He has a long history of success in life, including graduating from a top law school with excellent scores, making a large income, and having many friends and associates. He is gregarious and always seems to be the center of attention wherever he is. His new position is more stressful than his previous jobs were. He has been sleeping only 2 to 3 hours a night and then coming in to the office at 4 a.m. to keep up with the workload. He drinks heavily at night to try to sleep and uses stimulants in the morning to keep going. He has received a lot of attention in the office for a recent successful litigation. However, his assistant notes he is increasingly irritable and demanding, often changing from charming to angry at the slightest frustration. A woman in the office reports him to the superiors for inappropriate sexual advances. When he is brought into the office to discuss the allegations, he explodes and storms out of the office. Later that night he is arrested in a bar for fighting with a patron and tells the police he is friends with the chief of police and will get the officer fired.

Jonathan is brought to the ER by the police and acknowledges he had been diagnosed with bipolar disorder in college but stopped taking his lithium a year ago.

1. What other information would you need to know regarding what type of bipolar disorder he has?
2. What were the early signs that Jonathan was escalating into a manic phase?
3. What questions would you ask him regarding his history?

REFERENCES

Akiskai, H.S. (2009). Mood disorders: Treatment of bipolar disorder. In B.J. Sadock, V.A. Sadock, and P. Ruiz. (Eds.), *Kaplan & Sadock's Comprehensive textbook of Psychiatry*. 9th ed., pp. 1743–1813. Philadelphia: Wolters Kluwer/Lippincott Williams and Wilkins.

Carson, V.B., and Yambor, S.L. (2012). Managing patients with bipolar disorder at home. *Home health nurse 30*(5), 280–91.

Gorman, L.M. and Sultan, D.F. (2008). *Psychosocial Nursing for General Patient Care*. 3rd ed. Philadelphia: F.A. Davis.

Kessler, R.C., Chiu, W.T., and Demler, O. (2005). Prevalence, severity, and comorbidity of twelve-month DSM-IV disorders in the National Comorbidity Survey Replication. *Archives of general psychiatry, 62*(6):617–627.

McMurrach, S. (2012). Course outcomes and psychosocial interventions for first-episode mania. *Bipolar disorders 14*(6), 1–12.

National Institutes of Mental Health. Bipolar disorder. Retrieved from www.nimh.nih.gov/health/topics/bipolar-disorder/index.shtml

Sorrel, J.M. (2011). Caring for older adults with bipolar disorder. *Journal of psychosocial nursing and mental health services, 49*(7), 21–25.

Townsend, M.C. (2012). *Psychiatric Mental Health Nursing*. 7th ed. Philadelphia: F.A. Davis.

Ward, T. D. (2011). The lived experience of adults with bipolar disorder and comorbid substance abuse disorder. *Issues in mental health nursing 32*(1), 22–27.

Test Questions

Multiple Choice Questions

1. Mrs. A is admitted to the medical/surgical unit with a diagnosis of dehydration and pneumonia. She has a history of bipolar disorder and is controlled on lithium. As her nurse, you know you must:
  a. Treat her carefully because she may become catatonic.
  b. Observe for signs of lithium toxicity from dehydration.
  c. Alert the other staff of the "psych" patient on the unit.
  d. Treat the medical illness only.

2. Mrs. D has an appointment with the doctor. She began taking lithium one month ago as prescribed. She now states that her mouth and lips are constantly dry and she sometimes feels confused. She says, "I stagger like I'm drunk sometimes when I walk." You suspect:
  a. She is drinking to combat her depression.
  b. She is making it up to get different medications.
  c. She took too much lithium.
  d. She is dehydrated.

3. Marge is a 68-year-old woman with a long history of bipolar disorder I. She is brought to the emergency room by her sister, who reports that Marge has been increasingly agitated, is unable to sleep, and told her daughter that the mayor was calling her for advice on running the city. The behavior is an example of:
  a. Delusions of grandeur
  b. Delusions of persecution
  c. Auditory hallucinations
  d. Schizophrenia

4. The physician orders lithium carbonate 600 mg tid for a newly diagnosed bipolar patient. The therapeutic blood level for acute mania is:
  a. 1.0–1.5 mEq/L
  b. 10–15 mEq/L
  c. 0.5–1.0 mEq/L
  d. 5–10 mEq/L

5. Which of the following drugs is NOT classified as mood stabilizer?
  a. Carbamazepine
  b. Olanzapine
  c. Valproic acid
  d. Gabapentin

6. Your manic patient says, "Everything I do is great." How should you respond?
  a. "Yes, I am happy for you."
  b. "Is there a time in your life when things didn't go as planned?"
  c. "No one can be great at everything."
  d. "Keep it up."

7. Your manic patient has lost 5 pounds and is underweight. Which meal is most appropriate?
  a. Grilled chicken and baked potato
  b. Spaghetti and meatballs
  c. Chili and crackers
  d. Chicken fingers and French fries

8. A newly admitted patient in an acute manic state has a nursing diagnosis of risk for injury related to hyperactivity. Which nursing intervention is most appropriate?
  a. Place the patient in a room with another hyperactive patient.
  b. Have the patient sit in his room while you review all the rules of the unit.
  c. Administer antipsychotic medication as ordered prn by the physician.
  d. Reinforce previously learned coping mechanisms to calm the patient down.

9. Which statement is most true about bipolar disorder?
  a. Bipolar disorders all follow the same pattern of behavior.
  b. Bipolar disorders always include periods of major depression.
  c. Manic depression is the same as hypomanic disorder.
  d. Patients with bipolar II have major depression with hypomanic symptoms.

Test Questions

cont.

10. Which category of medication would not be given to a patient with bipolar disorder?
a. Stimulant
b. Antidepressant
c. Antipsychotic
d. Anti-anxiety

11. What is cyclothymic disorder?
a. A chronic mood disorder of at least 2 years
b. A one-time event of hypomania
c. A continuous state of hypomania for 2 years
d. A chronic depression for 2 years

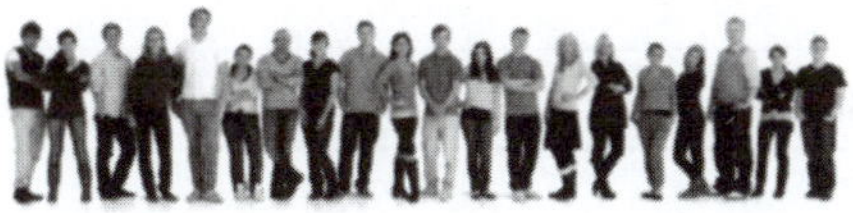

CHAPTER 13

Suicide

Learning Objectives

1. Identify main populations at risk for suicide.
2. Identify myths and truths about suicide.
3. Identify warning signs of suicide.
4. Identify nursing care for people who are suicidal.
5. Describe the management of a suicidal patient in the acute hospital.

Key Terms

- Lethality
- Suicide
- Suicide attempt
- Suicide contract
- Suicide ideation
- Suicide pact
- Survivor of suicide

■ The Reality of Suicide

Suicide is defined as self-inflicted death, with evidence that the person intended to die. Many people experience momentary self-destructive thoughts during a bout of depression or a setback in life, but they do not take action on these thoughts. Thinking about suicide does not mean the individual will act on those thoughts; however, anyone who talks about, threatens, or makes a **suicide attempt** must be taken seriously. Because suicide is viewed as unacceptable in Western culture, it generates anxiety that has led to a number of myths. See Table 13-1 for a list of common myths.

Here are some important facts about suicide in the United States:

- Suicide is the 10th leading cause of death in the United States, accounting for more than 1% of all deaths.
- More people die from suicide than from homicide.
- More years of life are lost to suicide than to any other single cause except heart disease and cancer.
- 37,000 Americans died by suicide in 2010, which included four times as many men as women; an additional 500,000 Americans attempt suicide annually.
- Suicide crosses all cultural, age, gender, race, and socioeconomic groups.
- The actual ratio of attempts to completed suicides is probably at least 10 to 1.
- A high percentage of people who complete suicide have made a previous attempt.
- The risk of completed suicide is more than 100 times greater than average in the first year after an attempt—80 times greater for women, 200 times greater for men, 200 times greater for people over 45, and 300 times greater for white men over 65.
- Suicide rates are highest in the age group of 45–54 years, with the over-85 group close behind (Fig. 13-1).
- Veterans returning from war have a higher rate of suicide than civilians.
- Suicide is the third leading cause of death among adolescents and young adults.
- **Suicide pacts** or copycat suicides among some adolescent groups have been seen in some communities.
- Single auto crashes are generally investigated as possible suicides.
- 8.3% of adults have serious thoughts of suicide during any year.
- The most common methods of suicide include firearms, hanging, and overdose. The **lethality** of suicide methods is a factor in the assessment of the patient. Men more commonly use the highly lethal methods of

Table 13-1 Clearing Up the Myths About Suicide

Myth	Truth
Asking people about their suicidal thoughts will make them more likely to act on them.	Most people are not afraid to talk about their thoughts of committing suicide and are usually grateful that someone is available and cares. Talking can reduce the sense of isolation.
All people who attempt suicide have a psychiatric disorder.	People can become overwhelmed with life circumstances without having a psychiatric disorder.
A person who talks about suicide will not do it.	Approximately 80% of individuals who attempt or complete suicide give some definite verbal or indirect clues. As many as 50% have seen their physician within the previous month, often with vague somatic complaints.
A person who attempts suicide will not try again.	Almost 75% of those individuals who complete suicide have attempted it at least once before.
People who attempt suicide are always determined to die.	Many individuals are ambivalent and are using the suicide as a cry for help.
People who attempt suicide just want attention.	Even if the suicide attempt is manipulative, the individual may go on to complete the suicide.
As the person becomes less depressed, the risk of suicide decreases.	As the depression begins to lift, the individual's energy level can increase before feelings of hopelessness are relieved. Once the individual makes the decision that suicide is an effective solution to the problems, his or her mood may even elevate.

Source: From Gorman and Sultan (2008). Psychosocial Nursing for General Patient Care, 3rd ed. Philadelphia: F.A. Davis Company, with permission.

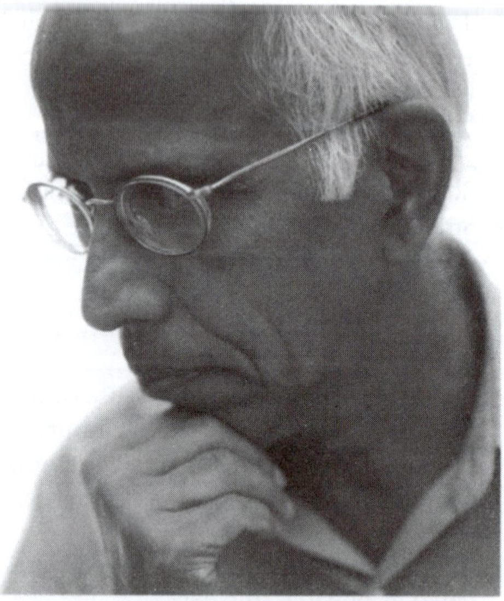

Figure 13-1 Older adults often have difficulty coping with loss, loneliness, and depression, and they have very high rates of suicide.

firearms and hanging, accounting for their higher death rate. Those who overdose have a greater chance of surviving because they receive treatment if found in time.

- For every person who commits suicide, six persons on average are left behind as **survivors of suicide.**

(References include: National Center for Health Statistics Suicide and Self-Inflicted Injury, 2012; Mental Health America: Suicide, 2012; National Health and Nutrition Examination Survey, 2010; Substance Abuse and Mental Health Services Administration Newsroom, 2012; CDC Morbidity and Mortality Weekly Report, 2013.)

Classroom Activity

- Discuss factors that contribute to suicide in today's society.
- Discuss the impact on yourself of suicide of well-known people.

Suicide remains a major public health problem, and all nurses must be familiar with risk factors, warning signs, and interventions to provide support to individuals at risk. Suicide can be a long-planned action or an impulsive act when the person is overwhelmed. People with a variety of psychiatric disorders, including depression, bipolar disorder, anxiety

Cultural Considerations

White males constitute the largest group of suicides. Native American males are also at high risk. African American females tend to have a lower rate (Goldston, 2008). Some groups are less prone to suicide based on religion; for example, Roman Catholics. Some cultures, however, are more tolerant than others of suicide.

disorders, personality disorders, and substance abuse, may consider suicide. Drugs or alcohol can contribute to accidental overdoses when the individual's judgment is impaired or be part of the self-destructive cycle. The *Diagnostic and Statistical Manual of Mental Disorders* (DSM-5) has created a new category, named Suicidal Behavior Disorder, for an individual who has initiated a behavior with the expectation that it would lead to the individual's own death within the last 24 months. Psychotic individuals can also experience hallucinations in which they believe they are being told to kill themselves by voices or powers outside of themselves. Being alert to signals that the patient is at risk for suicide requires good observation skills and communication with the patient and health-care team.

Critical Thinking Question

Your teenager tells you a friend swore her to secrecy that she was going to kill herself because her boyfriend rejected her. Your teen asks you not to tell anyone. What action should you take?

Etiology of Suicide

Research shows that the risk for suicide is associated with changes in brain chemicals called neurotransmitters, including serotonin. Decreased levels of serotonin have been found in people with depression, impulsive disorders, a history of suicide attempts, and suicide victims (National Institute of Mental Health Statistics on Suicide, 2012).

Psychological factors, such as anger turned on oneself; an overwhelming sense of hopelessness, shame, and guilt; and humiliation, have been linked to **suicidal ideation**. Suicide may be viewed by some as a relief from overwhelming suffering (physical or emotional); some see it as a way to reunite with a loved one who has died. A psychotic individual may view suicide as a way to stop hallucinations, or the hallucinations may be telling the patient to commit suicide.

See Box 13-1 for a list of common risk factors for suicide.

Box 13-1 Risk Factors for Suicide

Risk factors for suicide include the following:

- More than 90% of people who die by suicide have a mood disorder and/or a substance abuse disorder. Mood disorder can include depression or bipolar disorder.
- Suicide risk can increase at the beginning of treatment with antidepressants as the return of energy brings increased ability to act out self-destructive thoughts.
- Alcohol is involved in many suicides.
- Prior suicide attempt
- Family history of mental disorder, substance abuse, family violence, sexual abuse, or suicide
- Exposure to the suicidal behavior of others, such as family members, peers, or media figures
- Poor support system
- Grief from recent loss
- Untreated symptoms in terminal illness

Source: From U.S. Public Health Service (1999) and Centers for Disease Control and Prevention (2010).

Suicide crosses all age groups. See Chapter 19 for more information on suicidal behavior in children and adolescents. Older adults, especially those facing health issues and multiple losses, may be at risk for suicide. It is common for suicidal older adults to have seen a health-care provider in the prior year, so identifying any risk factors in elderly patients is an important part of the care plan. White elderly men are known to have one of the highest suicide rates.

The Warning Signs of Suicide

One of these signs does not necessarily mean the person is considering suicide, but several of them may signal a call for help. Eight out of 10 people considering suicide give some sign of their intentions, so these warning signs can save lives if recognized in time. People who talk about suicide, threaten suicide, or call suicide crisis centers are 30 times more likely to kill themselves. Suicidal people often reach out for help and generally retain some ambivalence or contradictory feelings experienced simultaneously. Consequently, getting help to someone who is considering suicide can save a life. Most people who consider suicide have some level of ambivalence.

The suicide warning signs from the National Center for Health Statistics on Suicide include the following:

- Verbal suicide threats, such as "You'd be better off without me," "Maybe I won't be around," or "I won't be here when you come back to work"
- Expressions of hopelessness and helplessness and the inability to see alternatives
- Previous suicide attempts
- Talking about suicide methods to which the person has access
- Saving pills
- Asking questions/researching about different methods of committing suicide
- Daring or risk-taking behavior
- Personality changes
- Depression
- Lack of interest in future plans

(National Center for Health Statistics Suicide and Self-Inflicted Injury, 2012)

Other warning signs may include the following:

1. *Noticeable improvement in mood occurs:* When this happens in a suicidal person, it is often a sign that the person has made the decision that has been causing personal conflict. The pain that is being experienced will soon be over for that person. The feelings of those who will be left behind may or may not be a consideration. It has been said that suicide is the ultimate controller. For some people, this may be the only situation they have felt they could control in their lives. Some people are not concerned about the survivors because their own pain overrides that of others. Some people, especially younger ones, may view death in a more romanticized way. Television, movies, and computer games that show death often do so in a way that is glamorous or humorous. Young people may not make the connection between the fantasy of the media and the reality of life, or they become so caught up in seeking revenge or making others suffer that they do not consider the finality of what they are attempting.
2. *Person starts giving away personal items:* When someone has made the decision to terminate his or her own life, it becomes no longer necessary to keep certain things. Some people will even attempt to give away a beloved pet. However, these individuals do want those items cared for. In an attempt to "tie up loose ends," they decide who will get certain items. The items will be given away for reasons other than "because I am going to kill myself," although people sometimes use that honest approach and are not taken seriously. Usually, these people will simply say that it is time to clean out a certain room or that they no longer need a certain item and they would like it to go to a special friend. Individuals may also write or change a will when contemplating suicide.
3. *Person starts talking about death and suicide or becomes preoccupied with learning about these things:* Curiosity about death is not unusual. People tend to be curious about what they do not know. When this curiosity becomes a preoccupation and a single thought for the patient, it signals that the patient has ideas of attempting suicide. Reporting this to the charge nurse and documenting the concerns are required.

> **Classroom Activity**
> Movies with suicide themes include *The Hours* and *Whose Life Is It Anyway?*

Treatment of Individuals at Risk for Suicide

Suicide is a major public health concern. Prevention is focused on identifying people who display the warning signs and risk factors, and providing them with support and interventions. Anyone who talks about suicide must be taken seriously and interventions instituted immediately to address her or his concerns and problems. Individual and group psychotherapy; emergency psychiatric care such as hotlines and on-call mental health professionals; pharmacological treatment for depression, psychosis, and anxiety; and inpatient hospitalization if the person is at high risk for suicide are some of the approaches. Patients who make multiple suicide attempts need ongoing psychotherapy to address their issues and impulses. Patients at low to moderate risk for suicide can be followed as outpatients with adequate support built in the treatment plan, such as family and friends, suicide contracts, medications, and regular mental health appointments.

Family and friends of anyone who commits suicide need special support. These individuals are referred to as survivors of suicide and are at risk for long-term emotional distress, especially related to guilt and anger and their elusive search for "why?" The stigma of suicide adds to the complexity of a lifetime of trying to recover. Support groups are available in many communities for survivors of suicide.

Tool Box

- Suicidology.org has many resources for suicidal patients, their families, and professionals, including support programs for survivors: www.suicidology.org/suicide-survivors
- National Suicide Prevention Lifeline offers a 24/7 free and confidential, nationwide network of crisis centers: 1-800-273-TALK (8255)
- Federal government mandated suicide prevention hotline number: 1-888-SUICIDE (1-888-784-2433)

Pharmacology Corner

Suicidal patients may benefit from taking anti-anxiety medication, such as lorazepam, to reduce feelings of intense anxiety or distress. In addition, antipsychotic and antimanic medications may be prescribed as needed for patients with bipolar or psychotic disorders. If antidepressants are being started, it is important to remember that it will take a number of weeks to lift depression, so other interventions must be used in the interim to prevent suicide. Antidepressants could actually increase suicide risk if the patient gets a sudden burst of energy to act out the plan before the depression lifts. However, untreated depression puts the patient at greater risk, so antidepressants are generally seen as protection against suicide.

Patients at high risk for suicide may need to have medications administered in liquid or parenteral form to avoid "cheeking" and hoarding pills that could be collected to use for an overdose. Outpatients should be given only a few days' supply of any medication that could potentially be used in a suicide attempt. Overdosing on antidepressants is a highly lethal method of suicide, so caution must be taken with how these are dispensed for someone at high risk.

Adequate symptom management for pain and other distressing symptoms must be provided to the patient with a serious or terminal illness. A patient's belief that his or her symptoms cannot be controlled could be a contributing factor in hopelessness and suicide.

Nursing Care of the Suicidal Patient

Common nursing diagnoses in those at risk for suicide include the following:

- Hopelessness
- Violence to self, risk for
- Anxiety
- Coping, ineffective
- Self-concept, disturbed
- Spiritual distress
- Thought processes, altered

Nursing responsibilities for patients who are suicidal are many. The goal, of course, is always to prevent the suicide. Because the nurse may not know when suicide potential exists, especially for a first attempt, using excellent observational skills and communication skills is mandatory. Nurses are bound (under the *Meier v. Ross General Hospital* case) to report any reasons they have to suspect the patient may be suicidal. Nurses must report their observations to their team and document actions in the health-care record. A nurse should never take the responsibility of helping a suicidal person on his or her own. Once a nurse suspects suicidal ideation, informing all members of the health-care team is essential so appropriate treatment and patient safety can be ensured. If a patient is considered suicidal, the following interventions can be helpful.

General Nursing Interventions

1. *Monitoring frequently:* Check on the suicidal patient frequently but avoid a predictable routine and ensure that the patient is checked during extra-busy times like shift change. If the patient is actively suicidal, a psychiatric consultation will be required and the patient may be placed on 1:1 precautions until the patient can be moved to an appropriate treatment setting. On 1:1 precautions the nurse will be required to accompany and remain with the patient in the bathroom. Nurses must follow their agency policies on providing safety for the suicidal patient.
2. *Safety:* Keep any potentially harmful items away from the patient, such as knives, scissors, glass, razor blades, belts, nail files, electrical cords, and even linens. Inform visitors of this so they do not bring items patient may request. Ensure that windows cannot be opened. The room may need to be searched periodically, and the patient may need a body search and close monitoring in the bathroom. It is common for patients who are at very high risk for suicide to wear paper gowns and to have paper bedding. Large objects that can be used to break a window also need to be removed. Plastic trash bags should not be used in the patient's room.

Tool Box |▶ American Association of Suicidology Guidelines for Inpatient and Residential Patients Known to Be at Elevated Risk for Suicide at:
http://www.suicidology.org/c/document_library/get_file?folderId=266&name=DLFE-613.pdf

Clinical Activity

- If your patient has been identified as suicidal, review the care plan for all the safety measures in place for this patient.
- Review policies from assigned hospitals on how to manage suicidal patients.

3. *Communication:* Ask outright if the patient is considering suicide and, if so, how and when. Asking a patient to talk about suicidal thoughts does not enhance the chance of completing a suicide. Rather, it demonstrates caring and acknowledges his or her value as a person. Ask if the patient has attempted suicide in the past. In addition, be prepared to talk to the patient about his or her feelings, work to reframe hopelessness, and assist in problem solving to identify alternative solutions to problems the patient views as insurmountable. When talking to someone who is suicidal, avoid platitudes like "think what this would do to your children." Often the suicidal person is so immersed in feelings of hopelessness and isolation that he is unable to identify with how others are feelings. In addition, the patient may view that the family will be better off without him. When working on problem solving, break down one problem into manageable steps rather than looking at the whole picture, which can be overwhelming. Most people who are suicidal have ambivalent or mixed feelings about taking action. Supporting the reasons the person does not want to commit suicide can help the person to reevaluate the situation.

Neeb's Tip

- If you suspect someone is suicidal, be direct in asking about his or her plans.
- Suicide is an emotional subject and great care must be taken with anyone who expresses suicidal ideation. Report any suicidal ideation or behavior immediately.
- The hopelessness experienced by a suicidal patient can be draining and overwhelming for the nurse. Recognize that team members need extra support when working with anyone who is suicidal.

Clinical Activity
If your patient has a history of suicide attempts, discuss any concerns with your instructor.

4. *Contract:* The treating team may want to consider making a **suicide contract** with the patient. This is a written agreement between the patient and the treating team where the patient agrees to inform the team before taking any action to harm him- or herself. See the Toolbox to access a sample contract. A contract is helpful for some patients who are wavering on what to do.

Tool Box Example of suicide contract at www.suicide.org/no-suicide-contracts.html

5. *Discharge planning:* Any patient with suicidal ideation needs close follow-up at time of discharge from the hospital. Mental health follow-up, hotline numbers, involving family/friends in the discharge plan, and ensuring that discharge prescriptions are dispensed in small amounts are some things to be incorporated in the plan. (Guptill, 2011; Puskar & Urda, 2011; Rittenmeyer, 2012; Sun, 2011).

See Box 13-2 for suggestions on talking with a suicidal patient to evaluate lethality.

Critical Thinking Question
Your 85-year-old patient is a recent widower. He is in the hospital for recovery from a recent fall. He tells you he wants to go home so he can be with his wife. How would you respond to that statement?

Critical Thinking Question
Your patient with multiple chronic health problems has been diagnosed by the psychiatrist as actively suicidal. She is too ill to be transferred to the psychiatric unit. Describe what actions the team should take to prevent a suicide attempt on your medical surgical unit.

Table 13-2 provides the nursing care plan for suicidal patients.

Classroom Activity
Obtain information about local suicide prevention programs such as counseling centers and hotlines.

Neeb's Tip
Patients who are terminally ill may verbalize vague suicidal thoughts such as "I would kill myself if my pain gets too bad." Encourage your patient to talk about fears and discomforts. Patients with good symptom management are much less likely to think about suicide.

Clinical Activity
When administering medications to suicidal patients, consider having a colleague with you to double-check that the patient has swallowed the pills.

Box 13-2 Talking With a Suicidal Patient to Evaluate Lethality

1. Do you think about hurting or killing yourself? If yes↓
2. Do you have a plan? How have you considered doing it? If yes↓
3. Do you think you may or will do something to act on your thoughts? If yes, where and when? Do you feel you have control over your own behavior?
4. Do you have the means available (such as rope, rolled-up sheet, gun, saved-up pills [note lethality of plan])?
5. Have you ever tried to harm yourself in the past? If yes, how? Did you expect to survive?
6. Are you willing to contract or notify staff whenever you feel you may act on these thoughts?

Our side of the contract is to be available and actively help you during these times.

If the patient denies having a suicide plan, ask about other plans for the future and support systems.

1. What do you see yourself doing in a week, in a month, and in a year from now?
2. Do you feel optimistic or pessimistic about the future?
3. Do you have family members or friends with whom you can freely discuss your problems?

Source: From Gorman and Sultan (2008). Psychosocial Nursing for General Patient Care, 3rd ed. Philadelphia: F.A. Davis Company, with permission.

Table 13-2 Nursing Care Plan for Suicidal Patients

Assessment/ Data Collection	Nursing Diagnosis	Plan/Goal	Interventions/ Nursing Actions	Evaluation
Patient describes hopelessness; unable to view the future in a positive manner; denies options to resolve dilemmas; verbalizes suicide as only alternative	Hopelessness	Verbalize possible solutions to current problems	Listen to patient's concerns and worries. Avoid minimizing them. Help patient identify one problem and discuss alternative ways to view it. Provide a different perspective on the problems. Appeal to the patient's ambivalence by stressing reasons he does not want to do this. Describe a recent situation where you observed the patient being successful.	Patient agrees to try one alternative solution to recent problem.

Key Concepts

1. Suicide is the 10th leading cause of death in this country and remains a serious public health problem. All nurses must be aware of risk factors and warning signs for suicide in their patients and take action as needed.
2. Caring for a suicidal patient requires excellent observation and communication skills, including working collaboratively with team members to keep the patient safe.
3. The most common psychiatric diagnoses for suicidal patients include depression and substance abuse.
4. Most people considering suicide have some ambivalence, so they will often leave clues as to their plans.

CASE STUDY

Jeff is a 54-year-old man who is recently divorced with four grown children. He is living alone in a furnished apartment and was recently laid off from his accounting job. He spends most days alone and has started drinking in the morning. He recently got a DUI and had to give up his driver's license. He has been a hunter all his life and has a variety of guns in a local storage unit. He has several close friends who report that Jeff is depressed, irritable, and much less sociable. They call him to go out, but he repeatedly declines. One friend calls Jeff's ex-wife to tell her that Jeff called him and was quite emotional, saying he feels guilty for the way he treated her and his children over the years. Jeff told the friend he feels like a failure in life and wonders if his kids would be better off if he were not around. The friend tells Jeff's ex-wife that he believes Jeff is thinking of moving away.

1. With the information presented, what signs would suggest that Jeff may be suicidal?
2. What suggestions would you give Jeff's ex-wife and his friend to address potential suicidal ideation?
3. If Jeff's ex-wife brought him to your mental health clinic, what information would you want to know initially?

REFERENCES

American Psychiatric Association. (2013). *Diagnostic and Statistical Manual of Mental Disorders 5*. Washington, DC, Author. (Known as DSM-5)

Centers for Disease Control and Prevention (2013). Suicide Among Adults Aged 35–64 Years United States 1999–2010. *Morbidity and mortality report* 6/13/13. http://www.cdc.gov/mmwr/preview/mmwrhtml/mm6217a1.htm?s_cid=mm6217_w

Centers for Disease Control and Prevention. (2010). Violence Prevention. Retrieved from www.cdc.gov/ViolencePrevention/suicide/riskprotectivefactors.html

Gelenberg A.J., et al. (2010). *Practice Guideline for the Treatment of Patients with Major Depressive Disorder.* 3rd ed. American Psychiatric Association. Retrieved from http://psychiatryonline.org/content.aspx?bookid=28&sectionid=1667485#654166

Goldston, D.B., et al. (2008). Cultural consideration in adolescent suicide prevention and psychosocial treatment. *American psychologist, 63,* 14–31.

Gorman, L., and Sultan, D. (2008). *Psychosocial Nursing for General Patient Care.* 3rd ed. Philadelphia: F.A. Davis.

Guptill, J. 2011. After an attempt: caring for the suicidal patient on the medical-surgical unit. *Medical-surgical nursing, 20*(4), 163–167.

Mental health America: Suicide. 2012. Retrieved from www.nmha.org/go/suicide

National Center for Health Statistics suicide and self-inflicted injury. 2012. Retrieved from www.cdc.gov/nchs.fastfacts/suicide.htm

National Health and Nutrition Examination Survey. 2010. Retrieved from www.cdc.gov/nchs/nhanes.htm

National Institute of Mental Health statistics on suicide. 2012. Retrieved from www.nimh.gov/health/publications/suicide-in-the-us-statistics-and-prevention/index.shtml

National Strategy for Suicide Prevention: Goals and Objectives for Action: A report of the U.S. Surgeon General and of the National Action Alliance for Suicide Prevention. 2012. Office of the Surgeon General (U.S.): National Action Alliance for Suicide Prevention (U.S.). Washington D.C.: US Department of Health and Human Services, September 2012. http://www.ncbi.nlm.nih.gov/books/NBK109922/

Puskar, K., and Urda, B. (2011). Examining the efficacy of no-suicide contracts in inpatient psychiatric settings: implications for psychiatric nursing. *Issues in mental health nursing, 32*(12), 785–788.

Rittenmeyer, L. (2012). Assessment of risk for in-hospital suicide and aggression in high-dependency care environments. *Critical Care nursing in clinics of North America, 24*(1), 41–51.

Substance Abuse and Mental Health Services Administration Behavioral Health, United States, 2012 at http://samhsa/gov

Sun, F.K. (2011). A concept analysis of suicidal behavior. *Public health nursing, 28*(5), 458–468.

U.S. Public Health Service. The surgeon general's call to action to prevent suicide. Washington D.C.: US Department of Health and Human Services, 1999. Retrieved from www.surgeongeneral.gov/library/calltoaction/default.htm.

Test Questions

Multiple Choice Questions

1. A nursing intervention that is appropriate for a patient who is suicidal is:
   a. Report the patient to the police.
   b. Ignore the patient's suicidal comments, considering them "attention getting."
   c. Tell the patient that he or she "has so much to live for!"
   d. Listen to the patient's concerns and worries

2. A person is more likely to commit suicide when he or she:
   a. Is in deepest depression
   b. Has a sudden lift from previous depressed mood
   c. Is confused
   d. Is feeling loved and appreciated

3. Your patient tells you, "I am just a burden. Everyone would be better off if I was dead." Nurses are aware that:
   a. Suicide talk is just an attention-getting device.
   b. Suicide is an impulsive act; it is not thought out.
   c. Suicidal talk or ideation can lead to suicidal behavior.
   d. Suicidal people seldom really attempt suicide.

4. Mr. P is brought to the hospital by his wife. She states that he has been treated for depression recently, but that tonight he said, "You and the kids don't need me messing up your lives." Mr. P tells you he has been thinking about suicide for some time now. A nursing diagnosis for Mr. P would be:
   a. Knowledge deficit related to family needs
   b. Ineffective individual coping as evidenced by manipulation of wife's feelings
   c. Anxiety related to hospitalization
   d. Potential for violence, self-directed, as evidenced by stating suicidal thoughts

5. Your charge nurse tells you that Mr. P must be placed on suicide precautions. The first intervention you begin is:
   a. Place Mr. P in a locked unit.
   b. Begin one-on-one observation at least every 15 minutes.
   c. Call the security code over the public address system.
   d. Allow Mr. P to shave and carry out his bedtime care.

6. Further discussion with Mr. P reveals he is of a religious sect that believes there is honor in dying for one's religion. He does not understand why everyone is so afraid to die in this country. As his nurse, you:
   a. Document the discussion and remove the suicide precautions, citing religious freedom.
   b. Encourage him to present his beliefs at group tomorrow.
   c. Document the discussion but tell him that the suicide precautions remain in effect.
   d. Thank him for his explanation and bring him his next dose of medication.

7. Which of the following people is at highest risk for suicide based on the information provided?
   a. Nancy is a 33-year-old mother of two who just lost her mother in a motor vehicle accident.
   b. Jim is a 68-year-old man who is a recent widower and has a long history of alcohol abuse.
   c. Carol, age 18, has a long history of sickle cell disease and is depressed over chronic pain and the inability to attend her prom.
   d. Hans is a 55-year-old man with end stage pancreatic cancer who is entering a hospice program.

Test Questions

cont.

8. Susan is 27 years old and has been admitted from the ED with an overdose of an antidepressant. She tells you, "My boyfriend broke up with me and I can't live without him." What is your best response?
- a. "You are young. You will find someone else."
- b. "Forget him. You can do better than him. He isn't worth losing your life for."
- c. "Why did he break up with you?"
- d. "You must have been feeling very sad when he told you."

9. The next day, Susan tells you that she has another plan to "finish the job when I get out of here. Please don't tell anyone." What would be your best response?
- a. "You are safe here."
- b. "What are you planning to do?"
- c. "I won't tell anyone if you promise not to do anything to yourself."
- d. "I was hoping you were feeling better."

10. The fact that Susan is telling you sh another plan indicates what?
- a. She is reaching out for help and ambivalent about wanting to die
- b. She is committed to her suicide
- c. She is psychotic.
- d. She needs antidepressants started right away.

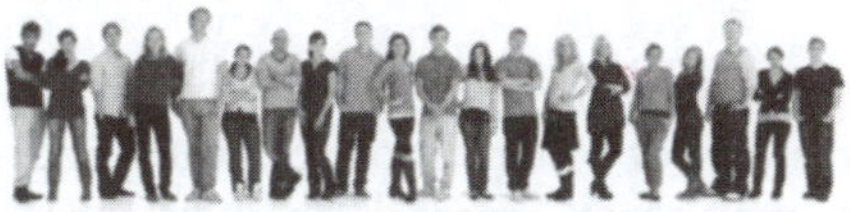

CHAPTER 14

Personality Disorders

Learning Objectives

1. Define and differentiate between personality and personality disorder.
2. Describe three personality disorders as designated by DSM-5.
3. Describe two behavioral symptoms of each of these three personality disorders.
4. Identify nursing interventions for these three disorders.
5. Discuss some of the challenges in caring for a patient with borderline personality disorder.

Key Terms

- Antisocial personality disorder
- Avoidant personality
- Borderline personality
- Dependent personality disorder
- Histrionic personality disorder
- Narcissistic personality
- Obsessive-compulsive personality disorder
- Paranoid personality disorder
- Personality
- Personality disorder
- Schizoid personality disorder
- Schizotypal personality disorder
- Self-mutilating behavior

Personality is defined as the complex characteristics that distinguish an individual. It includes one's thoughts, feelings, and attitudes. Personality traits are enduring patterns of perceiving, relating to, and thinking about the environment and oneself that are exhibited in a wide range of social and personal contexts. Personality development occurs in response to a number of biological and psychological influences. Theorists include Erik Erikson. **Personality disorders** occur when these traits become inflexible and maladaptive, and cause either significant functional impairment or subjective distress (Townsend, 2012). Most people display some traits of these disorders from time to time, but only when they are consistent behaviors that contribute to some dysfunction in different areas of life do they become personality disorders. Personality disorders are frequently seen in the general population and may coexist with other psychiatric disorders. It is common that more than one personality disorder exists in these patients. Patients with these disorders can present challenges for the nurse as maladaptive mechanisms including manipulation are used to cope with the stresses of their illnesses.

❃ Cultural Considerations

Personality development is impacted by culture. Thoughts, feelings, and attitudes are influenced by the cultural values surrounding people.

There are 10 personality disorders as described in DSM-5. These 10 disorders are grouped in 3 clusters based on their similarities.

1. **Cluster A** (Behaviors described as odd)
   - **Paranoid personality disorder**
   - **Schizoid personality disorder**
   - **Schizotypal personality disorder**
2. **Cluster B** (Behaviors described as dramatic)
   - **Antisocial personality disorder**
   - **Borderline personality disorder**
   - **Histrionic personality disorder**
   - **Narcissistic personality disorder**
3. **Cluster C** (Behaviors described as anxious or fearful)
   - **Avoidant personality disorder**
   - **Dependent personality disorder**
   - **Obsessive-compulsive personality disorder**

Generally, the personality disorders include one or more of the following traits:

- Negative affect: frequently experiences negative emotions
- Detachment: withdrawal from others
- Antagonism: difficult to get along with
- Disinhibition: impulsive
- Inflexible

Personality disorders often have their roots in difficult relationships with parental figures. Though each disorder has its own dynamics, this relationship is the thread that runs through all of them. Genetics may be a factor in some of these disorders as well.

> ■ ■ ■ Classroom Activities
> - Watch films that include people with personality disorders and discuss characteristics: *One Flew Over the Cuckoo's Nest* (antisocial), *Fatal Attraction* (borderline), *Wall Street* (narcissistic).
> - Share experiences of people you have known who exhibit various personality disorders.

■ Types of Personality Disorders

Cluster A

Paranoid Personality Disorder

Individuals with paranoid personality present with behaviors of suspiciousness and mistrust of other people. The person displays consistent mistrust of others' motives. These individuals may seem "normal" in their speech and activity, except for the fact that they feel people treat them unfairly. People with paranoid personality disorder are prone to filing lawsuits when they feel wronged in some way. They also seem to be hypersensitive to activity in their environment. They tend to be guarded and secretive since they can't trust others. They may have difficulty maintaining focused eye contact, for example, because they are so alert to other activity around them. People with paranoid personality disorder are not easily able to laugh at themselves; they take themselves very seriously. They may not show tender emotions and may seem cold and calculating in their relationships. They are reluctant to confide in others. They tend to take comments, events, and situations very personally. They have an excessive need to be self-sufficient which can create challenges if they become ill. As a general rule this person would probably avoid the health-care system if possible.

Patients with paranoid personality disorder are not psychotic and do not have hallucinations and delusions; they are, however, suspicious of other people and situations. The suspiciousness may cross into other areas of the person's life. For instance, it may be very challenging to enlist the cooperation of a person with this disorder when it comes to taking medications if the patient suspects ulterior motives.

Paranoid personality seems to have a high incidence of occurrence within families with schizophrenia, which supports the theories of the geneticists. Difficult parental relationships where the child is used as a scapegoat for parents' aggression can be a contributor as well.

> **❋ Cultural Considerations**
>
> Members of minority groups or immigrants may be prone to some paranoid traits due to their unfamiliarity with society's rules and expectations. This would not be considered a paranoid personality disorder unless it becomes pervasive and creates more problems for the person.

Schizoid Personality Disorder

People with schizoid personality disorder have a pattern of detachment from social relationships and a restricted range of expression of emotions in interpersonal settings. They may appear shy and introverted. They have trouble developing friendships. They tend to respond in a very serious, factual manner that is pleasant but not warm or inviting. They may be described by others as cold.

It is unusual to see patients hospitalized for this disorder because they are so quiet that the disorder often goes unnoticed. They often are described by others as "loners." It is common to see people with this type of personality become very engrossed in books. The books may be a substitute for human companionship. Partly because of this aversion to social interaction, people with schizoid personalities tend to be very intellectual and can be very successful in life if they choose a career that fits their personality. They may appear indifferent to the approval or criticism of others.

It is believed that ineffective and unemotional parenting may contribute to this disorder. A family history of schizophrenia or schizotypal personality disorder supports a genetic link.

Schizotypal Personality Disorder

Behavior in this disorder is often odd and eccentric but not to the level of schizophrenia (see Chapter 15). Although under stress, this person may decompensate with psychotic symptoms such as delusions and hallucinations. Aloof and isolated, these individuals often appear to be in their own world with language and gestures that only they understand and reduced capacity for close relationships. Often appearing blank and apathetic, their emotional responses may seem inappropriate. They also may display paranoia and social anxiety. Diagnosis is made by a mental health professional who looks at symptoms and life history.

Origins of this disorder may include poor relationships with parental figures where there is discomfort with affection and closeness, leading to distrust in personal relationships. In addition, this disorder is more common among first-degree relatives of people with schizophrenia, giving strength to genetic and biological factors.

> **Tool Box** ▶ Psych Central overview on schizotypal personality disorder: psychcentral.com/disorders/sx33.htm

Cluster B

Antisocial Personality Disorder

This group of people probably causes the greatest amount of trouble for society. Sometimes referred to as sociopathic, people with this disorder have a disregard for the rights of others. It often leads them to a path of violating rules, lying, stealing, participating in a variety of illegal activities, and other infringements of the law. The disorder seems to affect males more frequently than females and affects about 1% of the U.S. population (Lenzenweger, M. F., Lane, M. C., Loranger, A. W., & Kessler, R. C. [2007]). The serial killer Ted Bundy is one of the best-known sociopaths. As these individuals end up in the court systems, they may become part of the health-care system to avoid legal consequences or due to court order. These individuals have difficulty handling frustration and anger. They seldom feel affection, loyalty, guilt, or remorse and show very little concern for the rights or feelings of anyone else. It is rare that they display true remorse for their acts. People who have this disorder are also at high risk for substance abuse. In addition, a pattern of impulsiveness and irresponsibility are major features, with actions poorly planned. This type of person has difficulty with close relationships and may move from jobs and relationships frequently.

In spite of the inability to feel or show affection, patients with antisocial/sociopathic personality disorder are usually gregarious, intelligent, and likable but can quickly move to aggression if frustrated. Most people with this disorder are able to control their behavior out of fear of punishment; only those with extreme cases are unable to do so.

Because people with antisocial personality disorder are frequently highly intelligent, they learn the "jargon" of psychology and know how to manipulate it. Those with antisocial personality disorder are difficult to treat as the individual often has little motivation to change.

It is widely believed that the roots of this disorder stem from dysfunctional parenting and family life. This may be from a permissive or authoritarian parenting style that does not include guidelines for appropriate social behavior and includes abuse. A chaotic family life is often found. This personality disorder may be displayed in childhood with signs of callousness and lack of empathy. Some evidence also exists that there may be brain abnormalities in how the individual processes emotions. Childhood bullying and cruelty, animal abuse, as well as manipulative behaviors are seen at an early age. Individuals may have been diagnosed with conduct disorder before age 15 (see Chapter 19). These behaviors can run in families, so a genetic link is also suspected.

Neeb's Tip Patients with antisocial personality can be challenging as they can use unscrupulous means to accomplish their goals without the staff realizing it. Rather than telling the patient, "you shouldn't do that," reword to "you are expected to ..." to establish clear expectations that you are not negotiating.

Critical Thinking Question

You are working on a substance abuse unit. When you walk on the unit, you see a patient named Brad with a number of nursing staff. He is telling funny anecdotes about celebrities, and many of the nurses seem to be enjoying themselves. Brad is quite handsome and charming. After this occurrence, Brad asks one of the nurses for a special privilege to take a walk off the unit. How would you advise this nurse to handle this request?

When the nurse denies the patient's request, he quickly changes from charming to cruel as he insults the nurse and then knocks over a lamp. How should the staff respond?

Borderline Personality Disorder

This diagnosis is the most frequent personality disorder seen in the clinical setting, making up 2%–6% of the general population and 20% of psychiatric inpatients (BPD Resource Center, 2012). Borderline personality disorder (also known as BPD) is much more common in females. "Instability" is often the first word one thinks of when considering BPD. Individuals with this disorder often exhibit both clinging and distancing behavior as they struggle with fears of separation and abandonment. They are known for intense and chaotic relationships as well as self-destructive, impulsive, and dramatic coping. A chronic sense of emptiness, poor self-image, and excessive self-criticism are part of this disorder. These individuals operate using ingrained behavior patterns that involve manipulating others to achieve their goals to reduce anxiety. These patients may also utilize **self-mutilating behaviors,** including self-inflicted cuts (known as cutting), which usually are not performed with suicidal intent. The cutting can be a way to reduce tension, inflict pain to validate one's feelings and challenge a pervasive sense of emptiness, or seek attention. Substance abuse is also often a factor as the person tries to control the anxiety.

The origins of BPD can include coming from an abusive background and a childhood where one was dismissed by authority figures. Poor relationships with parental figures where the child grows up facing issues around abandonment and dependency are often seen. Defense mechanisms of denial, projection, and splitting (inability to integrate positive and negative feelings at the same time) are known to be commonly used. Splitting is manifested by a patient who needs to see others as all good or all bad. For example, a nurse who is caring during one shift may become to the patient the idealized "perfect" nurse, and then the nurse who sets limits on another shift is called "mean."

Neeb's Tip Recognizing staff splitting is essential for good care of the patient. If a patient complains about other staff members, never encourage him or her. Rather, point out that the patient needs to address the concerns with the individual and not complain about staff members to others. Avoid taking sides or acting as intermediary.

Tool Box |▶ AHRQ National Guidelines Clearinghouse on borderline personality disorder:
www.guideline.gov/content.aspx?id=14327&search=borderline+personality#Section420

■ ■ ■ Clinical Activity

When you are informed that your patient has a borderline personality, get specific information on interventions that the team has been using to avoid getting in the middle of conflict between the patient and staff.

Neeb's Tip Though cutting behaviors are more common in adolescents, they can occur in adults.

Tool Box |▶ Borderline Personality Disorder pamphlet for patients and families:
www.nimh.nih.gov/health/topics/borderline-personality-disorder/index.shtml
BPD Central with information for patients and families:
www.bpdcentral.com/

■ ■ ■ Critical Thinking Question

A 25-year-old woman is admitted from the ER to your unit with superficial cuts on both arms, a high blood alcohol level, and a complaint that she was attacked by her boyfriend. She is emotional and angry. As you sit with her to complete the admission, she shares with you that she cut her arms to get her boyfriend to "love" her. You are called out of the room. When you return, the patient yells at you and says she wants another nurse. She does not trust you.

This patient was diagnosed with borderline personality. Describe why she may have reacted so negatively to you when you returned to the room.

Histrionic Personality Disorder

This disorder is characterized by dramatic, excessive, extroverted behavior in someone who has a pattern of strong emotions. Excessive attention seeking, seductive and provocative behaviors are additionally seen. Some may describe the person as theatrical. They are known to be highly distractible and even flighty. Delaying gratification is difficult. Difficulty in maintaining close, intimate relationships is common despite the gregarious and seductive behaviors.

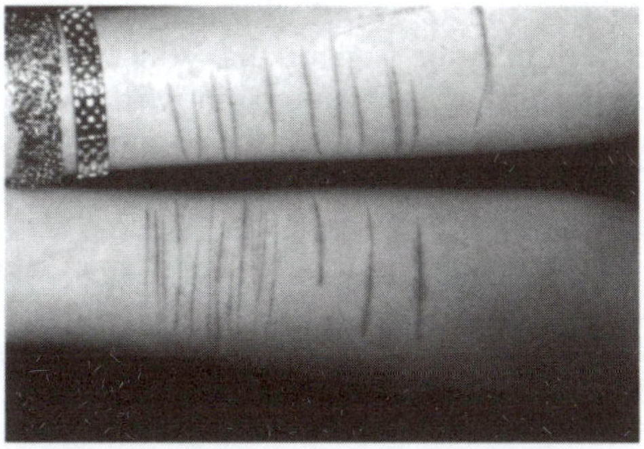

Figure 14-1 Self-inflicted lacerations on teenage girl's arms.

This disorder is more common in women. Childhood experience of needing to be dramatic to get recognition or needs met, lack of feedback from parents about appropriate behavior all contribute to the development of this disorder.

Neeb's Tip Histrionic traits do not mean the person has histrionic personality disorder. To have the disorder, the person would have consistent problems functioning in life as a result of these traits.

Narcissistic Personality Disorder

Those who have this disorder tend to display an exaggerated impression of self with an inflated sense of self-importance. They are preoccupied with fantasies of unlimited success. Another characteristic is limited ability to empathize with others' problems because they see everything through their own eyes. They also tend to be hypersensitive when they receive criticism. They have a tendency to overestimate their abilities, are attention

❁ Cultural Considerations

Cultural background can dictate social behavior. So this should be taken into consideration when a diagnosis of histrionic disorder is being made.

seeking, and are surprised if they do not receive admiration from others. While projecting an image of invulnerability, their deep sense of emptiness is hidden from others. These individuals have difficulty maintaining close relationships.

People with this disorder will seem to take criticism lightly. In reality, deep feelings of anger, resentment, and poor self-esteem are being repressed. Friends will be chosen according to how good they make the person with the narcissistic personality feel.

Often these people are children of narcissistic parental figures who were critical and demanding of their children. The children then model their behavior. Narcissistic traits are particularly common in adolescents though they will not necessarily have the personality disorder.

> **Critical Thinking Question**
> You are working on a psychiatric unit, and your patient with narcissistic disorder tells you that she plans to get the lead in a play once she leaves the hospital. She tells you she has always been successful in every audition she has had. What concerns would you have for this patient? How would you respond to her statements?

Cluster C

Avoidant Personality Disorder

These individuals are extremely sensitive and may avoid social situations to protect themselves from possible rejection. However, these people also have a strong need to be accepted. Often labeled shy, these individuals are awkward in social situations. They often view others as critical. They want a close relationship but avoid it because of fear of being rejected. Characteristics include low self-esteem, avoidance of close relationships, anxiety, and anhedonia, or lack of pleasure in life. They are very hesitant to engage in new activities due to fear of failure. Highly critical parental figures are believed to be the origin. There also may be a hereditary link.

> **Neeb's Tip** The patient with avoidant personality disorder desperately wants social contact but goes to lengths to discourage it out of fear of rejection.

Dependent Personality Disorder

Dependent personality is a pervasive and excessive need to be taken care of that leads to submissive and clinging behaviors and fears of separation. These behaviors tend to elicit caregiving response in others including nurses. People with dependent personality disorder want others to make decisions for them and tend to feel inferior and suggestible, with a sense of self-doubt. These individuals tend to appear helpless and to avoid responsibility. On the other hand, individuals with this disorder tend to take everything to heart and go out of their way to satisfy people they feel close to and try to change those personality traits that people criticize.

There seems to be an inordinate amount of fear among people who experience dependent personality disorder. It may be the fear of criticism that brings about the inability to make decisions. Inability to make decisions can be severe enough as to limit a person's ability to have meaningful social interactions. In addition recognition that overuse of dependency behaviors can lead to a disturbed nurse-patient relationship.

Seriously overprotective parents who discourage independence and promote dependence in the child for the parents' needs can be a contributing factor. Chronic physical illness in childhood can predispose to this disorder.

> **Cultural Considerations**
> Nurses must be cautioned here because the behaviors that have been discussed as symptomatic of dependent personality disorder are behaviors and conditions that are expected in certain cultures, especially among females.

Obsessive-Compulsive Personality Disorder

These individuals are disciplined and rigid to an extreme. They are meticulous and demand accuracy and discipline in others. They are preoccupied with details, rules, and order. They display a stubborn streak in order to maintain control so things are done their way. They may appear polite and formal but can be autocratic and critical with others. They demonstrate persistence at tasks long after the behavior has ceased to be functional or effective and continuance of the same behavior despite repeated failures or obvious annoyance by others. The fear of making mistakes can lead to an inability to make any decisions.

The origins include overcontrolling parents, and the disorder does run in families. This personality disorder differs from what is known as OCD (obsessive-compulsive disorder). OCD is a disorder that is characterized by obsessions and compulsions in an effort to maintain control (Chapter 10).

Psychiatric Treatment of Personality Disorders

Because these personality disorders become engrained early in life, treatment is often difficult. People with personality disorders may not seek treatment as part of their disorder until the disorder drains their coping reserves. At times they will demonstrate resistance to treatment. Treatment may be pushed on them after a crisis or due to entrance into the legal system. Psychotherapy, cognitive behavior therapy, and group therapy may be useful in some situations. Maintaining a long-standing trusting relationship with a therapist can be advantageous. Medications to treat anxiety, depression, and delusions are often used. Family members of people with personality disorders often benefit from family therapy and psycho-education around coping with them.

Neeb's Tip

Though people with personality disorders may not seek mental health treatment, they often use the health-care system for other problems. Patients with personality disorders present many challenges to nurses. These patients may display rigid behavior patterns and be socially inappropriate.

Pharmacology Corner

Many patients with these disorders experience anxiety, so anti-anxiety medications are often prescribed. Borderline patients have been treated with SSRIs (selective serotonin reuptake inhibitors) to manage impulsivity. Antipsychotics may be used with patients with psychotic features such as schizotypal disorders. For patients prone to violence, antipsychotics may also be needed. Because many of these patients are susceptible to substance abuse to self-medicate, close monitoring of drug abuse should be included in the treatment plan.

Neeb's Tip

Compliance with a prescribed medication regimen can be challenging. Some may have a tendency to avoid following instructions or act impulsively.

Critical Thinking Question

Your patient with a diagnosis of avoidant personality requests alprazolam before group therapy session. Describe what this medication accomplishes for the patient and alternative approaches in place of medication.

Nursing Care of Patients With Personality Disorders

Common nursing diagnoses with personality disorders include the following:

- Coping, defensive
- Personal identity, disturbed
- Self-esteem, disturbed
- Self-mutilation, risk for
- Social interactions, impaired
- Violence, self-directed, risk for

Neeb's Tip

Nurses need to display much patience and acceptance as part of the care plan.

General Nursing Interventions for Personality Disorders

See Table 14-1 for a summary of nursing interventions for each personality disorder and Table 14-2, which details the nursing care plan for patients with borderline personality.

Clinical Activities

- Be alert to possible manipulation or staff splitting; patients may view nursing students as being more vulnerable and try to take advantage of them.
- At the same time, make efforts to avoid stereotyping or judging such patients based on information that they have a personality disorder.

Table 14-1 Nursing Interventions for Personality Disorders

Type	Symptoms	Nursing Interventions
Antisocial	• Requires immediate self-gratification • Often in trouble with the law • Has difficulty handling frustration and anger • Seldom feels affection, loyalty, guilt, or remorse • Shows very little concern for the rights or feelings of others • Good at manipulating others for personal gain • High risk for substance abuse • Usually gregarious, charming, intelligent, and likable	• Promote positive, healthy interpersonal relationships • Monitor for violent behaviors • Provide feedback on negative behaviors • Encourage appropriate expression of angry feelings • Support analysis of feelings • Point out impact of manipulative behavior • Avoid negotiating rewards • Set limits
Avoidant	• Avoids social situations • Preoccupied with thoughts of being rejected or criticized • Low self-esteem • Avoids new activities for fear of being embarrassed	• Promote self-esteem by acknowledging any success • Encourage participation in supportive social situations • Provide emotional support • Teach calming techniques to use to deal with anxiety • Reinforce strengths
Borderline	• Moods unstable and changeable • Uncertainty regarding self-concept • Substance abuse • Suicide attempts • Anhedonia • Difficulty handling strong emotion • Bored and empty feelings • Fear of being alone • Self-destructive behaviors • Self-mutilation • Manipulative	• Remain calm in presence of patient's drama • Build trusting relationship • Set limits and establish clear ground rules that are followed by everyone • Establish therapeutic communication • Demonstrate positive role modeling • Monitor for self-destructive behaviors • Provide safety/security • Communicate a consistent plan of care among all staff • Encourage patient to verbalize feelings rather than act them out • Avoid power struggles • Involve family and friends in treatment plan

Table 14-1 Nursing Interventions for Personality Disorders—cont'd

Type	Symptoms	Nursing Interventions
Dependent	• Dependent and submissive • Want others to make decisions for them • Tend to feel inferior and suggestible and have a sense of self-doubt • Tend to appear helpless and avoid responsibility • Tend to take everything to heart—will go out of their way to satisfy people they feel close to and try to change those personality traits that people criticize • Inordinate amount of fear	• Allow patient to make some decisions for his or her treatment • Reinforce the patient's decisions • Encourage patient to make truthful, positive self-statements each shift • Recognize patient's insecurities and anxieties.
Histrionic	• Dramatic • Emotional • Provocative • Suggestible	• Support healthy coping • Reassurance • Support consistent healthy relationships • Give appropriate feedback
Narcissistic	• Exaggerated self-image • Appears self-centered • Lacks empathy for others' problems • Expresses need for self-importance • Takes criticism lightly but in reality represses feelings of anger and resentment • Sense of entitlement • Cheerful, carefree mood which can quickly change to distress if criticized	• Encourage patient to learn to accept limitations in self and others • Give patient feedback on how others are responding to patient • Prepare patient for possible setbacks • Recognize the patient is very sensitive to hurt feelings • Encourage the patient to talk about his or her vulnerabilities
Obsessive-Compulsive	• Rigid behavior • Preoccupied with rules • Formal • Perfectionistic • Intense fear of making mistakes • Though calm on outside, dealing with intense conflict and hostility	• Understand patient's fears and be flexible as to his/her needs • Allow patient to make simple decisions with limited choices • Establish trusting, supportive relationship • Discuss alternative strategies for dealing with new situations • Support healthy coping mechanisms to deal with stress
Paranoid	• Suspicious and mistrustful of other people • May seem "normal" in speech and activity • Believe that people treat them unfairly • Hypersensitive to activity in the environment • Difficult to maintain focused eye contact	• Avoid situation that the patient may perceive as demeaning • Encourage trusting relationship • Encourage verbalizing one's perceptions of the situations • Reinforce trusting behaviors • Acknowledge other possible explanations for others motives

Continued

Table 14-1 Nursing Interventions for Personality Disorders—cont'd

Type	Symptoms	Nursing Interventions
	• Not easily able to laugh at themselves • Take themselves very seriously • May not show tender emotions • May seem cold and calculating in their relationships • Tend to take comments, events, situations personally • Few social interactions • Loners • Appear to be shy and introverted	
Schizoid	• Detached • Chooses solitary activities • Avoids social situations • Loner • Often excel in fields where limited interaction needed	• Acceptance of behavior • Encourage appropriate brief social interactions • Meet patient on his/her own terms • Help patient understand how behaviors may contribute to satisfactory relationships
Schizotypal	• Eccentric behavior • Inappropriate affect • Aloof • Psychotic symptoms under stress	• Brief, concrete conversations that are focused on reality • Acceptance of behavior • Encourage appropriate social behaviors • Recognize need for personal space • Reinforce reality gently

Table 14-2 Nursing Care Plan for Patients With Borderline Personality Disorder

Assessment/ Data Collection	Nursing Diagnosis	Plan/Goal	Interventions/ Nursing Actions	Evaluation Criteria
After drinking heavily, got in physical fight with acquaintance, then made attempt at cutting wrists	Risk for self-directed violence	Verbalize alternative coping mechanisms when under stress	Provide safe, secure environment; Convey acceptance of patient as a person; Discuss alternative ways to express anxiety, irritation; Identify alternative actions to reduce destructive impulses	Able to describe alternative coping mechanisms; Able to utilize these coping mechanisms next time in a stressful situation

Key Concepts

1. Personality disorders are maladaptive responses to personality development.
2. People with personality disorders are seldom hospitalized for them. They do not see a need for obtaining help and are not always taken seriously by the medical community.
3. Borderline personality disorder is the most common one seen in the mental health setting.
4. People with personality disorders often present challenges to nursing staff when receiving care for physical ailments due to their challenging behaviors, which can include poor interpersonal skills, negative emotions, and inflexibility.
5. Common traits of people with personality disorders include socially inappropriate behavior, negative emotions, and difficulty with close relationships.

CASE STUDY

Marsha is a 25-year-old woman who is brought to the emergency room by her girlfriend after threatening to take sleeping pills when her boyfriend broke off their relationship. On questioning Marsha, she acknowledges a long history of problems. She has made multiple suicide attempts, which include cutting her arms and taking handfuls of sleeping pills. Each attempt occurred after a rejection by a boyfriend or in earlier years by her parents. Marsha describes falling in love easily and a history of intense relationships that often are discontinued by the man after Marsha becomes increasingly clinging and demanding.

She describes a chaotic childhood in which her mother was away a lot and Marsha moved around to live with a variety of relatives. She barely finished high school and has struggled to find unskilled jobs.

On interviewing her you find her cheerful and charming. She does not appear depressed. When you leave the room to attend to another patient, she cries out that she is being ignored. She calls multiple friends to visit in the ER so she will not be alone, thus creating a chaotic environment that must be monitored by security.

Her long-term psychiatrist comes to see her and tells you she is treating Marsha for borderline personality disorder.

1. Which behaviors in this case study are indicative of this diagnosis?
2. What treatment options are used to treat this disorder?
3. What medications would you expect her to have prescribed?

REFERENCES

American Psychiatric Association. (2013). *Diagnostic and Statistical Manual of Mental Disorders 5*. Washington, DC, Author. (Known as DSM-5)

ARHQ National Guidelines Clearing House, Borderline Personality Disorder. (2009). Retrieved from http://www.guideline.gov/content.aspx?id=14327&search=borderline+personality#Section420

BPD Resource Center. Retrieved from http://bpdresourcecenter.org/factsStatistics.html

Cloninger, C.R., and Surakic, D.M. (2009). Personality disorders. In B. J. Sadock, V.A. Sadock, & P. Ruiz (Eds.), *Kaplan & Sadock's Comprehensive Textbook of Psychiatry*. 9th ed. Philadelphia: Wolters Kluwer/ Lippincott Williams & Wilkins.

Lenzenweger, M.F., Lane, M. C., and Loranger, A. W. (2007). DSM-IV personality disorders

in the National Comorbidity Survey Replication. *Biological psychiatry, 62*(6), 553–564.
Puskar, K. R., et al. (2006). Self-cutting behavior in adolescents. *Journal of emergency nursing 32*(5), 444–446.
Townsend, M. (2012). *Psychiatric Mental Health Nursing.* 7th ed. Philadelphia: F.A. Davis.

Test Questions

Multiple Choice Questions

1. When setting limits with patients with personality disorders, the consequences to those limits should be set:
   a. When the behavior is done
   b. Just before the nurse anticipates the behavior
   c. When the staff or family complains about the behavior
   d. When the limit is set

2. David, 30 years old, comes to your unit for treatment of multiple broken bones following a car accident. He is friendly and flirtatious but very demanding. As you take your data from him, you learn that the police have been looking for him for petty theft. He laughs and says, "Like they don't have better things to do!" He states he has changed jobs three times in the past year and has just broken off his second engagement. His former fiancée is visiting and privately tells you that you need to be careful because "he doesn't always tell the truth." You suspect which of the following personality disorders?
   a. Paranoid
   b. Dependent
   c. Antisocial
   d. Schizoid

3. A primary mechanism used by people with personality disorders is:
   a. Manipulation
   b. Depression
   c. Projection
   d. Euphoria

4. For the patient with a personality disorder, which of the following behaviors would be the most difficult for the patient to comply with?
   a. Listening to music
   b. Abiding by the rules in the hospital
   c. Playing volleyball
   d. Developing a friendship

5. A patient who is in trouble with the law would probably have which of the following personality disorders?
   a. Narcissistic
   b. Schizoid
   c. Antisocial
   d. Borderline

6. Patients who display very bizarre behavior most likely have which of the following types of personality disorder?
   a. Narcissistic
   b. Schizotypal
   c. Antisocial
   d. Borderline

7. Which intervention describes an important component in treatment of personality disorders?
   a. Antidepressants are most effective with most personality disorders.
   b. Inpatient psychiatric hospitalization is particularly effective.
   c. Self-awareness by the nurse is necessary to ensure a therapeutic relationship.
   d. Long-term psychoanalysis is the treatment of choice.

8. Your patient has been admitted with a diagnosis of bilateral pneumonia. You have trouble communicating with this patient, who is pouty and is demanding of your constant attention. She talks for long periods about the smallest details of her life. Besides the pneumonia, you ask the physician if the patient has a history of which of the following personality disorders?
   a. Schizoid
   b. Antisocial
   c. Narcissistic
   d. Borderline

Test Questions

cont.

9. Nursing care for people with personality disorders includes all of the following *except:*

a. Unconditional positive regard
b. Trust
c. Limit setting
d. Vague communication (to decrease feelings of inferiority)

10. You are caring for a 25-year-old male who has been admitted for infections that resulted from self-inflicted burns. This is not the first admission for this young man, but he is new to you as a new nurse on the unit. You have not read his entire chart, but you suspect he has a history of which one of the following personality disorders?

a. Narcissistic
b. Borderline
c. Schizoid
d. Passive-aggressive

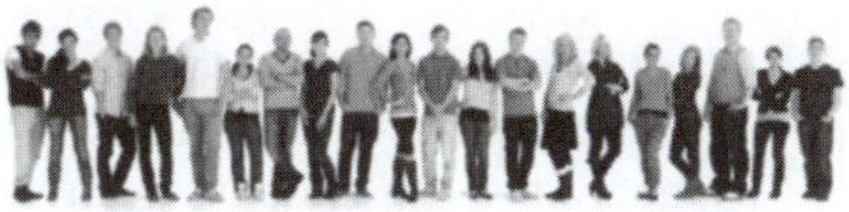

CHAPTER 15

Schizophrenia Spectrum and Other Psychotic Disorders

Learning Objectives

1. Define schizophrenia.
2. Differentiate between positive and negative symptoms seen in schizophrenia.
3. Identify two other psychotic disorders.
4. Identify treatment modalities for people with schizophrenia.
5. Describe catatonic features in schizophrenia
6. Identify nursing care for people with schizophrenia.

Key Terms

- Catatonia
- Delusions
- Echolalia
- Echopraxia
- Extrapyramidal symptoms (EPS)
- Hallucinations
- Illusions
- Psychosis
- Schizophrenia
- Schizoaffective disorder
- Schizophrenia spectrum disorder

The term *schizophrenia* (which literally means "split mind") was first used by Swiss psychiatrist Eugen Bleuler (Fig. 15-1). **Schizophrenia** is a serious, chronic, psychiatric disorder characterized by impaired reality testing, **hallucinations, delusions,** and limited socialization. It is a psychotic thought disorder where hallucinations and delusions dominate the patient's thinking, leading to confusing and bizarre behaviors. People with schizophrenia have a "split" between their thoughts and their feelings and between their reality and society's reality, which can lead to unusual and frightening behaviors. Schizophrenia is a frequent cause for long psychiatric hospitalizations. The suffering for a schizophrenic patient and his/her family can last a lifetime as this crippling condition continues. As a chronic illness, schizophrenia is characterized by remissions and exacerbations throughout one's life. The first psychotic break often responds well to treatment, but the relapse rate is high and the person may become increasingly disabled.

Schizophrenic individuals are vulnerable to substance abuse as they self-medicate to control their symptoms, contributing to co-occurring disorder (see Chapter 17). These patients can also be at risk for suicide, which may be manifested as voices telling the person to kill her/himself or a means to end suffering.

DSM-5 now categorizes schizophrenia under the global title of **schizophrenia spectrum disorders** (2013). In the past, schizophrenia was divided into five subtypes of catatonic,

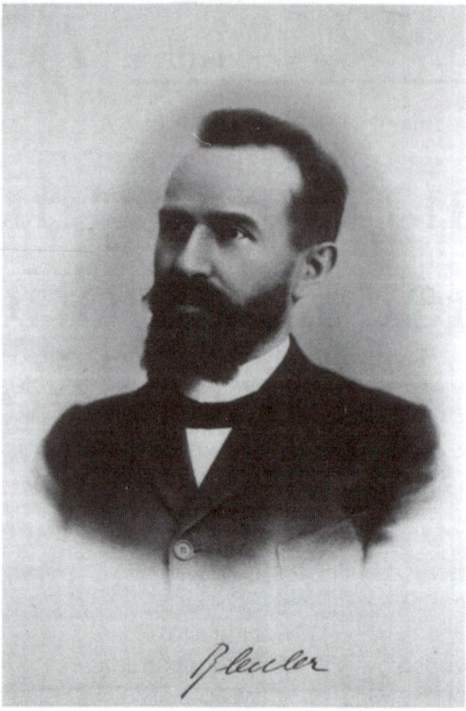

Figure 15-1 Eugen Bleuler (1857–1940) was a Swiss psychiatrist who coined the term *schizophrenia* and contributed to the understanding of the disorder.

delusional, disorganized, undifferentiated, and residual, but in 2013 these were eliminated. The new term of schizophrenia spectrum disorders reflects a gradient of psychopathology that a patient can experience from least to most severe. Disorders such as schizophreniform and schizoaffective would be the less severe forms. See Table 15-1 for other disorders with schizophrenic features.

In addition, **psychoses** can occur in bipolar disorder and major depression. Another psychotic disorder is brief psychotic disorder, which includes postpartum psychosis (see Chapter 20) as well as psychosis due to substance abuse or medical conditions. Medical conditions that can contribute to psychoses include brain tumors, CNS infections, delirium, and endocrine disorders. All of these disorders, though not schizophrenia, have some of the same symptoms but different etiology and duration of disability.

Neeb's Tip Sudden onset of hallucinations and delusions requires quick action to identify the cause. Causes can include medical conditions, metabolic changes, and drug reactions.

Classroom Activities

- View and discuss movies that feature schizophrenic characters, including *A Beautiful Mind* and *I Never Promised You a Rose Garden*.

Critical Thinking Question

Your patient has a diagnosis of schizophreniform disorder. How is this different from a diagnosis of schizophrenia?

Table 15-1 Other Disorders With Schizophrenic Features

Type	Characteristics
Delusional Disorder	Delusions without the other symptoms or disabilities of schizophrenia
Schizoaffective	Symptoms of schizophrenia along with symptoms of major depression or manic episode that requires treatment of both disorders
Schizophreniform	Schizophrenia symptoms without the level of impairment of functioning usually seen in schizophrenia and lasting more than 1 month and fewer than 6 months
Schizotypal	A personality disorder characterized by odd and eccentric behavior that does not decompensate to the level of schizophrenia (see Chapter 14)

Source: Adapted from Diagnostic and Statistical Manual of Mental Disorders, 5th Edition (Copyright 2013). American Psychiatric Association, Townsend (2012), and Goldberg (2007).

Frequently, schizophrenia is initially diagnosed in adolescents and younger adults between the ages of 16 and 35 with the occurrence of the first psychotic break, though later onset does occur. A common scenario is a young person who has left home for college or the military and suddenly exhibits psychotic behavior (Fig. 15-2), though premorbid personality may indicate this individual was withdrawn, had problems with social relationships, and exhibited possible antisocial behavior. Schizophrenia is rare in young children. The National Institute of Mental Health (NIMH) estimates that nearly 3 million Americans will develop schizophrenia during the course of their lives. That is about 1.1% of the U.S. population (National Institute of Mental Health, 2012).

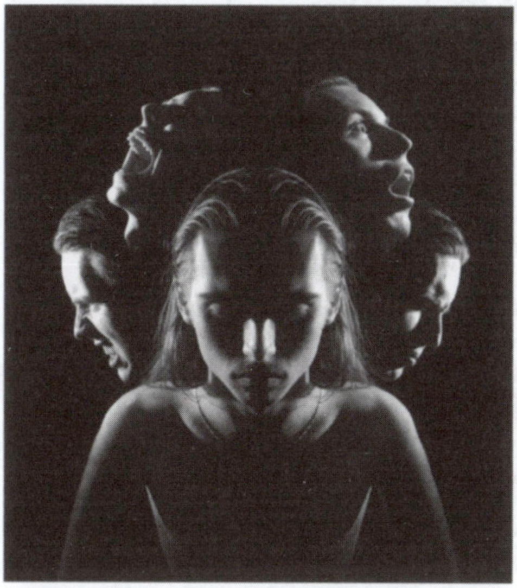

Figure 15-2 Schizophrenia can create extreme distress.

> **Classroom Activities**
> - Contact a local NAMI (National Alliance on Mental Illness) support group and attend a meeting if possible.

Symptoms

- The presence of delusions, hallucinations, and/or disorganized speech for a significant portion of time during a 1-month period. At least one of these must be present for the diagnosis.
- Grossly abnormal motor behavior and/or negative symptoms (see below for explanation)
- One or more areas of functioning, such as work, school, personal relationships, or self-care, are impaired. Some disturbance needs to be evident for at least 6 months.
- Schizophrenia can also have features of **catatonia,** which include any of the following: motor immobility to stupor, excessive motor activity, peculiar voluntary movements, and **echolalia** or **echopraxia.**

Schizophrenia's symptoms are typically described as "negative" or "positive." *Negative* symptoms are those found among people who do not have the disorder but are missing or lacking among individuals with schizophrenia and reflect a lessening or loss of normal functions. These may include avolition (a lack of desire or motivation to accomplish goals), lack of desire to form social relationships, inappropriate social behavior such as pacing or rocking, and blunted affect and emotion. These symptoms make holding a job, forming relationships, and other day-to-day functions especially difficult for people with schizophrenia.

Positive symptoms are those that are found among people with schizophrenia but not present among those who do not have the disorder. They reflect an excess or distortion of normal functions such as delusions, thought disorders, and hallucinations. People with schizophrenia may hear voices other people don't hear or believe other people are reading their minds, controlling their thoughts, or plotting to harm them. Other positive symptoms can include magical thinking (belief that one's thoughts can control others), neologisms (invents new words that only have meaning to the individual), concrete thinking (literal interpretation of the environment), loose associations (ideas shift from unrelated one to another), echopraxia (repeating movements of

> **Cultural Considerations**
>
> Schizophrenia crosses all races and cultures.

Cultural Considerations

One's culture often influences the content of hallucinations and delusions. Familiarity with the patient's culture can provide insight into the origin of some of these behaviors.

others), and echolalia (parrot-like repeating words spoken by others). Most schizophrenics have a mixture of both positive and negative symptoms.

See Tables 15-2 and 15-3 for lists of common delusions and hallucinations.

Neeb's Tip Schizophrenia is a debilitating and painful lifelong disease for the patient and family requiring long-term management and compassion.

Critical Thinking Question
Your schizophrenic patient tells you that his mother has communicated with him that he needs to leave the hospital right now to help save the mayor from peril. What type of delusions and hallucinations is this patient experiencing?

Table 15-2 Common Delusions

Delusion	Example
Grandeur (belief of exaggerated importance)	"I am Napoleon Bonaparte."
Paranoia (belief of deliberate harassment and persecution)	"The FBI is following me and wants to kill me."
Reference (belief that the thoughts and behavior of others is directed toward self)	"Those people on the TV show are talking to me."
Physical sensations (belief that parts of body are diseased, distorted, or missing)	"I have no blood in me."
Thought insertion	"The devil made me say that."

Source: Adapted from Gorman and Sultan (2008). Psychosocial Nursing for General Patient Care, 3rd ed. Philadelphia: F.A. Davis Company, with permission.

Table 15-3 Recognizing Hallucinations

Affected Sense	Example
Visual	"I watch gypsies bring different babies to my apartment each night."
Auditory (most common)	"The voices are calling me a prostitute."
Tactile	"When I touched my arm, I could tell my arm is made of stone."
Olfactory	"I don't want to stay in that room. I can smell the odors of the people who died there."
Gustatory	"I taste milk in my mouth all the time."
Kinesthetic (bodily movement or sense)	"It feels as if the rats in my head are eating up my brain."

Source: Adapted from Gorman and Sultan (2008). Psychosocial Nursing for General Patient Care, 3rd ed. Philadelphia: F.A. Davis Company, with permission.

Etiology of Schizophrenia

No single cause has been identified, but it is now known that schizophrenia is a brain disorder. Disruption of neurotransmitters, including dopamine, has been identified. Some dysfunction in neuron functioning has also been found. Some cerebral changes in the brain have also been suggested in the limbic system and prefrontal cortex. These factors may contribute to the problems with attention and information processing. The person

Cultural Considerations

Behaviors that may be normal in some cultures can be confused with psychotic behavior. For example, speaking in tongues and talking to spirits may be normal behavior in some cultures. If psychotic behavior is suspected, it is important to obtain information on what is normal behavior for the culture of your patient.

is unable to filter stimuli, leading to disorganization of mental functioning. While family dysfunction may exist, it appears that psychological factors by themselves do not cause this condition. There is also evidence of genetic predisposition, and the most significant risk factor is having a close relative with this disorder.

■ Psychiatric Treatment of Schizophrenia

A comprehensive, multidisciplinary treatment plan including pharmacotherapy, social support, social/life skills training, self-help groups, and family therapy can be helpful to maintain the patient effectively. Gaining life skills to deal with everyday challenges, occupational training, and family education have been helpful. Intensive individual psychotherapy is generally not as effective, but reality-based therapy to promote trust can be incorporated into the plan. Ongoing support can promote compliance with antipsychotic medications. Management of antipsychotic medications is generally the primary treatment. See Pharmacology Corner.

Tool Box ▶ Brief Psychiatric Rating Scale (BPRS)—Standardized tool to track response to treatment:
http://www.public-health.uiowa.edu/icmha/outreach/screening.html
Treating Schizophrenia Guideline from American Psychiatric Association:
http://psychiatryonline.org/content.aspx?bookid=28&sectionid=1663093

■ ■ ■ Classroom Activities

- Invite a local mental health professional to class to discuss the treatment approaches to schizophrenic patients in your community.

Most people respond to one of the typical or atypical agents to a degree at the first psychotic episode. *Typical antipsychotics* have been around since the 1950s and work by blocking postsynaptic dopamine receptors.

Pharmacology Corner

Antipsychotic medications are key to a patient's returning to a stable state. Once achieved, maintenance therapy is established to prevent exacerbations. Most schizophrenics will relapse once off their medications, so incorporating a plan for medication compliance is essential. Once established on appropriate medications, the patient is usually more open to counseling and supportive interventions. It can take time to establish the appropriate medication and dosages so the patient and family must be monitored closely. Some patients may require longer periods of trials for months or even years to find the best available medication, the right dosage, and manageable side-effect profile. A trial of any one medication should last for a substantial period, usually 6 to 8 weeks, unless intolerable side effects occur early.

These agents are generally used to treat the positive symptoms of schizophrenia. *Atypical antipsychotics* have been available since the 1990s and are weaker dopamine receptor antagonists but more potent antagonists of serotonin receptors. New atypicals are added to the market regularly. These drugs treat both the positive and negative symptoms and generally have fewer side effects. Even though the atypical agents have a better side-effect profile for long-term treatment, the typical or older agents may be chosen for short-term management of psychosis or long-term management of symptoms that do not respond to the atypical agents. See Table 15-4 for a list of the common typical and atypical antipsychotics with their side-effect profile. Most of these agents are available only in oral form. A few are available as a long-acting injection that is given every few weeks. These include haloperidol, fluphenazine, and risperidone. These can be effective if a patient refuses or is unable to take oral medications. Some medications come in liquid forms or quick dissolving tablets, which can also be useful if the patient is not cooperative with taking oral medication.

Table 15-4 Comparison of Side Effects Among Typical and Atypical Antipsychotic Agents

Class	Generic Name	EPS	Sedation	Anti-cholinergic	Orthostatic Hypotension	Weight Gain
Typicals	Chlorpromazine (Thorazine)	3	4	3	4	*
	Fluphenazine (Prolixin)	5	2	2	2	
	Haloperidol (Haldol)	5	2	2	2	
	Loxapine (Loxitane)	3	2	2	2	*
	Perphenazine (Trilafon)	4	2	2	2	*
	Pimozide (Orap)	4	2	3	2	*
	Prochlorperazine (Compazine)	3	2	2	2	*
	Thioridazine (Mellaril)	2	4	4	4	*
	Thiothixene (Navane)	4	2	2	2	*
	Trifluoperazine (Stelazine)	4	2	2	2	*
Atypicals	Aripiprazole (Abilify)	1	2	1	3	2
	Asenapine (Saphris)	1	3	1	3	4
	Clozapine (Clozaril)	1	5	5	4	5
	Iloperidone (Fanapt)	1	3	2	3	3
	Lurasidone (Latuda)	1	3	1	3	3
	Olanzapine (Zyprexa)	1	3	2	2	5
	Palperidone (Invega)	1	2	1	3	2
	Quetiapine (Seroquel)	1	3	1	3	4
	Risperidone (Risperdal)	1	2	1	3	4
	Ziprasidone (Geodon)	1	3	1	2	2

Key: 1=Very low, 2=low, 3=moderate, 4=high, 5=very high
+Weight gain occurs, but incidence is unknown.
Source: From Townsend (2012): Psychiatric Mental Health Nursing,7th ed. Philadelphia: F.A. Davis, with permission.

Critical Thinking Question
You realize your schizophrenic patient has been "cheeking" his risperidone (hiding the pill in his cheek). What might be some of the reasons the patient is doing this? Identify two alternatives for taking this medication.

Managing the side effects of antipsychotics can promote patient compliance. Typical antipsychotics are more prone to **extrapyramidal symptoms** (EPS) as well as anticholinergic effects, though the drugs can be particularly effective in controlling psychotic symptoms. See Box 15-1 and Table 15-5 for lists of extrapyramidal and anticholinergic side effects. Extrapyramidal symptoms are generally managed with anticholinergic drugs such as benztropine, biperiden, trihexyphenidyl, dopaminergic agonists such as amantadine, or antihistamines such as diphenhydramine.

The atypicals are generally less associated with extrapyramidal symptoms than the typical agents, but there is a wide range of other side effects, so close monitoring of the prescribed drug is essential. Some atypicals are prone to anticholinergic effects. Serious side effects in specific atypicals can include reduced seizure threshold, blood dyscrasias, and cardiac arrhythmias. One of the most serious is agranulocytosis, which is a rare blood complication of clozapine requiring close monitoring of the white blood cell count. The specific side effects of the atypicals must be reviewed and monitored whenever these drugs are ordered.

Neeb's Tip
Compliance to antipsychotics remains a lifelong challenge for the schizophrenic patient and his/her family. It is important to regularly monitor medication compliance and the current side-effect profile. Education must be reinforced each time the patient is seen in any health-care setting.

Neeb's Tip
Extrapyramidal symptoms can be devastating to quality of life. Close monitoring to treat these and prevent long-term consequences must be part of the treatment plan.

Tool Box Abnormal Involuntary Movement Scale (AIMS): This tool is a rating scale developed by the National Institute of Mental Health to measure involuntary movements associated with tardive dyskinesia (available at: www.atlantapsychiatry.com/forms/AIMS.pdf

Clinical Activity
- Review chart for CBC results if the patient is on clozapine.
- Review chart for evidence of side effects of antipsychotic medications.
- Discuss management of side effects with patient and his/her family.

Critical Thinking Question
Your patient with schizophrenia has been taking clozapine for 2 years. He is now in the hospital and is NPO awaiting an appendectomy. What concerns would you have that the patient has been without his medications for 2 days? Why is the MD monitoring his WBC counts closely?

Box 15-1 Extrapyramidal Side Effects

- Dystonia: muscle rigidity, torticollis (neck turned in awkward angle)
- Pseudoparkinsonism or dyskinesia: stiffness, tremors, shuffling gait
- Akathisia: restlessness, inability to sit still
- Tardive dyskinesia: late onset movement disorder that includes lip smacking, grimacing, tongue protrusion

Table 15-5 Anticholinergic Effects

Symptom	Action
Dry mouth	Offer sugarless candy, good oral hygiene, saliva substitute
Orthostatic hypotension	Instruct patient to get out of bed slowly, monitor BP
Constipation	Promote high-fiber diet, fluids, stool softeners, laxatives as needed
Urinary retention	Instruct patient to report symptoms promptly
Dry eye	Lubricant eye drops

Source: Adapted from Gorman and Sultan (2008). Psychosocial Nursing for General Patient Care, 3rd ed. Philadelphia: F.A. Davis Company, with permission.

Nursing Care of the Schizophrenic Patient

The nursing care of the schizophrenic patient requires knowledge and compassion. Common nursing diagnoses for the schizophrenic patient include:

- Self-care deficit
- Sensory perception, disturbed
- Social isolation
- Thought processes, disturbed
- Violence, risk for

General Nursing Interventions

- Watch for clues that patient is hallucinating, e.g., darting eyes, mumbling to self, staring at a vacant wall for long periods. You can also ask the patient if he is hearing voices.
- If the patient is hallucinating, your response could be, "I don't see the devil standing there, but I understand how upsetting this is for you." In this way you are acknowledging what the patient is experiencing without reinforcing it as your reality.
- If your patient is delusional, reinforce reality, "that man works for the hospital not the FBI," "Yes, there was a man at the nurse's station, but I did not hear him talk about you." Remind the patient he has some control to look at alternative ways to view reality.
- Work to slowly build trust in small ways. Avoid overreacting to patient's bizarre behavior or appearance
- Maintain a calm, consistent environment with a regular routine
- Even though he/she appears to be in another world, continue to include the patient in conversations and activities. Acknowledge his/her presence and importance.
- Focus on reality, e.g., rather than listen to a long monologue about a delusion, talk about the schedule for the day.
- Never argue with the patient about what he or she is experiencing.
- Incorporate Quality and Safety Education for Nurses (QSEN) competencies to maintain a safe environment for the psychotic patient (qsen.org), e.g., remove sharp objects, provide adequate supervision.
- Take action to provide medications before agitation escalates. Make sure there are orders for prn medications for agitation.
- Never reinforce hallucinations, delusions, or **illusions.** An example of an inappropriate response is, "Jesus wants you to take these pills," That response reinforces the delusion about Jesus.
- Avoid whispering or laughing when the patient cannot hear the whole conversation; such behavior can promote paranoia.
- Avoid putting the patient into situations that are competitive or embarrassing.
- Build trust by using therapeutic communication skills.
- If the patient is catatonic, provide for basic physical needs and safety, and make brief supportive contacts with the patient without pressuring the patient to communicate.

Table 15-6 provides the nursing care plan for patients with schizophrenia.

Neeb's Tip

It is important for the nurse to avoid reinforcing psychotic thinking, as in delusions. For example, avoid asking the patient what "they" are telling the patient. Rather, let the patient know you are concerned but do not hear these voices.

Neeb's Tip

Remember that schizophrenic patients are often very concrete thinkers, so it is important to speak clearly and plainly. Make only one request at a time.

Classroom Activity

- Have a mental health counselor from a local clinic present information on managing schizophrenia to your class.

See Table 15-7 for interventions for patients with schizophrenia who are hallucinating.

Tool Box |▶ National Institute of Mental Health information for Patients and Families on Schizophrenia:
http://www.nimh.nih.gov/health/topics/schizophrenia/index.shtml

Critical Thinking Question

Your 19-year-old patient with a new diagnosis of schizophrenia begins yelling "Stay away, don't touch me" as you walk into his room. His mother is in the room and is trying to comfort the patient. What approaches might be helpful for the patient and his mother?

Table 15-6 Nursing Care Plan of the Schizophrenic Patient

Data Collection	Nursing Diagnosis	Plan/Goal	Interventions/ Nursing Actions	Evaluation Criteria
Patient is mumbling to himself, looks suspiciously at staff, avoids contact with staff, other people avoid patient.	Social isolation	Patient will spend time in a social activity.	• Approach patient for brief periods in a non-threatening manner. • Avoid touching patient without asking permission. • Talk about concrete unit activities. • Demonstrate acceptance of patient's behavior and appearance by avoiding reacting to bizarre behavior. Point out possible alternative behaviors once relationship established.	Patient will participate in unit activity once a day.

Table 15-7 Suggested Interventions for Patients With Schizophrenia Who Are Hallucinating

Suggested Action	Rationale
1. "Mr. R, I don't see any bugs. It is time for lunch. I will walk to the dining room with you."	**1.** This lets the patient know you heard him but brings him immediately into the reality of time of day and the need to go to the dining room.
2. "I see a crack in the wall, Mr. R. It is harmless; you are safe. Susan is here to take you down to Occupational Therapy now."	**2.** This is in response to a probable illusion. It lets the patient know that you see something. It validates his fear but tells him what you see and then moves him into the here and now.
3. "I know that your thoughts seem very real to you, Ms. C, but they do not seem logical to me. I would like you to come to your room and get dressed now, please."	**3.** Again, you are validating the patient's concern without exploring and focusing on the delusion.
4. "Ms. C, It appears to me that you are listening to someone. Are you hearing voices other than mine?"	**4.** This is a method of validating your impression of what you see. This is as far as you will go into exploring what she may be hearing.
5. "Thank you, Ms. C. I want to help you focus away from the other voices. I am real; they are not. Please come with me to the reading room."	**5.** In this statement, you respond to her in the present and reinforce her response to you. This response attempts to redirect her thinking.

Source: Adapted from Gorman and Sultan (2008). Psychosocial Nursing for General Patient Care, 3rd ed. Philadelphia: F.A. Davis Company, with permission.

■■■ Key Concepts

1. Schizophrenia is a chronic, serious, often debilitating psychiatric disorder that impacts all aspects of the patient's life and his/her loved ones.
2. Schizophrenia is now known to be a brain disorder.
3. Not all psychoses are schizophrenia. Other psychotic disorders can include brief psychotic disorder, psychosis in bipolar disorder, substance abuse, and major depression.
4. Schizophrenia is now viewed as a spectrum disorder, which means there is a gradient of less to more severe conditions. Schizophrenia is usually diagnosed in a person's late teens and young adulthood but often continues for the rest of the patient's life.
5. Hallucinations and delusions are examples of positive symptoms that present challenges to all health-care professionals.
6. The main treatment for schizophrenia remains antipsychotic medications. Because of the side-effect profile of these medications, close monitoring is needed to achieve the best outcomes and patient compliance.

CASE STUDY

Ralph is a 20-year-old college student who is admitted to your psychiatric facility by his parents. Ralph is in his second year at an out-of-state college. Over the past 6 months, he has been exhibiting increasingly bizarre behavior, such as walking the halls of his dorm at night knocking on doors, asking strange questions, mumbling to himself, and sleeping on the floor during the day. He has also been exhibiting disruptive behaviors in class. Students report being afraid of him and he has become increasingly isolated. Most recently he became violent in the school cafeteria. Then the school counselor reported to his parents that he needed immediate hospitalization.

The parents report that Ralph had a normal childhood and never displayed any unusual behavior until the last year. The parents tell you they feel guilty that they did not monitor his behavior more closely in the last few months.

On meeting Ralph he avoids eye contact and appears to be talking to someone he sees in the corner of the room. When his parents walk into the room, he begins hitting his head repeatedly against the wall.

1. How should you respond to Ralph when first meeting him?
2. How would you respond to the parents' fears?
3. What medications might be useful for this patient?

REFERENCES

American Psychiatric Association. (2000). *Diagnostic and Statistical Manual of Mental Disorders IV-Text Revision.* Washington DC, Author. (Known as DSM-IV-TR)

American Psychiatric Association. (2013). *Diagnostic and Statistical Manual of Mental Disorders 5.* Washington, DC, Author. (Known as DSM-5)

Bauer, S.M., et al. (2011). Culture and the prevalence of hallucinations in schizophrenia. *Comprehensive psychiatry, 52*(3), 319–325.

Collier, E. (2011). Schizophrenia in older adults. *Journal of psychosocial nursing and mental health services, 49*(8), 17–21.

Goldberg, R J. (2007). *Practical Guide to the Care of the Psychiatric Patient.* 3rd ed. St Louis: Mosby-Elsevier.

Gorman, L., and Sultan, D. (2008). *Psychosocial Nursing for General Patient Care.* 3rd ed. Philadelphia: F.A. Davis.

Harris, B.A. (2012). Schizophrenia. A critical nursing perspective of pharmacological interventions for schizophrenia and the marginalization of person-centered alternatives. *Issues in Mental Health Nursing. 33*(2),127–132.

National Institutes of Mental Health. Schizophrenia. Retrieved from http://www.nimh.nih.gov/statistics/1SCHIZ.shtml

Townsend, M. (2012). *Psychiatric Mental Health Nursing.* 7th ed. Philadelphia: F.A. Davis.

Test Questions

Multiple Choice Questions

1. Brian, an 18-year-old with schizophrenia, has a negative attitude, is delusional, hears voices, and is withdrawing from others. A nursing intervention that is appropriate for promoting activity for Brian is:
a. Tell him "the voices" told you he should participate in the weekly party.
b. Remind him that he does not want to get worse by sitting alone.
c. Tell him he must join the party; it is part of his care plan.
d. Invite him to join in the party.

2. Shawna is a 22-year-old woman who has episodes of extreme muscle rigidity and hyperexcitability. She sometimes repeats a word or a phrase over and over. Attempts to move her are met with even more muscle resistance. What is she exhibiting?
a. Catatonia
b. Disorganized schizophrenia
c. Brief psychotic disorder
d. Schizotypal personality

3. Mr. G is calling out, "Nurse!" When you arrive in his room, he tells you to be careful of the snake in the corner. You do not see anything in the corner. Mr. G is experiencing a (an):
a. Hallucination
b. Attention-getting behavior
c. Illusion
d. Delusion

4. Of the following responses, which would be your *best* response to Mr. G regarding the snake?
a. "Don't worry; I'll get rid of it." (You pretend to remove the snake.)
b. "I don't see a snake; what else do you see that isn't there?"
c. "I don't see a snake. It is time for your group meeting. I'll walk with you to the meeting room."
d. "Where is it? I hate snakes. Let's get out of here."

5. Which of the following is *not* a sign of untreated schizophrenia?
a. Loss of reality
b. Living in one's own world
c. Maintaining satisfactory performance on the job
d. Delusions, hallucinations

6. A nursing intervention for a person with schizophrenia is to:
a. Reinforce the hallucinations.
b. Keep the person oriented to reality and to the present.
c. Encourage the patient to begin psychoanalysis.
d. Encourage competitive activities.

7. Mr. S states, "Look at the snakes on the ceiling." You see some cracks in the plaster. Mr. S is experiencing a (an):
a. Hallucination
b. Illusion
c. Delusion
d. Flashback

8. Your best response to Mr. S might be:
a. "How many snakes do you see, Mr. S?"
b. "Yes, I see them, too. Let's go to the dayroom."
c. "I see some cracks in the plaster, but I do not see snakes. Let's go to the day room."
d. "I don't think your medication is working. I'll call the doctor."

9. A patient who repeats a word or part of a word over and over might be said to have which of the following symptoms?
a. Echolalia
b. Echopraxia
c. Echocardia
d. Word salad

Test Questions

cont.

10. An individual stands on the train track with the train coming nearer. The person exclaims, "I am invincible! The train will not hurt me." This is an example of:
   a. Delusions of grandeur
   b. Echolalia
   c. Sensory hallucinations
   d. Extrapyramidal symptoms

11. Which of the following pairs of symptoms are closely associated with EPS?
   a. Muscle rigidity and protruding tongue
   b. Overly emotional, depressed
   c. Shuffling gait and depression
   d. Fatigue and painful joints

12. The primary goal in working with an actively psychotic, suspicious patient is to:
   a. Improve her relationship with her parents
   b. Encourage participation in individual psychotherapy
   c. Decrease her anxiety and increase trust
   d. Promote healthy living habits

13. The most current thinking on the cause of schizophrenia is:
   a. A brain disorder
   b. Primarily a disturbed mother/child relationship
   c. Brain damage caused by the mother's use of tranquilizers during pregnancy
   d. Alternation in opioid receptors

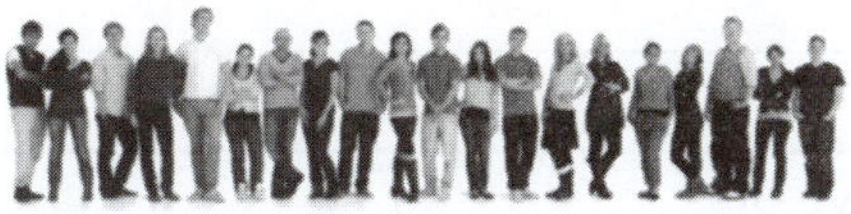

CHAPTER 16

Neurocognitive Disorders: Delirium and Dementia

Learning Objectives

1. Describe the differences between delirium and dementia.
2. Define neurocognitive disorders.
3. List the most common forms of dementia.
4. List common causes of delirium.
5. Describe effective treatments for each.

Key Terms

- Agnosia
- Agraphia
- Alzheimer's disease
- Apraxia
- Chemical restraint
- Delirium
- Dementia
- Mild neurocognitive disorder
- Neurocognitive disorder
- Nocturnal delirium
- Physical restraint
- Pseudodementia
- Vascular dementia

Neurocognitive disorder is the new global term that includes the diagnoses of delirium and dementia (DSM-5, 2013). In the past these were referred to as organic mental syndromes and disorders by the American Psychiatric Association. The disorders in this category all include deficits in cognitive function.

Delirium

Delirium is an acute reaction to underlying physiological (e.g., toxins, drug reactions, illness) or psychological stress (e.g., sensory overload). It is a temporary condition that is characterized by a disturbance in attention (i.e., reduced ability to direct, focus, sustain, and shift attention) and orientation to the environment. For example, the patient may need questions repeated due to inattention, is easily distracted, or needs repeated orientation to the situation. It can also include memory deficit, language disturbance, and/or perceptual disturbance. Delirium may include alterations in sleep-wake cycle, including hypervigilant state to stupor. The patient may exhibit **nocturnal delirium**, known as sundowning, when confusion and agitation increase at dusk. See Table 16-1 for types of delirium with common symptoms. Delirium usually develops quickly and often fluctuates throughout the day. The condition often resolves once the cause is identified and treated. Delirium should be considered when the person exhibits sudden onset of confusion, memory impairment, incoherence, fluctuating levels of consciousness, sleep-wake cycle disruption, hallucinations, and/or delusions.

Delirium is an extremely common condition seen in the acute hospital, nursing home, and home settings, particularly in the elderly. DSM-5 reports that delirium occurs in 15%–53% of older individuals postoperatively and 70%–87% of those in ICU. The condition also

Table 16-1 Types of Delirium

Assessments	Hypoactive-Hypoalert	Hyperactive-Hyperalert	Mixed
Level of alertness	Lethargic, falls asleep between questions, difficult to arouse	Overly attentive to cues	Alternates between hyperalert and hypoalert states within hours or days
Motor activity	Decreased activity	Moves quickly	Alternates within one episode of delirium
Ability to follow commands	Follows a simple command, e.g., lift your foot Is passively cooperative	May be combative, pulls at tubes, tries to climb out of bed	Alternates between hypoactive and hyperactive states, may be unpredictable
Thinking ability	Difficulty in focusing attention, disorganized	Easily distracted, Rambles May mumble, swear, or yell	Alternates between hypoactive and hyperactive states in an unpredictable manner

Source: Adapted from Forrest et al. (2007) and Gorman & Sultan (2008).

contributes to mortality. DSM-IV-TR reports that 15% of elderly people die within one month of an episode of delirium. Common causes can include electrolyte imbalance, poor oxygenation, medication side effects or misuse, urinary tract infections, and dehydration. See Table 16-2 for a more comprehensive list of causes. Identifying the cause can be challenging in people with complex medical conditions, as multiple factors may contribute to the delirium. Substance-induced delirium is a separate category when delirium developed during or within a month after severe intoxication or withdrawal from a substance capable of producing delirium.

Treatment of Delirium

Treatment of delirium must be focused on finding and treating the cause. Often symptoms of delirium can resolve quickly once the appropriate treatment for the cause is begun. Supportive interventions to maintain patient safety, control agitation, prevent further complications, and reorient can be very helpful.

Clinical Activity

If your patient has a delirium diagnosis or exhibits a sudden change in consciousness and/or behavior, review his or her medical record for possible causes, including medication side effects, recent lab results, and recent infections.

Pharmacology Corner

Prescribing medications to control delirium symptoms is risky because these medications can mask or compound the confusion and agitation. However, at times low-dose antipsychotic medications such as haloperidol, risperdal, and olanzapine may be needed to address agitation. The benefits of the medications must be weighed against the possible side effects. Generally, anti-anxiety medications like lorazepam should be avoided as they further confuse the picture of alterations in consciousness.

Neeb's Tip

Your patient with delirium needs to be monitored closely. He can appear normal at times and then suddenly become agitated and try to get out of bed unsupervised.

Critical Thinking Question

An 81-year-old woman is admitted from the ER with a diagnosis of delirium manifested by acute confusion, rambling speech, and new onset of incontinence. Her husband reports this all started 24 hours ago after several episodes of diarrhea. She had recently been in the hospital for complications from diabetes. List the possible causes of delirium that should be evaluated.

Table 16-2 Causes of Delirium

Biological Factors	Other Factors
Hypoxia	Medication side effect
Nutritional deficiencies, e.g., iron, B_{12}	Anesthesia reaction
Electrolyte imbalances, e.g., ↑ calcium	Overdose of medication
Hypoglycemia/hyperglycemia	Substance abuse/withdrawal, e.g., alcohol, cannabis, opioids, anxiolytics, sedatives
Renal failure, hepatic encephalopathy	Sensory overload and deprivation
Sepsis and other infections including UTI	Head trauma
Metabolic disorders, e.g., acid-base imbalance	
Medication or anesthesia reaction	
Hypothyroidism	
Cardiac insufficiency	
Primary brain disorders, e.g., brain tumors, Parkinson's disease	
Pain	

Source: Gorman & Sultan (2008) and Townsend (2012).

■ Dementia

Dementia is defined as a gradual loss of previous levels of cognitive functioning, which can include memory, language, executive functions (includes organizing), and attention in a state of being fully alert. In DSM-5 it is classified as a major neurocognitive disorder. In contrast to delirium, dementia is a slowly progressive condition that eventually impacts all aspects of mental and social functioning. Primary dementias, including Alzheimer's disease, are those where the dementia itself is the major cause. Secondary dementia, including vascular and HIV-related, is caused by another disease or condition.

Depression is a common disorder in the elderly. Sometimes depression can mimic dementia; in that case, it is referred to as **pseudodementia.** Depression in the elderly can be confused with dementia with the following symptoms:

- Forgetfulness
- Little effort to complete responsibilities
- Limited communication

One differentiation is that the depressed patient generally remains oriented to time and place, unlike the dementia patient.

Alzheimer's Disease

This most common form of dementia was initially recognized by Dr. Alois Alzheimer in 1906 as a form of impairment of brain function (Fig. 16-1). **Alzheimer's disease** accounts for 60%–80% of dementias. It is estimated that 13% of Americans over 65 years old have this diagnosis and incidence increases with age. The impact on society is a major one as people are living longer. It is not reversible. Alzheimer's disease is the sixth leading cause of death in the United States. The cause of death is often aspiration pneumonias, infections, and complications from falls, which are all outcomes

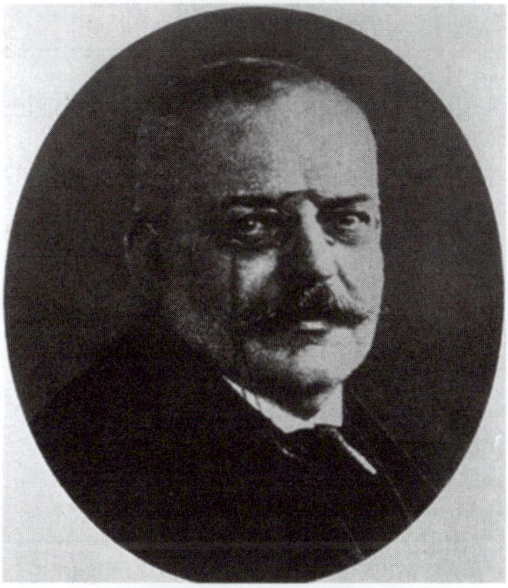

Figure 16-1 Alois Alzheimer (1864–1915) was a German neurologist who first identified Alzheimer's disease in 1906.

of immobility, swallowing disorders, and malnutrition that are present in late stages of the disease (Alzheimer's Association, Alzheimer's Disease 2013 Facts and Figures, 2013). See Box 16-1 for the symptoms of Alzheimer's disease and Box 16-2 for warning signs.

> **Tool Box** |▶ Review the government's National Plan to Address Alzheimer's Disease (2012) at http://aspe.hhs.gov/daltcp/napa/NatlPlan.shtml

In addition to symptom assessment, the diagnosis of Alzheimer's disease is made by MRI or PET scan, which can detect physical and chemical changes in the brain. The changes seen in the brain include development of plaque (chemical deposits made of degenerating nerve cells and proteins called beta amyloid) and tangles (malformed nerve cells). These plaques and tangles are greatly increased in someone with this form of dementia. As they increase, they create a toxic environment for normal brain cells. It is known that an enzyme used to produce the neurochemical acetylcholine is reduced as well. Some of the medications that are being used to slow the progression of this disease increase the level of acetylcholine. There are genetic markers for some forms of this disease. Research is ongoing as to the causes of these brain changes (Fig. 16-2). A rare form of the disease is genetic and accounts for less than 5% of cases. Other specific causes are still unclear.

The presence of the diagnosis of **mild neurocognitive disorder** (previously called mild cognitive impairment) is a risk factor. Mild neurocognitive disorder is a condition in which a person has mild deficits with memory, language, or another essential cognitive ability. The person begins making changes in his/her life to compensate for these, and it begins to affect daily living. Mild cognitive disorder is not normal aging.

Many people fear that forgetfulness is a sign of developing Alzheimer's disease. See Table 16-3 for the differences between Alzheimer's disease and normal aging.

Box 16-1 Symptoms of Alzheimer's Disease

- Memory loss that disrupts daily life
- Challenges in planning or solving problems (executive functions)
- Difficulty completing familiar tasks at home, at work, or at leisure
- Confusion with time or place
- Trouble understanding visual images and spatial relationships
- New problems with words in speaking or writing
- Misplacing things and losing the ability to retrace steps
- Decreased or poor judgment
- Withdrawal from work or social activities
- Changes in mood and personality
- **Agnosia**: loss of ability to recognize objects
- **Agraphia**: difficulty writing and drawing
- **Apraxia**: inability to carry out motor activities despite intact motor function

Source: Adapted from Alzheimer's Association and Townsend (2012).

Box 16-2 Warning Signs of Alzheimer's Disease

1. Asking the same question over and over again.
2. Repeating the same story, word for word, again and again.
3. Losing one's ability to pay bills or balance one's checkbook.
4. Getting lost in familiar surroundings, or misplacing household objects.
5. Relying on someone else, such as a spouse, to make decisions or answer questions they previously would have handled themselves.
6. Finding it hard to remember things.
7. Losing things or putting them in odd places.

Source: Adapted from National Institute on Aging (2012). Alzheimer's Disease Fact Sheet.

The Stages of Alzheimer's Disease

Alzheimer's disease has been divided into stages.

Stage 1: No Impairment (Normal function)

The person does not experience any memory problems. An interview with a medical

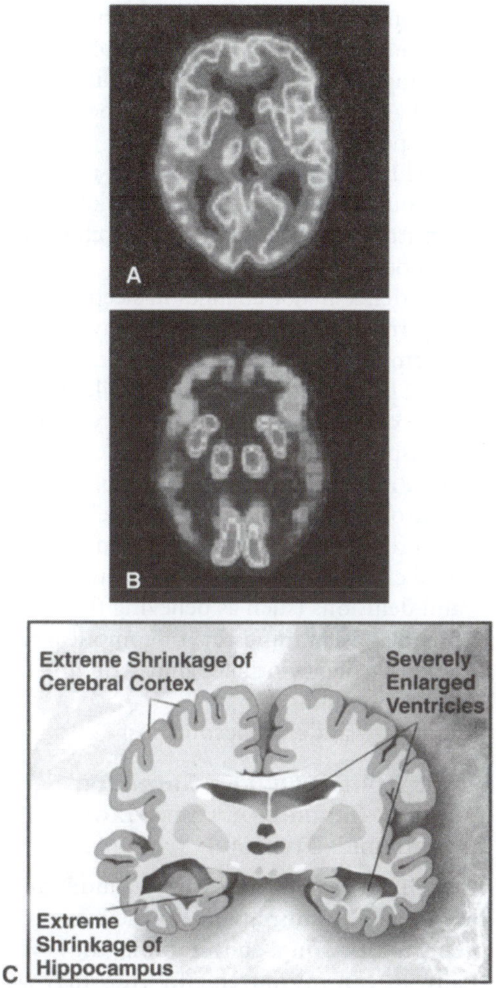

Figure 16-2 Changes in the Alzheimer's brain. A. Metabolic activity in a normal brain. B. Diminished metabolic activity in Alzheimer's diseased brain. C. Late-stage Alzheimer's disease with generalized atrophy and enlargement of the ventricles. *(Source: Alzheimer's Disease Education & Referral Center, A Service of the National Institute on Aging.)*

professional does not show any evidence of symptoms of dementia.

Stage 2: Very Mild Cognitive Decline (May be normal age-related changes or earliest signs of Alzheimer's Disease)

The person may feel as if he or she is having memory lapses—forgetting familiar words or the location of everyday objects. But no symptoms of dementia can be detected during a medical examination or by friends, family, or coworkers.

Table 16-3 Differentiating Alzheimer's Disease From Normal Aging

Alzheimer's Disease	Normal Aging
Making poor judgments and decisions a lot of the time	Making a bad decision once in a while
Problems taking care of monthly bills	Missing a monthly payment
Losing track of the date or time of year	Forgetting which day it is and remembering it later
Trouble having a conversation	Sometimes forgetting which word to use
Misplacing things often and being unable to find them	Losing things from time to time

Source: The National Institute on Aging. Retrieved from www.nia.nih.gov/alzheimers/publication/understanding-alzheimers-disease/what-are-signs-alzheimers-disease

Stage 3: Mild Cognitive Decline (Early-stage Alzheimer's can be diagnosed in some but not all individuals with these symptoms)

Friends, family, or coworkers begin to notice difficulties. During a detailed medical interview, doctors may be able to detect problems in memory or concentration. Common stage 3 difficulties include:

- Noticeable problems coming up with the right word or name
- Trouble remembering names when introduced to new people
- Having noticeably greater difficulty performing tasks in social or work settings
- Forgetting material that one has just read
- Losing or misplacing a valuable object
- Increasing trouble with planning or organizing

Stage 4: Moderate Cognitive Decline (Mild or early-stage Alzheimer's Disease)

At this point, a careful medical interview should be able to detect clear-cut symptoms in several areas:

- Forgetfulness of recent events
- Impaired ability to perform challenging mental arithmetic—for example, counting backward from 100 by 7s
- Greater difficulty performing complex tasks, such as planning dinner for guests, paying bills, or managing finances
- Forgetfulness about one's own personal history
- Becoming moody or withdrawn, especially in socially or mentally challenging situations

Stage 5: Moderately Severe Cognitive Decline (Moderate or mid-stage Alzheimer's Disease)

Gaps in memory and thinking are noticeable, and individuals begin to need help with day-to-day activities. At this stage, those with Alzheimer's may:

- Be unable to recall their own address or telephone number, or the high school or college from which they graduated
- Become confused about where they are or what day it is
- Have trouble with less challenging mental arithmetic; e.g., counting backward from 40 by subtracting 4s or from 20 by 2s
- Need help choosing proper clothing for the season or the occasion
- Still remember significant details about themselves and their family
- Still require no assistance with eating or using the toilet

Stage 6: Severe Cognitive Decline (Moderately severe or mid-stage Alzheimer's Disease)

Memory continues to worsen, personality changes may take place, and individuals need extensive help with daily activities. At this stage, individuals may:

- Lose awareness of recent experiences as well as of their surroundings
- Remember their own name but have difficulty with their personal history
- Distinguish familiar and unfamiliar faces but have trouble remembering the name of a spouse or caregiver
- Need help dressing properly and may, without supervision, make mistakes such as putting pajamas over daytime clothes or shoes on the wrong feet
- Experience major changes in sleep patterns—sleeping during the day and becoming restless at night
- Need help handling details of toileting (for example, flushing the toilet, wiping or disposing of tissue properly)
- Have increasingly frequent trouble controlling their bladder or bowels
- Experience major personality and behavioral changes, including suspiciousness and delusions (such as believing that their caregiver is an impostor) or compulsive, repetitive behavior like hand-wringing or tissue shredding
- Tend to wander or become lost

Stage 7: Very Severe Cognitive Decline (Severe or late-stage Alzheimer's Disease)

In the final stage of this disease, individuals lose the ability to respond to their environment, to carry on a conversation, and, eventually, to control movement. They may still say words or phrases. At this stage, individuals need help with much of their daily personal care, including eating or using the toilet. They may also lose the ability to smile, to sit without support, and to hold their head up. Reflexes become abnormal. Muscles grow rigid. Swallowing is impaired.

(Reprinted with permission, Alzheimer's Association.)

Neeb's Tip

Alzheimer's disease is a progressive illness that will eventually lead to the patient's death. The nurse should be aware of signs of late-stage Alzheimer's disease (Stage 7) when hospice care may be an appropriate referral. Signs such as bedbound, incontinent, multiple infections, aspirations can indicate the patient is appropriate for hospice care.

Classroom Activity
- View and discuss recent movies that address dementia, including *Iron Lady, The Savages,* and *The Notebook.*

Tool Box ▶ The mini-mental state exam (MMSE) is a widely used test of cognitive function. It is a 30-point questionnaire used extensively with dementia patients to track changes over time. Available online at http://en.wikipedia.org/wiki/Mini%E2%80%93mental_state_examination.

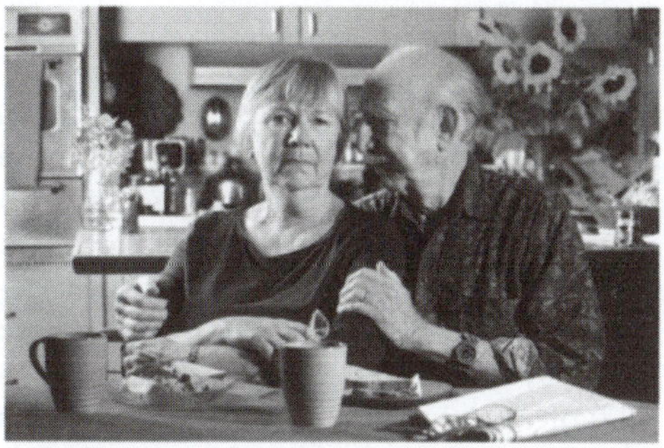

Figure 16-3 Alzheimer's disease makes a tremendous impact on the family.

Treatment of Alzheimer's Disease

No treatment is available to stop the deterioration of brain cells in Alzheimer's disease. The U.S. Food and Drug Administration (FDA) has currently approved five drugs that temporarily slow worsening of symptoms for about 6 to 12 months (see the Pharmacology Corner). However, researchers around the world are studying numerous treatment strategies that may have the potential to change the course of the disease. Approximately 75 to 100 experimental therapies aimed at slowing or stopping the progression of Alzheimer's are in clinical testing in human volunteers (Alzheimer's Association, *Alzheimer's Disease 2013 Facts and Figures, 2013).*

In addition to the medications, supportive care, maintaining safety, prevention of infections, and caregiver support are the major interventions. Once diagnosed, the patient and his/her family need to develop a plan to provide care as the disease progresses. This is important in the early stages so the patient can participate in decisions about future care while he/she still can. For example, identifying options for home caregivers or facilities in the area based on the patient's wishes can be documented early on. Family members of Alzheimer's patients need to be prepared for what to expect as it progresses (Fig. 16-3).

Clinical Activity
If your patient has dementia, talk with patient's family about how they are coping.

Neeb's Tip People with early-stage Alzheimer's disease should be encouraged to complete an advance directive so they can document their wishes for care and treatment as the disease progresses.

Pharmacology Corner

Cholinesterase inhibitors are the class of medications used in treatment of early to moderate Alzheimer's disease. They are effective for only about half of the individuals who take them. These drugs act by inhibiting acetylcholinesterase, which increases the concentrations of acetylcholine in the brain. They have been found to slow the process of dementia in some people but not control it. Another medication, memantine, is used in moderate to severe Alzheimer's disease. It works as a receptor antagonist of *N*-methyl-D-aspartate (NMDA) and has been shown to slow down progression of cognitive decline and daily functioning in some patients with more advanced disease. The two types of drugs may be given together in some cases. See Table 16-4 for the cholinesterase inhibitors used to treat Alzheimer's dementia. Early treatment with these medications with mild neurocognitive disorder may be helpful.

When extreme agitation requires the use of antipsychotic medications in dementia

Continued

Pharmacology Corner—cont'd

patients, it must be recognized that the FDA has ordered black-box warnings on atypical antipsychotics due to increased risk of death in the elderly with psychotic behaviors associated with dementia. These deaths were cardiovascular related. In 2008 all typical antipsychotics were added to this warning. Therefore close monitoring is required when any of these medications are used. This presents a dilemma to the clinician. These medications can control behavior and promote safety, but there is a risk for untoward effects. Generally, the adage "start low and go slow" when using any medications in this population is particularly true.

Other medications to treat depression, anxiety, and insomnia may be utilized. Because depression and anxiety are especially common if the person is aware of the decline, these medications can be very helpful. Be aware that paradoxical reactions (drug has opposite effect than what it is intended for) sometimes occur in the elderly with anti-anxiety medications.

Managing anxiety with these medications can be useful to reduce the patient's suffering and disruptive behaviors.

Table 16-4 Cholinesterase Inhibitors

Cholinesterase Inhibitor	Side Effects
Tacrine (Cognex)	Dizziness, headache, GI upset
Donepezil (Aricept)	Insomnia, dizziness, headache, GI upset
Rivastigmine (Excelon)	Dizziness, headache, fatigue
Galantamine (Razadyne)	Dizziness, headache, GI upset

Source: Adapted from Townsend (2012): Psychiatric Mental Health Nursing: Concepts of Care in Evidence-Based Practice, 7th ed. Philadelphia: F.A. Davis Company, with permission.

Neeb's Tip

It can be challenging to give oral medications to dementia patients. An effective strategy is to crush the pills and put them in sweet foods like pudding.

Neeb's Tip

Close monitoring of side effects of all medications can be challenging as the patient may not be able to tell you what he/she is experiencing e.g., dry mouth, itching, constipation.

Critical Thinking Question

Your 72-year-old patient with advanced dementia has been screaming all night, calling for her mother. All attempts to console her are ineffective. Every time someone walks by her room, her screaming increases. You have orders for several medications to control agitation, including haloperidol and lorazepam. Before administering one of these, what should you consider?

Clinical Activity

Monitor side effects of any medications your patient is taking. Your observation is most important as your patient may not be able to verbalize about symptoms.

Other Forms of Dementia

The second most common form of dementia is vascular and is caused by small strokes which over time result in interruption of blood flow to the brain. **Vascular dementia** is sometimes referred to as multi-infarct dementia. Progression of this form of dementia can vary from Alzheimer's disease depending on the occurrence of vascular events, i.e., progression of dementia occurs with each new stroke. So an individual with vascular dementia can remain stable for longer periods if there are no new strokes. There are a number of other forms of dementia including dementia associated with Parkinson's disease, Lewy bodies, substance abuse, HIV, and traumatic brain injury among others. These dementias can also exist in the mild neurocognitive disorder forms as in mild neurocognitive disorder due to HIV infection as an example. Each of these forms of dementia has its own unique components in addition to core diagnostic features of dementia.

Differential Diagnosis of Delirium and Dementia

A new patient presenting with confusion and agitation can sometimes be misdiagnosed. Symptoms of delirium and dementia can seem similar, especially on first meeting a patient. See Table 16-5 and Box 16-3 to differentiate between delirium and dementia and common factors leading to misdiagnosis.

■ Nursing Care of Patients With Delirium and Dementia

Common nursing diagnoses in patients with delirium and dementia include the following:

- Anxiety
- Injury, risk for
- Memory, impaired
- Self-care deficit
- Sensory perception, disturbed
- Sleep pattern, disturbed
- Thought processes, disturbed

Table 16-5 Characteristics of Delirium and Dementia

Delirium	Dementia
• Fluctuating levels of awareness and symptoms • Sudden onset • Clouding of consciousness • Perceptual disturbances (hallucinations, illusions) • Memory disturbance, more often for recent events • Highly distractible • Reversibility possible with treatment	• Slow, insidious onset with less fluctuation of symptoms • Deterioration of cognitive abilities • Impaired long- and short-term memory (memory impairment always present) • Personality changes • May focus on one thing for a long time • Often irreversible

Source: Adapted from Gorman and Sultan (2008). Psychosocial Nursing for General Patient Care, 3rd ed. Philadelphia: F.A. Davis Company, with permission.

Box 16-3 Factors That Contribute to Misdiagnosis in Dementia and Delirium

- Some symptoms of dementia and delirium are similar.
- Several causes may occur simultaneously to bring about dementia.
- Delirium occurring in a patient with a dementia can exacerbate already existing symptoms.
- Health-care personnel may harbor unfounded beliefs that serious memory deficits, confusion, and other progressive intellectual deficits are a normal part of the aging process.
- Health-care personnel may harbor unfounded beliefs that confusion always indicates Alzheimer's disease in an older patient.
- Confusion and behavioral changes may be the first signs of medical illness in the elderly.
- Head injuries and other conditions causing brain tissue trauma may present with symptoms similar to those of dementia.
- Confusion is an adverse reaction to many medications.

Source : Gorman, L., Raines, M., & Sultan, D. (1989): Psychosocial Nursing for the Nonpsychiatric Nurse. Philadelphia: F.A. Davis Company. Table 8.1, page 131.

General Nursing Interventions

The nursing interventions for patients with either or both of these diagnoses are based on the patient's symptoms.

1. *Collect data:* Collect information on vital signs, medications used by the patient, circumstances immediately preceding symptoms, and any other information the patient or person who may be accompanying the individual can provide. Note anything that is considered to be a change in the patient's condition. Question family/caregivers on interventions that have been useful in the past.
2. *Stay calm:* Be ready for anything. Patients with symptoms of delirium and/or dementia can be very changeable. No matter what the situation, nurses must diffuse the situation calmly and return the situation to safety. It is very important to make every attempt to maintain the patient's dignity during periods of excitability. Due to memory deficits, these patients can exhibit impulsive behaviors and labile emotions as they forget the context of the situation. The nurse remaining calm will reinforce maintaining a calm environment.

Neeb's Tip A patient with early to moderate dementia may suffer intense anxiety due to confusion and awareness of losing his/her memory. This can be the cause of agitation and paranoia.

3. *Do not argue:* Patients with dementia and/or delirium have cognitive impairment. They do not have the capacity to make rational decisions during the agitated episode. Attempting to model the desired behavior or simply waiting a few minutes and attempting the verbal instruction again may prove to be successful techniques. These patients may no longer have the filters to control their behavior or act in a socially acceptable manner. Distraction can be helpful in some cases. Be aware that patients may use disruptive behaviors such as swearing, insulting others as a way to express frustration.
4. *Use clear, simple verbal communication:* Sensory overload is a common experience for patients experiencing delirium and dementia. To avoid a behavioral "short circuit," it is a good idea to use simple communication and activity in the room. Keep the area quiet. Keep curtains drawn or partially open; keep televisions and radios off or at a very low volume. The stimulation can be adjusted according to the patient's tolerance. Focus on one task at a time. Do not give the patient two to three instructions at the same time.
5. *Allow time for patient to respond:* The ability to function cognitively and physically is diminished when a person is in delirium or dementia. Nurses and other health-care workers must remember to plan to allow more time for performing care. Patience is an important intervention. This can be frustrating for caregivers, but by following this plan the patient will have more opportunities to remain independent and reduce his/her anxiety. This will make the nurse's job easier with better outcomes.
6. *Use touch when appropriate:* It is impossible not to touch this group of patients. There is a danger for misinterpretation of that touch, however. People who have a threat to their ability to process and understand information may not remember the situation as it actually happened. They may have forgotten the episode of incontinence and not understand why "that nurse had to touch me there!" Having a second person—another nurse or a family member—in the room can be a helpful protection for both the nurse and the patient. Documenting all actions and patient responses very carefully is also necessary.
7. *Wandering:* Patients in a state of delirium or dementia may wander. This is a major safety risk that frequently encourages nurses to request restraint orders from the physician. Restraints should only be used as last resort when alternative interventions are

unsuccessful. Interventions to use earlier include:

- Providing a safe environment where the patient can walk or pace
- Distracting patient to other activities
- Putting up large signs in the area reminding patient of his room or areas off limits
- Using alarms on the patient or to off-limit areas (e.g., exit door to stairwell)
- Engaging family and volunteers to closely watch the patient's movements

When the physician has ordered restraints, the nursing responsibilities include careful observation and documentation of alternative interventions that have been tried. **Physical restraints** are defined as any physical method of restricting an individual's freedom of movement, activity, or normal access to his/her body and cannot be easily removed. For physical restraints, each state has guidelines for how often to check, release, and reposition or exercise the patient. Assessing for signs of dermal ulcers and stiffness of muscles helps to maintain skin integrity and full range of motion. **Chemical restraints** are defined as the use of a medication as a restriction to manage the patient's behavior or restrict the patient's freedom of movement, and are not a standard treatment or dosage for the patient's condition. Again, each state may have guidelines on the use of chemical restraints. For chemical restraints, the nurse must document the effect of the medication and any possible side effects. Many medications have side effects, such as confusion, restlessness, and forgetfulness, and may be counterproductive for people with delirium and dementia. Medications should not be used as a substitute for appropriate activities, programming, and personal interaction.

8. *Assist with ADLs as appropriate to the situation:* The nurse will be doing as much for the patient physically as the individual condition requires. For temporary delirium and early stages of dementia, the nurse may only have to use some verbal cues as to what the patient needs to do. For deeper delirium and later stages of dementia, performing total care for the patient may be necessary. Always maintain the patient's dignity and allow him or her to do as much independently as able.
9. *Provide adequate stimulation:* It is as detrimental to understimulate people with cognitive disorders as it is to overload them. The brain needs some encouragement to activate. This will be a "trial-and-error" situation between the nurse and the patient, and it will be different for every patient. Some success has been made with music, pets, art, and physical therapies.
10. *Maintain appropriate milieu:* People living with irreversible, progressive dementia require special attention to the milieu. Acceptance is mandatory. In dementia, nurses should not emphasize "reality orientation" such as repeated attempts to ask or remind patient of his name, the year, and current location—especially in later stages of the disease. Changes in the brain will not allow the memory to function successfully and may, in fact, cause the patient to experience frustration, feel agitation, and increase acting-out behaviors if "reality orientation" is emphasized. Reality orientation may be helpful in delirium and early stages of dementia where the patient gains a sense of comfort from being reoriented, but with short-term memory gaps this may be helpful only for a brief time.

    Having old photos of the patient or familiar smells such as perfume or favorite foods in the environment can have a reassuring effect. Many dementia facilities ask families to bring in special personal items such as photos or mementos that can be housed in a "memory box" in the patient's room to provide a calming influence from familiar items.
11. *Emotional support:* The patient often experiences anxiety as he/she realizes loss of mental abilities. The person can become panicky when disoriented. A consistent, calm environment is important. Patients can also suffer from depression, especially in early stages when the full impact of the progressive disease is made. Family caregivers also need much support as caring for this patient is exhausting. They

often need assistance in identifying support groups and resources for additional caregivers and facilities.

See Table 16-6 for the nursing care plan of confused patients.

Cultural Considerations

The type of care the family wants for the dementia patient will be influenced by culture. In some cultures the family will maintain the patient in the home no matter how difficult the care. Incorporating important cultural values in the discharge plan is essential.

Language barriers can also add to complications in understanding the dementia patient's needs, especially if the patient is in a facility. It is important for these patients to have access to people who speak the same language and have similar cultural experiences to enhance reality orientation and correctly assess cognitive function.

Neeb's Tip Family members must be provided information on being a caregiver and how to cope with the long-term emotional strain.

Tool Box The 36-Hour Day: A Family Guide to Caring for Persons With Alzheimer Disease, Related Dementing Illnesses, and Memory Loss in Later Life (3rd Edition) by Mace and Rabin is a must read for family caregivers.

Neeb's Tip Review agency policies on use of restraints. Be aware of alternatives to restraints that are useful with the patient.

Classroom Activity
- Arrange a visit to a local dementia facility. Interview the staff to learn how they do this work every day.
- Identify local resources such as support groups or adult day care for people with dementia.

Table 16-6 Nursing Care Plan of the Confused Patient

Data Collection	Nursing Diagnosis	Goal	Interventions	Evaluation
Confused as to time, place Becomes agitated when efforts made to reorient patient	Disturbance in sensory perception	Reduced episodes of agitation	• Encourage family to provide familiar items in patient's room, e.g., old photos, mementos. • Place a large sign on door to identify patient's room, bathroom. • Spend time with patient to reminisce about an important event in the past. • Play music or TV shows that are meaningful from patient's past. • Judge whether reorienting patient regularly is effective. If it increases agitation, then avoid this. • Distract the patient with concrete activities like sorting papers of the same color.	Patients will have periods of calmness.

Critical Thinking Question

In report you are told that your 90-year-old patient with moderate dementia has been awake all night, pacing the floor. In the morning you find him sound asleep at 10 a.m. What should be your plan for the day shift?

The next day, this patient is very agitated and repeatedly insists on walking out the unit door. The MD leaves an order for soft restraints to prevent wandering. Before applying these, what interventions should you try?

Key Concepts

1. Delirium is a frequent diagnosis in the acute hospital setting due to complex medical conditions, medication side effects, and sensory overload.
2. Delirium is usually reversible once the cause is identified; dementia is usually irreversible.
3. Alzheimer's disease is by far the most common form of dementia.
4. Alzheimer's disease is a terminal illness which has a tremendous impact on the patient's family and society.
5. Other causes of dementia include vascular insufficiency, substance abuse, and Parkinson's disease.
6. Medications such as anti-anxiety and antipsychotics often have a side effect of confusion and should be chosen carefully in people with dementia. Medications are chosen to treat specific behaviors; they are not a substitute for more direct interventions.
7. Care of the dementia patient should focus on maintenance of safety, prevention of infection, and family support.

CASE STUDY

Mrs. G is 84-year-old widow who lives alone. She has episodes of anxiety and paranoia in her apartment. She calls her son at odd hours, telling him that a neighbor is spying on her. Despite these episodes she seems to function normally and is able to care for herself. Her son reports that her memory seems to be getting poorer, and he notices that she leaves notes to herself around the apartment reminding her to lock the door, brush her teeth, or water the plants. He also notices that she looks as though she has lost weight recently, though she tells him she is eating well. He looks in her refrigerator and sees very little food. He asks her what she eats, and she says "yogurt." She cannot think of anything else. She reports fear of using the stove so she only eats cold foods. He looks at her mail and notices a past due notice on her water bill. She says she is sure she paid that. He is getting concerned and takes her to a geriatric physician for an evaluation. Mrs. G has been a widow for 2 years.

The physician does a complete assessment in the office and orders an MRI. A diagnosis of early to moderate stage Alzheimer's disease is made.

1. What actions would you suggest the patient and her son institute at this time?
2. How would you differentiate between dementia and depression?
3. What safety measures need to be implemented?

REFERENCES

Alzheimer's Association. (2013). *Alzheimer's Disease 2013 Facts and Figures* (Vol. 2). Chicago: Alzheimer's Association. www.alz.org/alzheimers_disease_facts_and_figures.asp

Alzheimer's Association. Stages of Alzheimers disease. Retrieved from alz.org/alzheimers_disease_stages_of_alzheimers.asp

American Psychiatric Association. (2000). *Diagnostic and Statistical Manual of Mental Disorders IV-Text Revision.* Washington DC, Author. (Known as DSM-IV-TR)

American Psychiatric Association. (2013). *Diagnostic and Statistical Manual of Mental Disorders 5.* Washington, DC, Author. (Known as DSM-5)

Forrest, J., Willis, L., and Holm, K. (2007). Recognizing quiet delirium. *American Journal Nursing, 107*(4), 35–39.

Gorman, L., Raines, M., and Sultan, D. (1989). *Psychosocial Nursing for the Nonpsychiatric Nurse.* Philadelphia: F.A. Davis.

Gorman, L., & Sultan, D. (2008). *Psychosocial Nursing for General Patient Care.* 3rd ed. Philadelphia: F.A. Davis.

National Institute on Aging. (2012). Alzheimer's Disease fact sheet. Retrieved from www.nia.nih.gov/alzheimers/publication/alzheimers-disease-fact-sheet

Rabins, P., et al. (2007). *Practice Guidelines for the Treatment of Patients With Alzheimer's Disease and Other Dementias in Late-Life.* 2nd ed. Retrieved from http://psychiatryonline.org/guidelines.aspx

Stanley. M., Blair, K.A., and Beare, P.G. (2005). *Gerontological Nursing: Promoting Successful Aging With Older Adults.* 3rd ed. Philadelphia: F.A. Davis.

Townsend, M.C. (2012). *Psychiatric Mental Health Nursing.* 7th ed. Philadelphia: F.A. Davis.

Test Questions

Multiple Choice Questions

1. You are working the night shift in your surgical unit. Ms. Y, one day postoperative for total hip replacement, is taking several medications for pain, along with an antibiotic. She is 70 years old and presented as alert and oriented prior to surgery. She lives independently. Ms. Y suddenly begins screaming and thrashing in bed, begging you to "Get the spiders out of my bed!" What is the best explanation for Ms. Y's behavior?
   a. Delusions
   b. Delirium
   c. Dementia
   d. Sepsis

2. The best nursing intervention for you, the LPN/LVN, to help Ms. Y is:
   a. Inform the charge nurse and doctor immediately.
   b. Turn on the light and ask her where the spiders are.
   c. Stop her pain medications.
   d. Check her medical record for a diagnosis of mental illness.

3. Mr. H has been admitted to your nursing home in Stage 6 Alzheimer's disease. His wife is crying and says to you, "Nurse, when will he get better? I don't know what I will do without him home. Why can't the doctor fix him?" Your best response to Mrs. H is:
   a. "Hopefully with time he will improve."
   b. "Maybe you should stop visiting for a few days and then you'll feel better."
   c. "You sound really worried. Tell me what the doctor has told you about his condition."
   d. "Mrs. H, your doctor has explained that Mr. H will not get better. You need to make a plan for the future."

4. Donepezil (Aricept) is a medication approved for the treatment of symptoms of Alzheimer's-type dementia. Nurses must be alert to which of the following side effects?
   a. Tachycardia
   b. Insomnia
   c. Mania
   d. Weight gain

5. Which statement is *not* true about Alzheimer's disease?
   a. It is a dementia disorder.
   b. It may occur in middle to late life.
   c. It is a chronic disease.
   d. It is caused by hardening of the arteries.

6. Which of the following would you expect to see in a patient who is diagnosed with neurocognitive disorder?
   a. Intact memory
   b. Appropriate behavior
   c. Disorganization of thought
   d. Orientation to person, place, and time

7. Ms. P has been admitted to your unit with a diagnosis of right tibial fracture. Her emergency department notes say that she fell at home. She admits to having "a lot to drink" over the past week. She is disoriented to time, forgets where she is momentarily, is easily distracted, and has a short attention span. She does not answer questions appropriately. Her family reports that her behavior has been more and more erratic over the past 6 months with periods of confusion. Her son reports she has been a heavy drinker all her life. She is probably experiencing:
   a. Delusions
   b. Delirium
   c. Dementia
   d. Dilemma

Test Questions

cont.

8. Your patient, who is recovering from an exacerbation of an AIDS-related infection, is opting to be treated by family and friends at home. The family has expressed concern because they sense a change in the patient's cognitive abilities. Part of the discharge teaching for this family might include:

a. "It's nothing, really. Patients sometimes get confused in the hospital."
b. "Keep an eye on him. You don't want him to start wandering."
c. "You're concerned about the change in his ability to remember things? Let me call the doctor for you. This is something that you need to discuss together."
d. "I thought something was strange!"

9. Mr. F is brought in by a family member who expresses concern over his memory loss. The physician diagnosed the patient with vascular dementia (multi-infarct dementia). You realize this disorder:

a. Is irreversible
b. May progress rapidly or slowly
c. Indicates the patient has most likely experienced more than one CVA
d. All of the above

10. The use of reality orienting techniques is usually helpful with which patient?

a. Patient in Stage 7 Alzheimer's disease
b. Patient with advanced vascular dementia
c. Elderly patient who is confused and screaming out for her mother
d. Patient who is recovering from delirium and seems more relaxed when reminded of where she is

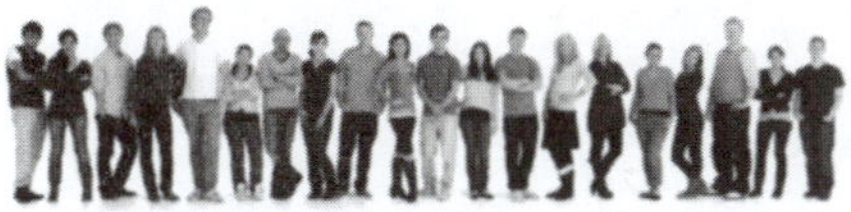

CHAPTER 17

Substance Use and Addictive Disorders

Learning Objectives

1. Describe substance use disorder and how it impacts society.
2. Define co-dependency.
3. Define co-occurring disorders.
4. Identify common medical treatments for addictive disorders.
5. Identify nursing interventions for patients with addictive disorders.

Key Terms

- Addiction
- Alcohol abuse
- Alcohol dependence
- Alcoholism
- Binge drinking
- Co-dependency
- Co-occurring disorder
- Detoxification
- Dysfunctional
- Psychoactive drugs
- Substance abuse
- Substance dependence
- Tolerance
- Withdrawal

Mind- or mood-altering substances have been used throughout human history. Today these include alcohol, sedatives/hypnotics, narcotic analgesics, stimulants, hallucinogens, and cannabis as well as **psychoactive drugs.** Most of these categories of substances can be and are used legally and therapeutically. They all have the strong potential to be abused and to become addictive. These substances taken in excess activate the brain's reward system and can lead to neglecting normal activities in favor of seeking out this substance again and again.

People use these substances for a variety of reasons: to relieve physical and emotional pain, relax, elevate mood, enhance socialization, improve alertness, and alter perceptions of reality. Alcohol and caffeine are probably the most used socially acceptable substances. Tobacco was also part of that group, but in recent years its use has become much less acceptable in U.S. society (Fig. 17-1).

Substance abuse is a major health problem in the United States. Overall 14.6% of the population has had a substance abuse disorder at some time in their lives (Kessler, Berglund et al., 2005). Substance abuse contributes to higher health-care costs, significant disability, and suicide attempts (Cook & Alegría, 2011). The National Survey on Drug Abuse and Health conducts an annual survey of Americans' use of alcohol and other substances and provides the following data from 2011.

- 8.7% of Americans age 12 or older were current (past month) illicit drug users, meaning they had used an illicit drug during the month prior to the survey interview. Illicit drugs include marijuana/hashish, cocaine (including crack),

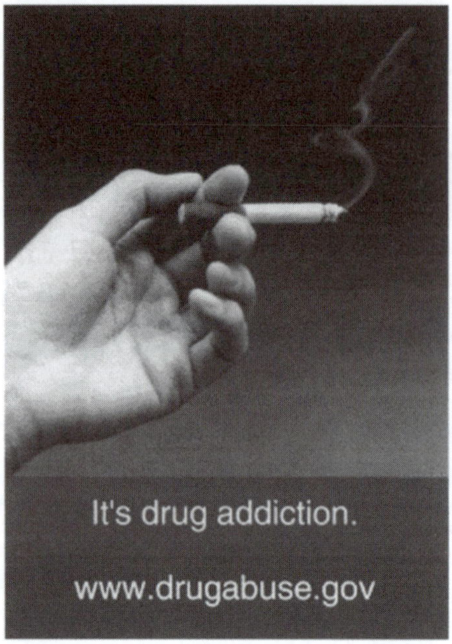

Figure 17-1 As this poster says, nicotine is an addiction, and it can be the most difficult one to overcome. *(Courtesy of the National Institute on Drug Addiction, National Institutes of Health, Bethesda, MD.)*

heroin, methamphetamines, hallucinogens, inhalants, or prescription-type psychotherapeutics used nonmedically; marijuana remains the most widely used illegal drug.

- An estimated 20.6 million persons (8% of the population age 12 or older) were classified with substance dependence or abuse in the past year based on criteria specified in the *Diagnostic and Statistical Manual of Mental Disorders*, 4th edition (DSM-IV-TR).
- Of these, 2.6 million were classified with dependence or abuse of both alcohol and illicit drugs, 3.9 million had dependence or abuse of illicit drugs but not alcohol, and 14.1 million had dependence or abuse of alcohol but not illicit drugs.

Tool Box |▶ National Survey on Drug Use and Health: Summary of National Findings: www.samhsa.gov/data/NSDUH/2k11Results/NSDUHresults2011.pdf

Generally, substance use becomes a problem when it:

1. Interferes with normal functioning
2. Continues despite negative consequences
3. Hurts others

Substance abuse and **substance dependence** have been traditionally separated as two distinct diagnoses. Because these two designations are sometimes confusing and difficult to differentiate, the DSM-5 (2013) has combined abuse and dependence into *substance use disorder* with a graded clinical severity of mild, moderate, and severe. In addition to substance use disorder, there are diagnostic categories for substance-induced intoxication and **withdrawal.** Each category has specific criteria to be met to be given the diagnosis for each substance. At least two criteria are required to make a diagnosis for a particular substance use disorder. However because the terms "abuse" and "dependence" are so common in today's culture, they will still be used throughout this chapter along with substance use disorder.

People with psychiatric disorders commonly abuse many drugs and alcohol as a way to self-medicate to reduce feelings of anxiety, insomnia, depression, loneliness, rapid thoughts, frightening hallucinations, and other distressing symptoms. Commonly referred to as a **co-occurring disorder** (also called dual diagnosis), this form of substance use disorder adds additional complications to the psychiatric diagnosis in terms of daily management, treatment, and recovery. Co-occurring disorders are the rule rather than exception when working with a patient with a psychiatric disorder. Co-occurring disorders can start with self-medicating to treat symptoms of a psychiatric diagnosis, or substance abuse can be the initial diagnosis that leads to other psychiatric disorders as a complication. See Figures 17-2 and 17-3 on pages 263 and 264. Outcomes for treatment are more effective when the substance use treatment is integrated into the treatment for the psychiatric disorder (Clark, 2012).

Health-care professionals are not immune to problems with alcohol and drugs. In fact, they tend to abuse alcohol or prescribed drugs. Since they do not fit the image of a

Critical Thinking Question

You are working in an outpatient mental health clinic. A new patient with a long history of schizophrenia tells you he needs to leave the clinic for an hour to meet someone who gives him "special medicines" that he calls herbs to help him sleep. What concerns would you have? What action would you take?

Neeb's Tip All psychiatric patients should be screened for substance abuse disorders.

substance abuser, it can be easier for healthcare professionals to deny the problem. Many states have developed drug diversion programs to provide confidential treatment and rehabilitation.

Classroom Activity

- Movies that address substance abuse include *Days of Wine and Roses, Lost Weekend, I'm Dancing as Fast as I Can, 28 Days,* and *Flight.*
- Obtain information on how your state addresses substance abuse in nurses.

Some of the characteristics of progressive substance use disorder include (American Psychiatric Association, 2000, 2013):

- A need for markedly increased amounts of the substance to achieve intoxication or desired effect (**tolerance**)
- Markedly diminished effect with continued use of the same amount of the substance (tolerance)
- There is a characteristic withdrawal syndrome for the substance
- The same (or a closely related) substance is taken to relieve or avoid withdrawal symptoms (e.g., alcohol and tranquilizers to sleep)
- The substance is often taken in larger amounts or over a longer period than was intended (analgesics originally used for pain relief then continued when source of pain resolved)
- There is a persistent desire or unsuccessful effort to cut down or control substance use
- A great deal of time is spent in activities necessary to obtain the substance (e.g., visiting multiple doctors or driving long distances to a source), in use of the substance, or to recover from its effects
- Important social, occupational, or recreational activities are given up or reduced because of substance use (e.g., quitting school, giving up a favorite sport)

Cultural Considerations

Substance abuse crosses all cultures and ethnic groups. Some groups are known to have a higher incidence that may reflect genetic risk and/or cultural patterns. For example, Native Americans have a high rate of alcoholism. Genetic factors that predispose them to poor metabolism of alcohol as well as other factors such as unemployment and poverty are contributors. Asians have a lower rate of substance abuse. Genetic intolerance for alcohol creating an unpleasant sensation may be a factor in the lower incidence of alcoholism (Townsend, 2012).

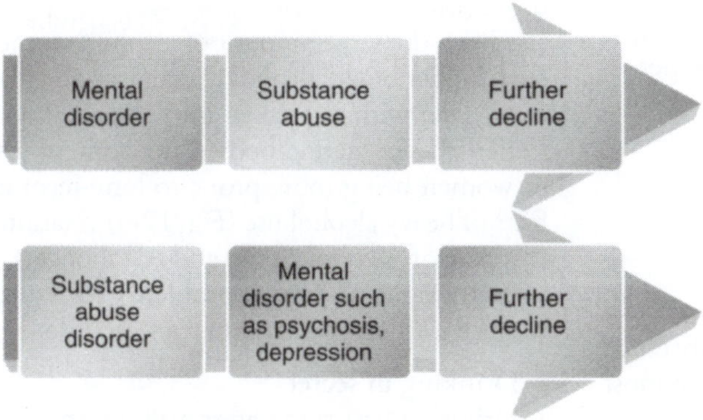

Figure 17-2 Common pathways in co-occurring disorders.

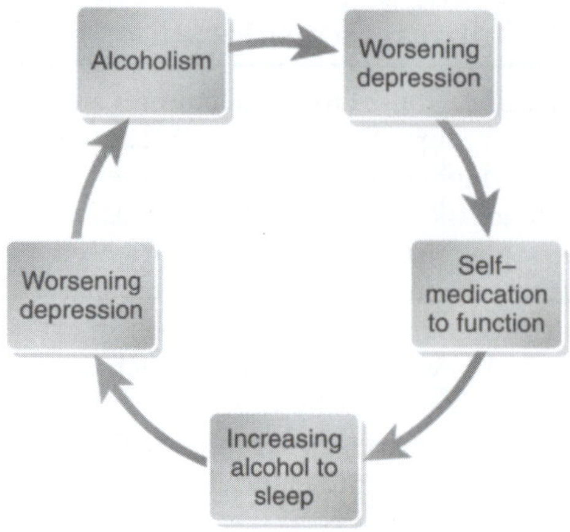

Figure 17-3 An example of the cycle of decline in co-occurring disorders.

- The substance use is continued despite knowledge of having a persistent or recurrent physical or psychological problem that is likely to have been caused or exacerbated by the substance (e.g., current cocaine use despite recognition of cocaine-induced depression, or continued drinking despite recognition that an ulcer was made worse by alcohol consumption)
- Failure to fulfill major role obligations at work, school, or home (e.g., repeated absences or poor work performance related to substance use; substance-related absences, suspensions, or expulsions from school; neglect of children or household)
- Recurrent substance use in situations in which it is physically hazardous (e.g., driving an automobile or operating a machine when impaired by substance use)
- Recurrent substance-related legal problems (e.g., arrests for substance-related disorderly conduct)
- Continued substance use despite having persistent or recurrent social or interpersonal problems caused or exacerbated by the effects of the substance (e.g., arguments with spouse about consequences of intoxication, physical fights)

Alcohol

As the most commonly abused substance worldwide, alcohol is readily available in most cultures and is often included in important occasions and religious ceremonies. Eight percent of Americans are dependent on alcohol at any one time (Kessler, Berglund et al., 2005). It is quickly absorbed in the body with initial effects of intoxication producing relaxation, euphoria, and loss of inhibition. The legal blood level of intoxication is 0.08–0.10 g/dL in most states (known as blood alcohol level). Higher levels of alcohol produce the central nervous system depressant qualities that lead to staggering gait, labile emotions, incoherent speech, poor judgment, and belligerent/aggressive behavior, and eventually can lead to coma and respiratory depression in extremely high levels (greater than 0.4 g/dL). Alcohol content varies with the type of beverage. The same amount of alcohol is present in:

- 12 ounces of most beers
- 5 ounces of wine
- 1.5 ounces of 80-proof distilled spirits such as whiskey or vodka

Neeb's Tip For most adults, low risk alcohol use —up to fourteen drinks per week for men and seven drinks per week for women and older people—causes few, if any, problems (National Institute of Alcohol Abuse and Alcoholism "Rethinking Drinking").

Alcoholism is defined as a chronic illness characterized by compulsive and uncontrolled consumption of alcoholic beverages usually to the detriment of the drinker's health, personal relationships, and social standing. **Addiction** to alcohol has been referred to as **alcohol dependence, alcohol abuse,** and now alcohol use disorder.

Given the same amount of alcohol, women have higher blood alcohol concentrations than men, even with size taken into consideration. Differences in fat and body water content lead to women being more prone to long-term effects of heavy alcohol use (Fig. 17-4) (National Institute of Alcohol Abuse and Alcoholism).

Early signs of serious problems with alcohol use in men and women can include:

- Drinking in secret
- Drinking first thing after waking up

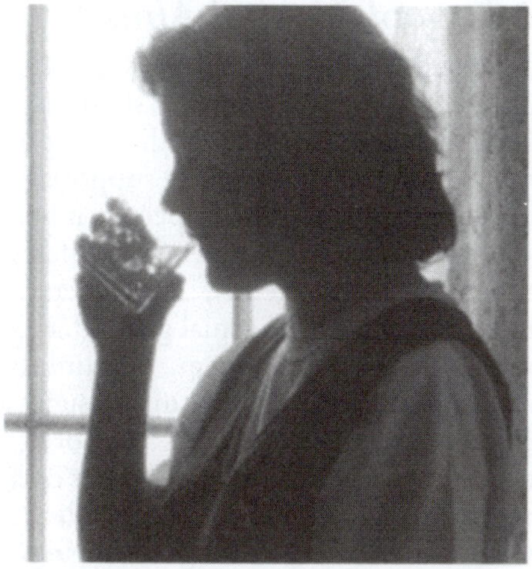

Figure 17-4 The use—and abuse—of alcohol occurs in person of all ages, races, and cultural backgrounds, and in women as well as men. *(Courtesy of the National Institute on Alcohol Abuse and Alcoholism, National Institutes of Health, Bethesda, MD.)*

- Gulping the first drink
- Preoccupation with alcohol
- Onset of blackouts (lapses in memory resulting from persistent heavy drinking)

In 2011, nearly one-quarter (23.1%) of persons aged 12 or older participated in binge drinking (National Survey on Drug Use and Health by Substance Abuse and Mental Health Services Administration, 2011). **Binge drinking** is defined as having five or more drinks (four drinks for women) on the same occasion on at least one day. Binge drinking can lead to serious health consequences from alcohol poisoning when alcohol reaches toxic levels, as well as risky behaviors when under its influence.

Neeb's Tip

Binge drinking in college age adults may be seen as a rite of passage for many, but it can lead to serious damage and even death. Students and parents need to be advised of the effects of toxic levels of alcohol. Many colleges now provide specific information to students about the risk of alcohol poisoning from binge drinking.

Neeb's Tip

Any alcohol use in children and teens is a cause for concern. They may access alcohol from their homes or homes of acquaintances, at parties, or by buying it with fake identification or from older friends. Seeing their parents drinking may give a double message to children or teens who are eager to be grown up. Experimenting with alcohol by adolescents is common, and it is difficult to know which ones will move to a lifetime of struggles with alcohol. A high percentage of adult alcoholics started drinking as teenagers, so any sign of alcohol use by a child or teen must be addressed and needs parental intervention.

Impact on the Family

Family members and friends often develop protective behaviors, sometimes called **codependency** or enabling to control, hide, or deny the alcoholic's behavior to maintain a sense of normalcy for the family. These can include finding excuses for the drinker's alcohol use, covering up the drinker's unacceptable behavior, and self-blame for the drinking. Codependency may be seen with use of other substances besides alcohol.

Alcoholism is a family disease. More than half of all adults have a family history of alcoholism or problem drinking, and one in four children grow up in a home where someone drinks too much (National Institute of Alcohol Abuse and Alcoholism).

Critical Thinking Question

Your patient is a 16-year-old girl admitted from the ER with moderate injuries from a car accident. She was the driver. The other teens in the car were also injured. The patient is awake and tells you that her parents cannot know that she had had a "couple of drinks" at a party just prior to driving her friends home. How would you respond? Should the parents be told? Does that make you an enabler if you choose not to share this?

Tool Box |▶ Adult Children of Alcoholics (ACOA) has support groups for people who grew up in a **dysfunctional** family related to alcoholism:
www.adultchildren.org/

Alcohol's Impact on Health

Alcoholism is the third leading cause of preventable death in the United States (Kessler, Berglund et al., 2005; Kessler, Demler et al., 2005). It can become a chronic medical illness. Heavy drinking contributes to heart disease, some cancers, liver failure, and stroke as it affects most organs in the body. It leads to more complications in the presence of diabetes. It also contributes to countless traffic accidents, falls, domestic violence, suicides, participating in risky activities, industrial accidents, and other unsafe activities as judgment is impaired. Alcohol abuse is often unrecognized and undertreated in the over 65 age group. Whether a lifelong pattern or a new coping mechanism in facing problems, heavy drinking can be confused with dementia, mask depression, and contribute to falls or fires in the home. Alcohol can also contribute to adverse reactions to many medications. Fetal alcohol syndrome includes physical, mental, and/or learning disabilities in a child exposed to alcohol in utero.

Tool Box |▶ The National Institute on Alcohol Abuse and Alcoholism has information on research and the current picture of alcohol use in the United States.
http://niaaa.nih.gov/

Neeb's Tip Long-term alcohol abuse can contribute to a form of dementia in later life.

Tool Box |▶ Use the CAGE questionnaire as a four-question tool to identify problems with alcohol use. CAGE questionnaire is found at:
http://www.integration.samhsa.gov/clinical-practice/sbirt/CAGE_questionaire.pdf

Etiology of Alcohol Abuse

Alcoholism runs in families. Biological offspring of alcoholic parents have a significantly greater incidence of alcoholism than offspring of non-alcoholic parents. This supports the genetic theories. The genes a person inherits partially explain this pattern, but lifestyle is also a factor. Currently, researchers are working to discover the actual genes that put people at risk for alcoholism. The link between depression and alcoholism also suggests biological factors. These facts support the view of alcoholism as a disease. Recent developments in medications to treat alcoholism demonstrate the role of biological cravings to induce a sense of well-being (see Pharmacology Corner for Alcohol Abuse). Disturbance in neural pathways that establish a biological craving to induce well-being is one of the theories. Social factors, stress, and how readily available alcohol is also are factors that may increase the risk for alcoholism. Growing up in a home where alcohol is used as a major coping mechanism for stress also puts a person at risk. But, just because alcoholism tends to run in families does not mean that a child of an alcoholic parent will automatically become an alcoholic too. Some people develop alcoholism even though no one in their family has a drinking problem.

Alcohol Withdrawal

It is estimated that about 25% of admissions to the acute hospital are alcohol related (National Institute of Alcohol Abuse and Alcoholism). Nurses will see patients who are known alcoholics and those where the diagnosis is not known. Awareness of the signs of alcohol withdrawal is essential for all nurses. Signs include:

- Autonomic hyperactivity (high blood pressure, tachycardia, fever)
- Hand tremor
- Insomnia
- Nausea and/or vomiting
- Anxiety
- Transient visual, tactile, or auditory hallucinations or illusions
- Early signs of delirium
- Grand mal seizures

Withdrawal symptoms can occur as early as 8 hours after the last drink in a heavy drinker. Analgesics and recovery from anesthesia can precipitate a withdrawal reaction. It may look like a classic delirium. Screening patients about alcohol use is increasingly common as part of the routine admission assessment in the general hospital.

Neeb's Tip The U.S. Preventative Services Task Force (2012) recommends that primary care providers screen for alcohol abuse in all adults and pregnant women to identify problem drinkers earlier.

Questions that can be asked routinely on admission to identify patients at risk for withdrawal include:

- How often do you drink alcohol?
- How much do you usually drink?
- When was the last time you used alcohol or any drug?
- Have you had any problems because of drinking or drug use?

Neeb's Tip The routine admission questions noted above can also be used to screen for use of other substances.

Withdrawal symptoms are generally most intense on the second day of abstinence. The physician can order a detoxification regimen that will prevent or reduce the alcohol-induced delirium. Withdrawal from alcohol is very uncomfortable but generally not life threatening. Generally, withdrawal is managed with longer acting CNS depressants such as diazepam and chlordiazepoxide, which have anticonvulsant actions and are relatively safe. These are administered routinely and tapered down over several days. Fluids, vitamins, and electrolyte replacement are also part of the treatment plan.

Withdrawal can induce an extreme form of delirium sometimes referred to as delirium tremens or "DTs," evidenced by impaired consciousness and memory as well as hallucinations and severe tremors.

Classroom Activity

- Role-play with classmates how to ask patients about their alcohol and drug use.

Clinical Activity

Any patient who indicates a history of problems with alcohol should be monitored for withdrawal.

Tool Box ▶ The Clinical Institute Withdrawal Assessment for Alcohol Scale, known popularly at CIWA-Ar, is a useful tool used by many hospitals to monitor patients at risk for withdrawal syndrome. Available at Sullivan, J. T., et al. (1989). Assessment of alcohol withdrawal: The revised Clinical Institute withdrawal assessment for alcohol scale. *British Journal of Addiction, 84,* 1353–7 and at: http://ireta.org/sites/ireta.sitesquad.net/files/CIWA-Ar.pdf.

Critical Thinking Question

Your 80-year-old patient is two days post-op recovering from a fractured hip. Until now, her recovery has been routine. She calls you to her bedside and looks anxious and tremulous. She tells you that a glass of wine would help make her more comfortable. What would you do?

Neeb's Tip An individual desperate for alcohol may take alcohol-based medications like cough syrup to control withdrawal.

Treatment of Alcoholism

Perhaps the single most effective treatment for alcoholism is Alcoholics Anonymous (AA). AA is a nationwide organization begun in 1935 by two alcoholic men who bonded and vowed to support each other through recovery. AA has groups in most communities and internationally. It is run by alcoholics, but there is no leader in the group.

One of the main tenets of AA is anonymity. People identify themselves by first names only. Someone usually starts the topic or introductions or asks an opening question, but the group runs itself. It is based on twelve steps, and frequently one step is discussed each week or on a designated week per month. AA meetings are closed—that is, nobody except the alcoholics themselves are allowed to attend. There is usually a group that has an open meeting monthly or quarterly. If the meeting is listed as open, any interested person may attend.

There are corresponding groups for families of the alcoholic (Al-Anon) and a special group for teenagers (Alateen). Adult Children of Alcoholics (ACoA) is a branch of AA formed for people who are now adults but grew up in an alcoholic home and were not able to get help at the time. These groups all follow a similar model.

Table 17-1 lists the twelve steps of AA (Alcoholics Anonymous, 1981). Other twelve-step groups serving other dependency needs, including narcotics, cocaine, and gambling, have modeled themselves after the AA model.

Neeb's Tip AA is usually a lifetime commitment. It is known internationally and the person can reach out to any group when away from home

Tool Box A Brief Guide to Alcoholics Anonymous is available at http://aa.org/lang/en/catalog.cfm?origpage=18&product=8 t

Classroom Activity

- Attend an open meeting of Alcoholics Anonymous and identify how the meeting provided support to the attendees.

One of the slogans of AA is "One Day at a Time." Members of AA believe that they are always in a state of *recovery,* not that they have *recovered.* Recovery from alcoholism is a process. With very few exceptions, an alcoholic who is recovering cannot ever have another drink, or he or she risks returning to the abusive patterns.

Other forms of treatment often include family therapy, short-term hospitalization for detoxification, and individual and group therapy to learn new coping mechanisms. Life without alcohol presents many challenges to

Table 17-1 The Twelve Steps and Twelve Traditions of Alcoholics Anonymous

The Twelve Steps of Alcoholics Anonymous	The Twelve Traditions of Alcoholics Anonymous
1. We admitted we were powerless over alcohol—that our lives had become unmanageable. **2.** Came to believe that a Power greater than ourselves could restore us to sanity. **3.** Made a decision to turn our will and our lives over to the care of God *as we understood Him.* **4.** Made a searching and fearless moral inventory of ourselves. **5.** Admitted to God, to ourselves and to another human being the exact nature of our wrongs. **6.** Were entirely ready to have God remove all these defects of character. **7.** Humbly asked Him to remove our shortcomings. **8.** Made a list of all persons we had harmed and became willing to make amends to them all.	**1.** Our common welfare should come first; personal recovery depends upon A.A. unity. **2.** For our group purpose, there is but one ultimate authority—a loving God as He may express Himself in our group conscience. Our leaders are but trusted servants; they do not govern. **3.** The only requirement for A.A. membership is a desire to stop drinking. **4.** Each group should be autonomous except in matters affecting other groups of A.A. as a whole. **5.** Each group has but one primary purpose—to carry its message to the alcoholic who still suffers. **6.** An A.A. group ought never endorse, finance, or lend the A.A. name to any related facility or outside enterprise, lest problems of money, property, and prestige divert us from our primary purpose.

Table 17-1 The Twelve Steps and Twelve Traditions of Alcoholics Anonymous—cont'd

The Twelve Steps of Alcoholics Anonymous	The Twelve Traditions of Alcoholics Anonymous
9. Made direct amends to such people wherever possible, except when to do so would injure them or others. **10.** Continued to take personal inventory and when we were wrong promptly admitted it. **11.** Sought through prayer and meditation to improve our conscious contact with God, *as we understood Him,* praying only for knowledge of His will for us and the power to carry that out. **12.** Having had a spiritual awakening as the result of these steps, we tried to carry this message to alcoholics and to practice these principles in all our affairs.	**7.** Every A.A. group ought to be fully self-supporting, declining outside contributions. **8.** Alcoholics Anonymous should remain forever non-professional, but our service centers may employ special workers. **9.** A.A., as such, ought never be organized; but we may create service boards or committees directly responsible to those they serve. **10.** Alcoholics Anonymous has no opinion on outside issues; hence the A.A. name ought never be drawn into public controversy. **11.** Our public relations policy is based on attraction rather than promotion; we need always maintain personal anonymity at the level of press, radio, and films. **12.** Anonymity is the spiritual foundation of all our traditions, ever reminding us to place principles before personalities.

Source: The Twelve Steps and Twelve Traditions are reprinted with permission of Alcoholics Anonymous World Services, Inc. (A.A.W.S.). Permission to reprint the Twelve Steps and Twelve Traditions does not mean that A.A.W.S. has reviewed or approved the contents of this publication, nor that AA agrees with the views expressed herein. AA is a program of recovery from alcoholism only—use of the Twelve Steps and Twelve Traditions in connection with programs and activities that are patterned after AA but address other problems, or in any other non-AA context, does not imply otherwise.

the alcoholic. It can include reorganizing one's life around different friends and social activities and repairing family relationships. Pharmacological therapy is also part of treatment. See Pharmacology Corner under Alcohol.

Critical Thinking Question

Your friend stopped drinking about one year ago after she was in a car accident in which she was driving impaired with her three-year-old in the car. She has been attending AA regularly. She is now going through a divorce and tells you she is so stressed and depressed that she has no more energy to get to the AA meetings. What would be your concerns? How can you help her?

Critical Thinking Question

Your 35-year-old patient is being treated for alcohol-related liver disease. He tells you he stopped drinking last month but is worried about his relationship with his fiancée, who is a heavy drinker. What would be your concerns? What suggestions can you make?

Pharmacology Corner

Three drugs have been approved by the Food and Drug Administration to treat alcoholism. Many other approaches are being researched.

1. Disulfiram (Antabuse) was the first medicine approved for the treatment of alcohol abuse and alcohol dependence. It works by causing a severe adverse reaction when someone taking the medication consumes alcohol. This reaction includes palpitations, nausea and vomiting, severe headache, and shortness of breath with exposure to any alcohol.
2. *Naltrexone* is sold under the brand names Revia and Depade. An extended-release form of naltrexone is marketed under the trade name Vivitrol. These drugs works by blocking the "high" that people experience when they drink alcohol or take opioids like

Continued

Pharmacology Corner—cont'd

heroin and cocaine so it blocks the "reward" when taking a drink or the opioid.

3. *Acamprosate (Campral)* works by reducing the cravings for alcohol for someone who is in recovery.

See Table 17-2 for medications commonly used to manage withdrawal.

Neeb's Tip

Any patient on Antabuse must be advised to avoid taking any substance with an alcohol base, including cough syrups and mouthwashes. The patient should carry information so emergency personnel know this information.

Critical Thinking Question

Your 50-year-old patient on Antabuse tells you he is thinking of having a drink to test his response when he goes out on pass. What would you advise this patient? What actions should you take after hearing this information?

Table 17-2 Commonly Used Medications for Withdrawal Management of Alcohol and Other Substances

Alcohol Withdrawal
Chlordiazepoxide (Librium)
Diazepam (Valium)
Oxazepam (Serax)
Nutritional supplements (vitamins, magnesium, thiamine)
Anticonvulsants such as carbamazepine, valproic acid
Serotonin reuptake inhibitors (SSRIs) such as paroxetine, sertraline to treat anxiety and depression
Opioid Withdrawal
Naltrexone (Revia)
Naloxone
Nalmefene (Revex)
Buprenorphine
Buprenorphine and naloxone (Suboxone)
Clonidine (Catapres)
Heroin Withdrawal and Maintenance
Methadone hydrochloride (Dolophine)
Stimulants
Chlordiazepoxide (Librium)
Haloperidol (Haldol)

Other Substances

There are a wide variety of substances that are abused. See Table 17-3 for a summary of the effects of commonly abused substances. Signs and symptoms of substance use disorders vary as to the type of drug. Poly-drug use is common and can create a confusing clinical picture. The individual may use one drug to counteract or enhance the effects of the first drug. Drugs are often combined with alcohol. For example, cocaine users commonly use alcohol to get to sleep or calm down. Many drug and alcohol combinations have a synergistic effect that can be life threatening. Patterns of drug use vary as new substances are discovered. Nurses should be aware of newer drugs that may be used by their patient population. For example, in some communities methamphetamines has been a problem as are "club drugs," including ecstasy, ketamine, and rohypnol (Fig. 17-5). Club drugs are short-acting benzodiazepines that are slipped into an alcoholic drink, causing the unsuspecting victim to become incapacitated and unable to resist a sexual assault. The form of methamphetamine known as crystal meth is produced illegally from ephedrine and creates a highly addictive stimulant that is usually smoked. A new drug referred to as "bath salt" has recently been receiving national attention. This stimulant can produce a paranoia reaction.

DSM-5 now categorizes each substance by substance-induced intoxication and withdrawal disorders. Each disorder has its own criteria for diagnosing based on the specific substance used. A diagnosis of substance use

(Text continued on page 276)

Table 17-3 Comparing Commonly Abused Substances

Drug	Intoxication	Overdose	Withdrawal	Nursing Considerations
Amphetamines, including Dexedrine, methamphetamine (crystal meth)	*Signs:* Euphoria, high energy, impaired judgment, anxiety, weight loss, anorexia, increased libido, aggressive behavior, paranoia, panic disorders, insomnia, and delusions (often seen with long-term use)	*Signs:* Ataxia, high temperature, seizures, hypertension, arrhythmias, respiratory distress, cardiovascular collapse, coma, brain damage, death *Treatment:* Supportive	*Signs:* Depression, agitation, insomnia, confusion, vivid dreams followed by extreme lethargy *Treatment:* Antidepressants, counseling, suicide precautions	• Crystal meth made from ephedrine & pseudoephedrine products • Tolerance can develop fairly rapidly • User often also uses alcohol and other substances to relax • May cause a paradoxical reaction in children • May be used initially to lose weight • Crystal meth users prone to dental problems • Withdrawal is difficult and relapse is common • Remains in urine for up to 3 days
Cannabis, including marijuana and hashish	*Signs:* Euphoria; intensified perceptions; impaired judgment and motor ability; increased appetite; weight gain, sinusitis, and bronchitis with chronic use; anxiety, paranoia; red conjunctiva	*Signs:* Extreme paranoia, psychosis, delirium *Treatment:* Antipsychotics	*Signs:* Irritability, anxiety, insomnia, anorexia, restlessness, tremors, fever, headache *Treatment:* Supportive	• Most widely used illicit drug • Impaired judgment may contribute to accidents • Respiratory damage from inhaled substances can occur • Legal in some states for medical reasons • Remains in urine for up to 7 days • May exacerbate psychiatric symptoms in mentally ill patients • May negatively affect fertility • May therapeutically reduce nausea and vomiting, intraocular pressure, and stimulate appetite

Continued

Table 17-3 Comparing Commonly Abused Substances—cont'd

Drug	Intoxication	Overdose	Withdrawal	Nursing Considerations
Cocaine, including crack	*Signs:* Euphoria, grandiosity, sexual excitement, impaired judgment, insomnia, anorexia; nasal perforation associated with inhaled route; psychosis associated with long-term abuse	*Signs:* High temperature, pupil dilation, tachycardia, seizures, arrhythmias, transient venospasms possibly causing MI or CVA, coma, death *Treatment:* Supportive	*Signs:* Fatigue, vivid dreams, depression, anxiety, suicidal behavior. bradycardia *Treatment:* Support counseling, antidepressants	• Crack is smoked or injected IV; has a rapid onset and high dependency rate • Tolerance develops rapidly • Cocaine is inhaled, snorted, or injected IV • High risk of acquiring HIV, hepatitis, bacterial endocarditis, and osteomyelitis from shared IV needles or promiscuous sexual relations • May be used to control appetite
Hallucinogens, including LSD, psilocybin, and mescaline	*Signs:* Dilated pupils, diaphoresis, palpitations, tremors, enhanced perceptions of colors, sounds, depersonalization, grandiosity	*Signs:* Panic, suicidality, psychosis with hallucinations, cerebral tissue damage, seizures, hyperthermia, death *Treatment:* Diazepam or chloral hydrate; quiet environment antipsychotics	*Signs:* re-experiencing perceptual symptoms	• Flashbacks can occur for up to 5 years • Could precipitate a psychiatric disorder in susceptible persons
Inhalants, including glue, gasoline, cleaning solutions, aerosol propellants like deodorants or hair spray, and paint thinner	*Signs:* Euphoria, impaired judgment, blurred vision, unsteady gait, nausea/vomiting, wheezing, hypoxia	*Treatment:* Supportive	*Signs:* None	• Most available substance for younger children • Intoxication period is brief (15–45 minutes) • Can cause permanent CNS camage • Death from aspiration of emesis can occur • May be difficult to detect specific substance used • Particularly irritating and/or flammable substances can cause trauma and burns in nose, mouth, and airways

Nicotine, including cigarettes, chewing tobacco, and nicotine gum or patch	*Signs:* Produces a sense of anxiety reduction, relief from depression, and satisfaction	*Signs:* Tachycardia, hypertension, abnormal dreams	*Signs:* Insomnia, depression, irritability, anxiety, poor concentration, increased appetite *Treatment:* Transdermal nicotine patches in decreasing doses, nicotine gum, nicotine nasal spray, and clonidine for severe anxiety, behavioral modification. Long-term smokers may need to remain on nicotine therapy for some time. New medications now available (see Pharmacology Corner)	• Monitor for weight gain • Monitor for hypotension with clonidine • Hospitalized smoker may need nicotine replacement to control withdrawal
Opioids, including heroin, morphine, meperidine, OxyContin, propoxyphene, hydrocodone, and codeine	*Signs:* Euphoria, analgesia, slurred speech, drowsiness, impaired judgment, constricted pupils	*Signs:* Dilated pupils, respiratory depression, seizures, cardiopulmonary arrest, coma, death *Treatment:* Naloxone, supportive	*Signs:* Yawning, insomnia, anorexia, irritability, rhinorrhea, muscle cramps, chills, nausea, and vomiting, feelings of doom and panic *Treatment:* Detoxification, possibly with clonidine for severe anxiety and methadone, naloxone, and/or buprenorphine to block euphoria	• High risk of acquiring HIV, hepatitis, bacterial endocarditis, and osteomyelitis from shared IV needles • May be obtained illegally or through prescription abuse • At high risk for overdose after detox if the same pre-detox dose is taken • Monitor for hypotension with clonidine • Abuse of Suboxone is a growing problem

Continued

Table 17-3 Comparing Commonly Abused Substances—cont'd

Drug	Intoxication	Overdose	Withdrawal	Nursing Considerations
Phencyclidine (PCP, angel dust)	*Signs:* Impulsive behavior, impaired judgment, belligerent behavior, assaultive behavior, ataxia, muscle rigidity, nystagmus, hypertension, numbness or diminished response to pain	*Signs:* Hallucinations, psychosis, seizures, respiratory arrest, stroke *Treatment:* Gastric lavage; cranberry juice or ammonium chloride to acidify urine (if awake); quiet environment; haloperidol or diazepam; fluids	*Signs:* None	• Have adequate staff available because behavior is unpredictable and patient may become violent. • Drugs remain in urine for several weeks • Avoid using phenothiazines because they can potentiate the effects of PCP
Sedatives, hypnotics, and antianxiety drugs including barbiturates and benzodiazepines	*Signs:* Relaxation, Slurred speech, labile mood, inappropriate sexual behavior, loss of inhibitions, drowsiness, impaired memory	*Signs:* Hypotension, nystagmus, stupor, cardio-respiratory depression, renal failure, seizures (barbiturates) coma, death *Treatment:* Benzodiazepine antagonist (flumazenil); induce vomiting, if awake; activated charcoal; cardio-respiratory support	*Signs:* Insomnia, tachycardia, hand tremor, agitation, panic disorder, nausea and vomiting, anxiety, tinnitus (with benzodiazepines), seizures, and cardiac arrest *Treatment:* Detoxification using gradually reduced dosages of a similar drug, anticonvulsants, and support and counseling	• Abrupt barbiturate withdrawal can be life-threatening • Alcohol will potentiate drug effects and can contribute to overdose • Cross-tolerance may develop between alcohol and other CNS depressants. • Shorter-acting benzodiazepines have a greater risk of producing addiction and more severe rebound anxiety than longer-acting ones

Club Drugs including ecstasy (MDMA), rohypnol, ketamine	*Signs:* Euphoria, muscle relaxation, poor judgment	*Signs:* Confusion, hallucinations, severe anxiety, hypertension, seizures, high temperature *Treatment:* Supportive	*Signs:* Not physiologically addictive, but psychological dependence can cause depression, flashbacks	• Can cause memory loss and brain damage
Steroids (anabolic), including testosterone, stanozolol, oxymetholone	*Signs:* Dramatic increase in muscle mass, irritability, increased blood sugar, acne, edema from fluid retention, unwanted secondary sex characteristics	*Signs:* Liver damage, increased cholesterol, hypertension, paranoia, hostility, hyperactivity, manic symptoms *Treatment:* Supportive	*Signs:* Depression, fatigue, anorexia, decreased libido	• Masculinization of women and feminization of men is common • May be self-injected • Repeated use can produce dependence symptoms

Source: Adapted from Gorman & Sultan (2008) and Townsend (2012, DSM-5).

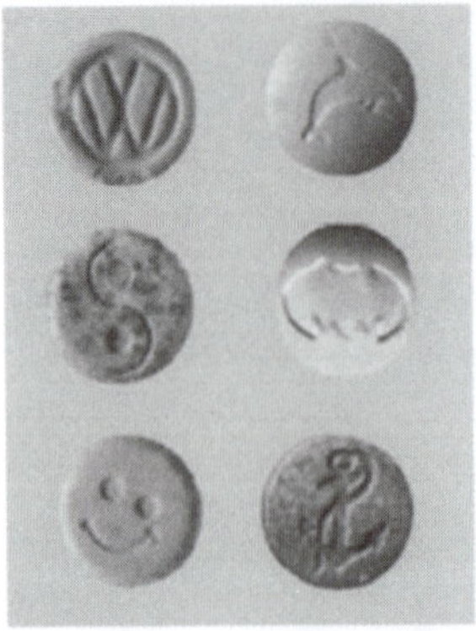

Figure 17-5 "Homemade" methamphetamine tablets. (*Courtesy of Drug Enforcement Agency, U.S. Department of Justice, Washington, D.C.*)

disorder is based on a pattern of continued use despite substance-related problems.

Use of opioid drugs for nonmedical use is a growing problem. This can include the use of pain medication to achieve a high or to relax rather than for physical pain relief. Desperate actions such as stealing drugs from family/friends, forging prescriptions, and doctor shopping are signs that the person needs help. People with chronic pain who regularly take analgesics may be at increased risk to misuse prescribed analgesic at times of stress, new onset of more medical problems, and mental health issues. They need to be educated on the appropriate use of these medications and monitored closely (Pergolizzi et al., 2012). Older adults are more likely to abuse prescription tranquilizers, sedatives, and analgesics.

Substance Use in Children and Teens

Children and teens can also be at risk for substance disorders. The use of inhalants, including household items such as hair spray and aerosol whipped cream, is most common in children. These easily obtained substances can contribute to sudden changes in behavior. Cough syrups and prescription drugs from parents are other sources for children and teens. Signs of substance use in children and teens can include:

- Change in functioning at school
- Loss of interest in sports
- Change in sleep patterns
- Increased isolation
- Irritability
- Mood swings

Lifelong struggles with substance use often begin in childhood and adolescence. Younger brains are thought to be more vulnerable to the addiction cycle. Therefore, intervention with young people is essential to prevent addiction. Children and teens are still developing judgment and decision-making skills, so they may be swayed to try things as part of peer pressure or to self-medicate.

> **Critical Thinking Question**
> Your 15-year-old nephew has been arrested for possession of a prescription analgesic that he stole from a friend's parent's medicine cabinet. You had noticed that recently he had more mood swings than usual, had been doing poorly in school, and was increasingly irritable. What other signs would you look for that he is using these drugs? What concerns would you have for his future?

> **Tool Box** | The Drug Abuse Screening Tool, known as DAST, is used in some settings. The 20-question self-screening tool is available at www.integration.samhsa.gov/clinical-practice/screening-tools

Etiology of Substance Use Disorders

The causes of substance use disorders are similar to those of alcohol abuse, but with the wide variety of drugs abused, there are some differences. Biological theories look at the role of specific brain dysfunction and view addiction as a brain disease. A drug will stimulate a specific brain pathway that includes an altered state and brain changes leading to craving this drug again. Cocaine has been studied the most, and it is believed that cocaine abusers have a deficiency of dopamine and norepinephrine that creates more craving. Other mind-altering drugs may be influenced by different pathways.

Psychological factors include use of drugs to relieve feelings of depression, anxiety, and low self-esteem. Sociocultural theories look at the impact of peer group and culture on the use of specific drugs.

Treatment of Substance Use Disorders

As with alcoholism, the twelve-step program provides an important treatment and support for the individual with substance abuse. The same philosophy of acknowledging one's powerlessness over a substance and the importance of group support are the foundation of these programs.

In addition, some people benefit from inpatient drug rehabilitation programs, which can include detoxification depending on the drug. Family therapy, individual psychotherapy, peer counseling with former addicts, and group therapy can also be helpful in many cases. Cognitive behavior therapy (CBT) can also be useful. This approach is a short-term therapy that emphasizes learning the connection between stressors and symptoms, teaching new coping skills, and challenging distorted thinking. Most substance abuse programs involve the family in the treatment plan. Heroin addiction may be treated with methadone maintenance when a long-acting opioid is taken daily to avoid the withdrawal symptoms without the high from taking other opioids. See the Pharmacology Corner for other medications used to treat addictions and withdrawal.

It is now commonplace for employers to request a drug screening of a urine or hair sample as a condition of employment or as a routine test while employed. Many companies have struggled with drug abuse with their employees and have found this to be a deterrent.

In the hospital setting, awareness of a patient's past substance abuse history is important information to prevent/control withdrawal syndromes. In addition, a recovering substance abuser may be hesitant to take analgesics or tranquilizers for fear of returning to a past lifestyle. It is important to work with the patient to address these fears and identify alternative interventions if possible.

Cultural Considerations

Disparities in availability of treatment for substance-related disorders for some ethnic groups and those of lower socioeconomic status have led to greater problems in some communities (Cook & Alegría, 2011).

People who take drugs intravenously are at risk of HIV, sexually transmitted diseases, and hepatitis from infected needles. Treatment for substance abuse should include a medical work-up for these potential problems as well as education on prevention.

Clinical Activity

- Review the medical record for what substances your patient was abusing, the last time they were used, and the potential complications.
- Your patient who is an IV drug abuser should be screened for HIV, sexually transmitted diseases, and hepatitis.
- Education may need to be provided on prevention of these diseases.

Classroom Activity

- Identify resources for drug abusers in your community, such as methadone maintenance programs and halfway houses for recovering addicts.

Critical Thinking Question

You work at a methadone clinic and see the same patients daily for their medication dose. You notice that one patient arrives disheveled with slurred speech. What actions should you take?

Critical Thinking Question

You are asked to submit a urine test as a condition of employment for a new job at a local hospital. What is your response to this request? What are the pros and cons of this for employer and employee?

Pharmacology Corner

A variety of medications are used in the treatment of substance use disorders. Pharmacology can be used in some cases to replace the illicit substance, as in methadone (see below), or to reduce the drug cravings by interacting with the receptor system in the brain affected by the substance. Examples include buprenorphine and naloxone for opioid addiction. These substances also reduce the physical signs of withdrawal.

Medications are used in detoxification programs for many drugs, including opioids, barbiturates, sedatives, and tranquilizers. They are used to control withdrawal symptoms and discourage continued use of the abused substance. Most are used for only short periods until withdrawal is complete; however, in some cases, they may be used for longer periods to control cravings for the drug.

Methadone, a synthetic narcotic that resembles morphine and heroin but does not produce the euphoric effects, is used daily on a long-term basis to treat heroin addiction. Both physical and psychological dependence are maintained on methadone, but the euphoric effects of heroin are blocked. Patients usually make daily trips to a methadone clinic to obtain the drug. Buprenorphine, an opioid with agonist and antagonist action, has been used as an alternative to methadone. Naltrexone also reduces the euphoric sensation from narcotics, and clonidine decreases discomfort during narcotic withdrawal. The newest opioid withdrawal treatment uses Suboxone (buprenorphine and naloxone). Addiction specialists must be certified to prescribe this regimen. Patients on this medication must be monitored closely if they have conditions that require use of analgesics. Administering analgesics could precipitate a withdrawal syndrome.

Benzodiazepines and sedative withdrawal is more risky because of the risk for seizures and delirium. Tapering the dose of the identified or similar drug, along with anticonvulsants and antidepressants, is usually used.

Withdrawal from stimulants may require use of tranquilizers and antidepressants. Bupropion and varenicline (Chantix) work in combination with behavioral treatments to help with nicotine withdrawal in addition to nicotine replacement in the form of lozenges or patches.

Herb and plant products to treat distressing symptoms may be helpful and include chamomile, valerian, kava kava, and St. John's wort. The last is contraindicated if the patient is taking antidepressants, narcotics, or amphetamines.

Commonly used medications to treat withdrawal are covered in Table 17-2.

Neeb's Tip The Clinical Institute Withdrawal Assessment for Alcohol Scale, known popularly at CIWA-AR, is also a useful tool used by many hospitals to monitor patients at risk for withdrawal syndromes from opioids and benzodiazepines.

Clinical Activity

- Review agency policy on the management of drug withdrawal regimens.
- Identify coping mechanisms your substance abusing patient uses to cope with stress now that he/she is not using.
- Monitor for potential complications during detoxification.

Critical Thinking Question

Your 19-year-old patient is admitted for surgery after he broke his ankle in a car accident. His sister confides in you that he has been taking frequent doses of the tranquilizer lorazepam that he was taking from his mother's prescription. He has asked her to bring these to the hospital. The patient's sister has them but now wonders if that is the right thing to do. What concerns would you have about this drug? What action should you take?

Nursing Care of Patients With Substance Use Disorders (Including Alcohol)

Common nursing diagnoses in patients with substance-related disorders include the following:

- Coping, ineffective
- Denial, ineffective

- Family coping: compromised
- Injury, risk for
- Sleep pattern, disturbed
- Thought processes, disturbed
- Violence, risk for

People who abuse drugs, alcohol, and other substances often use similar coping mechanisms to deal with their problems. See Table 17-4 for a list of common coping styles used by substance users. Understanding these coping mechanisms can help professionals understand behaviors and identify appropriate interventions.

General Nursing Interventions

Caring for patients with a variety of substance use disorders requires patience, knowledge, teamwork, and compassion. These patients present many challenges as there can be many complications related to the substance itself and/or the withdrawal process. In addition, the same coping mechanisms the patient has used for years to hide the addiction and problems it created are often still in use. These can include denial, manipulative behavior, and rationalization. The nurse may be in a role of limit setter and rule enforcer, which can be challenging.

Table 17-4 Common Coping Styles of Substance Abusers

Coping Style	Definition	Behaviors
Denial	Person minimizes or does not acknowledge the problem or the results of the problem even when strong evidence is presented.	• "I only have two drinks a day; I could stop any time." • Refuses to admit drug problems that are obvious to others. • Family may participate in denial by covering up the problems created by the abuser.
Projection	Blames others for his or her drinking and substance abuse.	• Avoids taking responsibility for own unacceptable behavior. • "My brother is the one with the problem. He drinks more than I do." • "I'd stop if everyone would leave me alone."
Rationalization	Justifies intolerable behavior by giving plausible excuses.	• Excuses reinforce denial. • "My kids are always in trouble. They make me take these pills" • "I only drink beer."
Minimizing	Avoids conflict by reducing the impact of the behavior.	• Places less value on the behavior and the impact of the problem. • "You worry too much." • "I'm not hurting anyone."
Manipulation	Plays one person against another in order to get one's way or cover up or avoid a problem.	• Convinces one or two people that he or she will improve if they will help. • If he or she fails, it is the fault of the helper.
Grandiosity	Maintains a sense of superiority and irresponsibility particularly evident when intoxicated.	• Lacks concern for others' feelings.

Source: Adapted from Gorman and Sultan (2008): Psychosocial Nursing for General Patient Care, 3rd ed. Philadelphia: F.A. Davis Company, with permission.

The nurse may also be faced with patients who are intoxicated on the substance. This can mean dealing with offensive, abusive behaviors that require maintenance of safety for all involved as well as limit setting.

See Table 17-5 for specific interventions related to alcohol and drug abuse disorders.

Neeb's Tip Patients with a substance abuse history often refuse analgesics for fear this will lead to abusing the substance again. Working with the patient to try alternate methods of pain control as well as appropriate ordering of analgesics by the physician (e.g., use of long-acting opioids rather than injectable to reduce the high) can be helpful.

Neeb's Tip Recognize that maintaining sobriety or abstinence from drugs or alcohol is a lifelong process. During periods of stress or illness, the urge to use these substances can increase. The patient needs added supports at these times

Neeb's Tip People with a drug abuse past may have learned to use charm and manipulation to get the drugs they are seeking. Family, friends, and health-care providers may have difficulty trusting them in recovery because of being taken advantage of in the past.

Table 17-5 Problems With Substance Abuse: Symptoms and Nursing Interventions

Types	Symptoms	Nursing Interventions
Alcohol Abuse	• Inability to cut down or stop using • Daily use common • Binges that last 2 days or more • Blackouts, which increase • Impaired social function • May use drugs in addition to alcohol to manage symptoms • Increase in alcohol tolerance • Drinking in "secret" • Preoccupation with alcohol • Gulping first drink • Inability to discuss problems • Loss of control • Rationalization of drinking • Failure in efforts to control drinking • Grandiose and aggressive behavior • Trouble with family, employer • Self-pity • Loss of outside interests • Unreasonable resentment • Neglecting food • Tremors (hands) • Morning drinking • Prolonged intoxication • Physical and moral deterioration • Impaired thinking	• Communicate honestly • Assist patient in identifying thoughts and feelings • Convey acceptance of individual • Challenge rationalizations or denial with reality • Encourage participation in support groups and maintain consistency with new behaviors learned in group • Confront use of maladaptive defense mechanism • Support any acknowledgement of the abuse • Support and give positive reinforcement of progress • Set firm limits as needed • Provide information about substance abuse, causes, and treatment • Monitor for withdrawal syndromes and complications from substance abuse • Support of drug/alcohol-free lifestyle • Recognize that patient may have setbacks with drinking but encourage to restart treatment • Avoid any enabling of patient's bad behavior

Table 17-5 Problems With Substance Abuse: Symptoms and Nursing Interventions—cont'd

Types	Symptoms	Nursing Interventions
	• Free-floating anxiety • Obsession with drinking • Constant use of alibis	
Substance Use	• Similar to alcohol abuse with addition of: • Red, watery eyes • Runny nose • Hostility • Paranoia • Needle tracks on arms or legs • Erratic, unpredictable behavior • Risky behaviors including stealing, lying to obtain drug • May use alcohol too to self-medicate for symptoms • Other symptoms depending on drug being used	• See "Alcohol Abuse" • Encourage patient to be tested for HIV if drug use included use of needles • Monitor drug testing if ordered • Be aware of attempts to manipulate you
Co-dependence	• Significant others beginning to lose their own sense of identity and purpose, existing solely for the abuser • Actions of significant others taking away opportunity for user to take responsibility for his or her own actions • Lowered self-esteem • Taking part in actions that are self-destructive and reinforce drug seeker's/drinker's problems	• Encourage participation in assertiveness classes • Promote self-care and problem solving • Encourage attendance at support groups • Challenge rationalizations/denial about substance abuser • Help person identify self-destructive patterns • Encourage activities to promote self-esteem and individuality

The nursing care plan for a patient abusing alcohol is provided in Table 17-6.

Critical Thinking Question

Your 45-year-old patient is admitted to the hospital with multiple injuries that she states she sustained in a fall at home. When the husband of the patient arrives, he smells of alcohol, is belligerent, and demands his wife be released. After security asks him to leave, the wife tells you that he has never acted like this before and she is sorry she upset him by telling him their son acted out in school. She denies he hurt her and says that she tripped down the stairs because she left some of the younger son's toys there. You wonder if the wife is covering up her husband's drinking problem as an enabler. What would you consider as possible nursing diagnoses for this patient? If the husband comes back, what actions should you consider?

Neeb's Tip

Denial is a powerful coping mechanism common in alcohol and substance use disorders that gets reinforced by the effects of the substance. Patients may minimize the effects of the substance abuse even when presented with objective data like a blood alcohol level or toxicology screen. Look for slightest indication of insight and emphasize that rather than support the denial.

Table 17-6 Nursing Care Plan for Patients Abusing Alcohol

Assessment/ Data Collection	Nursing Diagnosis	Plan/Goal	Interventions/ Nursing Actions	Evaluation Criteria
• History of heavy drinking • Minimizes negative effects of drinking • Denies concern about recent erratic behavior • Blames his spouse for recent argument	Ineffective denial	Acknowledges drinking is out of control Asks for help	Demonstrate acceptance by avoiding criticism or judgment of his behavior Identify recent inconsistencies in his behavior Help patient identify feelings/events that lead to recent binge Foster problem solving to identify new ways to cope with stress Provide information about Alcoholics Anonymous Set limits on manipulative behavior Promote taking responsibility for hurting spouse's feelings	Patient acknowledges need for help Patient attends AA meeting Patient shares one emotion

Key Concepts

1. Substance abuse and dependence are growing disorders in the United States with wide ranging impacts on health, safety, and family life.
2. Poly-drug use is common as the person tries to self-medicate to decrease discomforts from another drug. This contributes to more complications and possible synergistic effects that can be life-threatening.
3. Dependency on a substance occurs when one is unable to control its use, even while knowing that it interferes with normal functioning and more of the substance is required to produce the desired effects.
4. The presence of substance abuse with a psychiatric disorder is called a co-occurring disorder or dual diagnosis. It is commonly seen in the psychiatric population and needs to be included in the screening.
5. Co-dependency is often seen in family and friends of substance abusers as they try to help the person by covering up or enabling addictive behaviors.
6. Longer-acting tranquilizers are used as the initial treatment to detoxify from alcohol.
7. Serious complications from alcohol abuse include heart disease, liver failure, and some cancers.
8. Acute withdrawal is commonly seen in the acute hospital setting when the patient is without the abusing substance for hours or days.
9. Nursing management of patients with substance use disorders requires keen observation, setting limits, involvement of the family, and compassion.

CASE STUDY

Jim is a 26-year-old first-year resident in medicine at a large university hospital. His father and mother are both physicians, and he felt pressure to graduate from medical school with high honors. He struggled throughout medical school to maintain passing grades but achieved more success in his last year as he realized how much he wanted to be a doctor when he was working with patients. After graduation, he ranked high enough to be selected for a residency at a prestigious hospital. During medical school, he was in a car accident that left him with residual back pain, which he managed with yoga and occasional ibuprofen.

Once his residency began, he was working long hours. Often on his feet for long hours, his back pain increased. He no longer had time for yoga and ibuprofen was no longer helping. He had an old prescription for Vicodin, which he took at night when he was not on call. It helped him sleep and be more rested to function well at the hospital. He obtained a prescription for more Vicodin from a doctor friend based on his back pain. As time went on, he needed more pain medication to sleep and then started taking a pill during his shift when he felt jumpy.

Colleagues reported Jim was irritable and at other times almost euphoric. He was called in by his supervisor when he made a prescribing error. Jim felt he needed more Vicodin to function and then he would not make errors. Then Jim's friend said he could not write any more prescriptions for him. This friend suggested he pursue pain management referral. Jim was not interested and pursued other routes to get pain medication, including writing his own prescriptions to a fake patient. He had a minor car accident when he fell asleep at the wheel. When he returned home from work one day, the police arrived with a warrant for unlawful prescription writing. A local pharmacist had become suspicious and reported it to the police.

Jim is now in police custody. Jim's father and his hospital supervisor arrived and proposed a drug treatment program. Jim agreed.

1. Upon entering your drug treatment facility, what information would you want to know in the admission profile about Jim's drug use?
2. In reviewing Jim's case study, at what point did the Vicodin use turn from therapeutic to substance abuse?
3. Identify two interventions you would use initially to support Jim.

REFERENCES

American Psychiatric Association. (2000). *Diagnostic and Statistical Manual of Mental Disorders IV-Text Revision.* Washington DC, Author. (Known as DSM-IV-TR)

American Psychiatric Association. (2013). *Diagnostic and Statistical Manual of Mental Disorders 5.* Washington, DC, Author. (Known as DSM-5)

Clark, H. Prevention and impact of co-occurring disorders. Retrieved from www.nami.org/MSTemplate.cfm?

Cook, B.L., and Alegría, M. (2011). Racial-ethnic disparities in substance abuse treatment: The role of criminal history and socioeconomic status. *Psychiatric Services, 62*(11), 1273–1281.

Gorman, L., and Sultan, D. (2008). *Psychosocial Nursing for General Patient Care.* 3rd ed. Philadelphia: F.A. Davis.

Kessler, R.C., Berglund, P., and Demler, O. (2005). Lifetime prevalence and age-of-onset distributions of DSM-IV disorders in the National Comorbidity Survey Replication. *Arch Gen Psychiatry, 62*(6), 593–602. doi: 62/6/593 [pii] 10.1001/archpsyc.62.6.593

Kessler, R.C., Demler, O., and Frank, R.G. (2005). Prevalence and treatment of mental disorders, 1990 to 2003. *N England Journal of Medicine, 352*(24), 2515–2523.

Ling, W., Mooney, L., and Wu, L.T. (2012). Advances in opioid antagonist treatment for opioid addiction. *Psychiatric Clinics of North America, 35*(2), 297–308.

Lingford-Hughes, A.R., Welch, S., and Peters, L. (2012). Evidence-based guidelines for the pharmacological management of substance abuse, harmful use, addiction and comorbidity: recommendations from BAP. *Journal of Psychopharmacology, 26*(7) 899–952.

National Institute of Alcohol Abuse and Alcoholism. (2010). Rethinking drinking. Retrieved http://niaaa.nih.gov/publications/brochures-and-fact-sheets

National Survey on Drug Use and Health. (2012). Results from the 2011 National Survey on Drug Use and Health: Summary of national findings. Retrieved from www.samhsa.gov/data/NSDUH/2k11Results/NSDUHresults2011.pdf

Pergolizzi, J.V., Gharibo, C., and Passik, S. (2012). Dynamic risk factors in the misuse of opioid analgesics. *Journal of Psychosomatic Research, 72*(6), 443–451.

Stewart, S., and Conrod, P. (2008). *Anxiety and Substance Abuse Disorders: The Vicious Cycles of Comorbidity.* New York: Springer.

Townsend, M. (2012). *Psychiatric Mental Health Nursing.* 7th ed. Philadelphia: FA Davis.

U.S. Preventive Services Task Force. (2012). U.S. Preventive Services task force issues draft recommendation on screening & behavioral counseling to reduce alcohol misuse. Retrieved from www.uspreventiveservicestaskforce.org

Test Questions

Multiple Choice Questions

1. The defense mechanism most frequently demonstrated by the chemically dependent person is:
   a. Undoing
   b. Rationalization
   c. Denial
   d. Reaction formation

2. Nurses know that alcohol functions as a:
   a. CNS depressant
   b. CNS stimulant
   c. Major tranquilizer
   d. Minor tranquilizer

3. The patient who is experiencing delirium tremens is most likely to exhibit which of the following symptoms?
   a. Tremors
   b. Auditory hallucinations
   c. Confusion
   d. All of the above

4. Sally and Susie are twins. They are 20 years old. Susie has a habit of drinking too much when they go out, and this has been more frequent. They were out celebrating their birthday last night, and this morning Susie is vomiting. Sally calls her sister's teacher. "Susie is really ill. I think she has the flu; anyway, she can't come to school today. She said she has a test today and an assignment that she was supposed to pick up. I can come in and get the assignment for her. When can she make up the test?" Sally's behavior might indicate:
   a. Collaboration
   b. Compensation
   c. Lying
   d. Co-dependency

5. You are Sally and Susie's friend. A therapeutic response to them might be:
   a. "Sally and Susie, you are really going to get in trouble if you keep partying like that. It's bad for you."
   b. "Sally and Susie, I care for you both, but Susie, you misuse alcohol. You both need help. Sally, you are not helping Susie by 'taking care' of her; she needs to do it herself."
   c. "Sally, why do you keep lying for Susie? Just because she's in trouble doesn't mean you have to cover up for her."
   d. "Susie, this is just a stage you're going through. Everybody does it; it's not a big deal. You're young! Have fun!"

6. Sally and Susie seek treatment. Susie is treated as an inpatient and Sally as an outpatient. The nurse planning discharge teaching from their programs will encourage them to:
   a. Attend weekly AA and Al-Anon meetings.
   b. Check back into the hospital unit weekly.
   c. Attend weekly sessions with the psychologist.
   d. Attend weekly Adult Children of Alcoholics meetings together.

7. Your patient admits to using an illegal substance daily, thinking about it when not actually using it, and spending a lot of time figuring out where to get it. This patient could have:
   a. A delusion
   b. DTs
   c. An addiction
   d. Dementia

8. One of the major skills a person/family can learn during substance abuse treatment is:
   a. Honest communication
   b. Co-dependency
   c. Denial
   d. Scapegoating

9. Your spouse has been an alcoholic for many years. She/he has been sober for the last two years but has begun drinking again. She/he drives drunk. You fear for your spouse's life, so you begin driving him/her places. You are displaying what kind of behavior?
   a. Dry drunk
   b. Co-dependent
   c. Compassionate
   d. Tough love

Test Questions

cont.

10. Which of the following medications is most likely to be ordered for a patient experiencing alcohol withdrawal?
   a. Haloperidol
   b. Chlordiazepoxide
   c. Methadone
   d. Chlorpromazine

11. Your patient just attended her first AA meeting. Which statement reflects she understands the purpose of AA?
   a. "Once I dry out, I know I can have an occasional drink."
   b. "If I lose my job, AA can help me find another one."
   c. "AA is only for people who have hit bottom."
   d. "AA can help me stay sober."

12. A patient is suspected of methamphetamine abuse. What symptom would you be most likely to see?
   a. Weight loss
   b. Incontinence
   c. Weight gain
   d. GI bleed

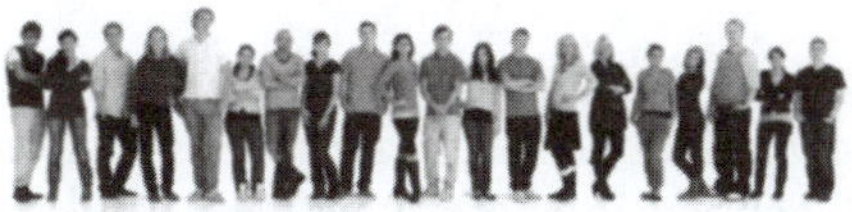

CHAPTER 18

Eating Disorders

Learning Objectives

1. Define anorexia.
2. Describe the similarities and differences between anorexia and bulimia.
3. Define morbid obesity.
4. Discuss bariatric or "weight loss" surgery.
5. Identify populations at risk for eating disorders.
6. Identify possible causes of eating disorders.
7. Describe nursing interventions for patients with eating disorders.

Key Terms

- Anorexia nervosa (also called *anorexia*)
- Binge eating disorder
- Body image
- Body mass index (BMI)
- Bulimia
- Morbid obesity
- Obesity
- Purging

Dieting is a national obsession, especially with women. Numerous fitness clubs are filled with individuals trying to attain the idealized thin, muscular body. The Barbie doll became the idealized female body shape for several generations. Extreme thinness is increasingly common in models and celebrities. It seems that it has become accepted behavior to be obsessed with body weight and shape and to view food as a source of stress. Self-esteem and happiness in young girls are often linked to weight and body shape. When this social influence is combined with certain biological, psychological, and family dynamic factors, it could be the beginning of an eating disorder, including **anorexia nervosa** and **bulimia** nervosa (Yager & Andersen, 2005). **Obesity** and **morbid obesity** are not considered eating disorders, but their effects often lead to emotional distress. Eating disorders have little to do with simply not eating enough or overeating. Rather, they are psychiatric disorders with substantial emotional and physical consequences.

Tool Box ▶ The National Eating Disorders Association Information and Referral hotline is 800-931-2237 and web site at: www.nationaleatingdisorders.org

■■■ Classroom Activity

- Discuss with classmates their experiences with eating disorders in themselves or friends.

■ Anorexia Nervosa

The term *anorexia* (as used in anorexia nervosa) is really a misnomer because this condition has very little to do with reduced appetite. It has more to do with the person's morbid fear of obesity causing anxiety and obsessive fear of losing control of food intake. In fact, the person is often hungry and views the discomfort of hunger as a reminder of the deprivation he or she needs to inflict on himself or herself. Only in the late stages is appetite actually lost. The distorted **body image** causes the patient to have a personal view as fat even though appearing emaciated (Fig. 18-1). No amount of weight loss relieves the anxiety, causing this deadly cycle to continue. Complications can continue for years, even after successful treatment.

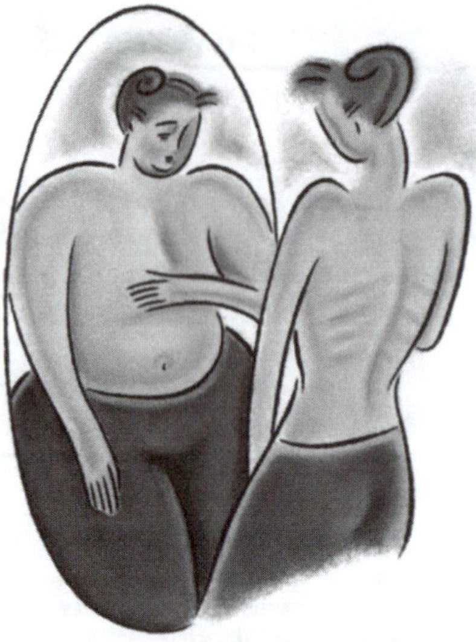

Figure 18-1 In anorexia nervosa, patients view their bodies in a distorted way. (Photograph by Stockbyte.)

Neeb's Tip Body image is a very personal perspective. When working with patients with eating disorders, take the time to learn about how they view their bodies. Avoid stereotyping and reacting emotionally to their appearance. The fact that they look thin to you does not mean that is how they see themselves.

Women have a 0.3%–1.0% lifetime risk of suffering from anorexia nervosa. Men have a prevalence of 1/10th of that risk (Hoek & van Hoeken, 2003; Yager & Andersen, 2005). Anorexia nervosa is viewed by many experts as representing struggles with autonomy and sexuality. Onset generally peaks in the early to late teens (Anderson & Yager, 2009). Poorer prognosis is associated with an older age of onset, a lower minimum weight, and vomiting.

Anorexic patients will go to great extremes to deprive themselves of food and use methods such as excess exercise to burn up calories and purging. **Purging,** which causes electrolyte imbalance and arrhythmias through inducing vomiting or overuse of laxatives, is usually combined with compulsive exercise to accelerate weight loss, making a lethal combination. Successful treatment is measured by weight gain, return of menstruation (usually absent in anorexic women), and reduced number of compulsive behaviors. Full recovery of weight, growth and development, menstruation, and normal eating behavior occurs in at least 50%–70% of treated adolescents (Yager & Anderson, 2005). The increased awareness of this disorder is leading many to receive earlier treatment, which improves the prognosis.

Symptoms of Anorexia Nervosa

Some of the behaviors, signs, and symptoms associated with anorexia nervosa are listed in Box 18-1.

Tool Box Four questions to help screen for eating disorders by Cotton, Ball, & Robinson are available at: www.ncbi.nlm.nih.gov/pmc/articles/PMC1494802/.

Cultural Considerations

Anorexia nervosa is most common in higher socioeconomic classes.

Box 18-1 Behaviors, Signs, and Symptoms of Anorexia Nervosa

- Excessive weight loss, usually more than 25% of body weight prior to dieting
- Refusal to maintain normal weight
- Intense fear of being fat
- Restricting food intake often to only 200–300 calories per day
- Excessive exercise
- Obsessive thoughts
- Perfectionist
- Absence of menstrual cycle
- Distorted body image
- Physical signs can include slow pulse rate, electrolyte imbalances, fatigue, dry skin and lanugo (fine body hair)

Source: Adapted from Gorman & Sultan (2008), Townsend (2012), and Anderson & Yager (2009).

Extreme weight loss is usually hidden to avoid exposure of the illness. Some ways the individual achieves this are by wearing baggy clothes, moving food around on the plate to give the impression of eating, exercising in secret, not eating unless certain demands about food combinations are met, or giving excuses for not eating, such as snacking before dinner. Once weight loss is exposed, the individual often objects to treatment and denies the seriousness of the condition in an effort to continue to control the illness.

Etiology of Anorexia Nervosa

Causes of anorexia nervosa include genetic and biological factors along with psychological ones. Dopamine regulation and dysfunction of the hypothalamus are viewed as important contributors. Psychological theory suggests that the core of anorexia is the child's fear of maturing and unconscious avoidance of developmental tasks. By not eating, the person forestalls sexual development and remains a child in the family. Other dynamics include overly demanding parents and profound disturbance in the mother/child relationship. Anorexia can represent a way to maintain control over parental figures. Anorexia requires a strong need to control one's intake, which counteracts feelings of loss of control and avoidance of conflict.

Treatment of Anorexia Nervosa

Treatment generally focuses on a collaborative approach between the following: internal medicine; behavioral approaches; nutrition counseling; individual, group, and family therapy; and pharmacological management. Specialized inpatient treatment programs are available in some areas.

Mortality rate for anorexia can be high, with serious complications including bone loss, heart failure, serious arrhythmias, and electrolyte imbalances. Close medical monitoring is essential for the patient with this disorder. A patient with severe anorexia may require long-term hospitalization with some form of artificial nutrition if severely malnourished. Some anorexics do better with this approach as they are relieved they no longer have to make decisions about food; however, the team must consider the ethics of involuntary re-feeding. Every effort must be made for the patient to eat voluntarily (American Psychiatric Association, 2006). Others become more anxious and resentful with forced re-feeding and need to try to take more drastic measures to take control of their intake by, for example, hiding weights in clothes to feign weight gain or changing drip rates on tube feedings. Total parenteral nutrition can be associated with many complications, so is usually avoided if possible.

Behavior programs often include building in rewards for weight gain and restrictions for weight loss as well as keeping a food diary. Therapeutic approaches should focus on increasing socialization and self-esteem. Successful treatment has focused on the goals of returning to normal weight, stopping abnormal eating behaviors, dismantling unhealthy thoughts, treating comorbidities, and planning for relapse prevention (Anderson & Yager, 2009). The dietary regimen generally promotes slow, steady weight gain of no more than 3 pounds per week (Yager & Anderson, 2005).

Neeb's Tip

Patients with anorexia often have a strong need to control their environment, leading to power struggles with the nurses.

Neeb's Tip

It is very stressful to care for a patient who refuses to eat. Nurses caring for these patients may experience frustration and anxiety as no matter what they do, the patient will not eat. Collaborating with the interdisciplinary team is essential.

Classroom Activity

- Obtain information about local eating disorders treatment programs and review and discuss with classmates.

Clinical Activity

Monitor electrolytes of your patient with anorexia nervosa.

Critical Thinking Question

Parents bring in their 14-year-old daughter, Amanda, to your primary care office to seek help. Amanda appears pale and thin despite being dressed in a long, baggy dress. As you prepare her for her physical exam by the nurse practitioner, you are shocked by her thin body. Her spine and ribs are most prominent, she has no breasts, and her skin is dry with a fine layer of hair over her body. Amanda asks you if you think she is fat. How would you respond?

Bulimia

Bulimia (also called *bulimia nervosa*) is binge eating followed by purging in an effort to control weight. Binging is eating large quantities of food at one sitting. The binge eating is followed by purging, usually in the form of self-induced vomiting, though laxatives and diuretics can also be used. The purging is often a result of the shame and guilt of the binge. Bulimia was officially designated as a psychiatric disorder in 1980 and is harder to diagnose than anorexia. Many of the behaviors are in private, and the person may appear to be a normal weight to others (Fig. 18-2).

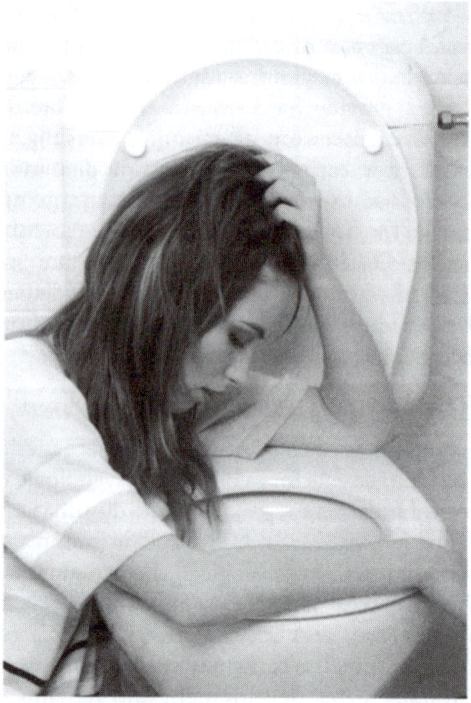

Figure 18-2 Bulimic woman vomiting after eating a large meal.

It is common that these behaviors are hidden for years. It affects a larger cross section of the population than anorexia does. Those with bulimia rapidly consume huge amounts of food—as much as 8,000 calories in a 2-hour period several times daily. Bulimia, like anorexia, tends to be manifested during adolescence. The binge may be triggered by a stressful event, feelings about weight and appearance, hunger from dieting, or negative self-image. Many celebrities have acknowledged a history of bulimia which has given this disorder more public attention. This disorder is much more common in females though does exist in males.

Pharmacology Corner: Anorexia

There are no medications to specifically treat anorexia, but medications can be useful to help manage some of the behaviors, for example, anxiety and depression as well as obsessive-compulsive behaviors, which can be seen in some anorexics. Fluoxetine (Prozac) as well as other SSRIs have been used in some cases; however, side-effect profiles can be high due to the patient being underweight. Anti-anxiety medications given prior to meals have been useful for some.

Cultural Considerations

Bulimia tends to occur in cultures where thinness is highly valued and where there is an abundance of food.

Binge eating disorder is recognized by psychiatry as a disorder on its own. Individuals with this disorder are more often obese or exhibit fluctuations in weight. This diagnosis is believed to be more common than anorexia or bulimia. Binge eating disorder is characterized by eating large amounts of food rapidly when not hungry, eating alone, and experiencing feelings of disgust and guilt after overeating. The person with binge eating disorder generally does not purge. To receive this diagnosis the binging must occur at least once per week for 3 months.

Neeb's Tip People with bulimia often keep their disorder secret and are only found out when a friend or relative finds evidence of purging behaviors such as vomiting or laxatives.

Symptoms of Bulimia

Box 18-2 lists the most common symptoms of bulimia. Bulimic individuals often are very self-conscious about their weight and appearance, and may focus a lot of their time on dieting and how to control their weight. Their self-concept is closely tied to their appearance.

Box 18-2 Behaviors, Signs, and Symptoms of Bulimia

- Extreme dieting
- Use and abuse of laxatives or syrup of ipecac (to induce vomiting)
- Use and abuse of diuretics
- Obsession with food and eating
- Poor self-concept
- Thoughts of harming self
- Routine use of bathroom immediately after eating
- Erosion of tooth enamel or hoarseness from vomiting
- Extreme sensitivity to body shape and weight
- Poor self-concept
- More likely to appear normal weight or slightly overweight
- Impulsive
- Feeling depressed, guilty, worthless

Source: Adapted from Gorman & Sultan (2008) and Townsend (2012).

Etiology of Bulimia

Because bulimia has close ties to depression, bulimics may have abnormalities in levels of serotonin. An impaired satiety mechanism also could be a factor as the person may not recognize when he/she has had enough to eat. Psychological theories include low self-esteem, presence of conflict in parental relationships, and family history of alcoholism and abuse. These individuals are more likely to have comorbid psychiatric disorders, such as borderline personality disorder, panic disorder, substance use disorder, and major depression. Childhood obesity may be a contributing factor.

Treatment of Bulimia

The patient must acknowledge the disorder. Bulimics may suffer in silence for years before acknowledging the need for treatment. Individual, group, and family therapy are important components of treatment to gain insight into feelings that lead up to the need to binge as well as to treat depression or other disorders. Keeping a food diary with associated feelings is a common behavioral approach. Complications of bulimia include electrolyte imbalance, dehydration, and tears in the gastric or esophageal mucosa that require involvement of internal medicine and dentistry. The support group Overeaters Anonymous has been helpful for bulimics.

Critical Thinking Question

Your friend Carole constantly talks about her weight. She needs frequent reassurance that she is attractive, but then criticizes herself for being fat. She is not overweight in your opinion. She is part of group that meets monthly at a restaurant for drinks and dinner. You notice that she eats a very large, high-calorie meal each time but visits the restroom two to three times during the evening. You are wondering if she has bulimia. What else would you look for to consider bulimia? What concerns would you have for her?

Pharmacology Corner: Bulimia

Because of the high correlation with depression, patients with bulimia are often on SSRI antidepressants. Some antidepressants, including fluoxetine, paroxetine, and fluvoxamine, are particularly helpful if there are obsessive-compulsive features with the bulimia. Other medications to treat additional psychiatric disorders such as anxiety disorder, substance abuse, and bipolar disorder may be used as well.

Similarities Between Anorexia and Bulimia

There are many similarities between these two eating disorders, and long-term anorexics may develop bulimia in later life. See Table 18-1 for a summary of the differences between them.

Morbid Obesity

Morbid obesity often leads to a lifetime of emotional, social, and physical problems. Potential health problems include a wide range of chronic conditions, including hypertension, cardiac problems, diabetes, respiratory insufficiency, and joint and back disorders. Risk of death increases with a **body mass index (BMI)** greater than 30. (See Box 18-3 to determine BMI.) Nutritional deficiencies are also extremely common because the obese person may lack a well-balanced diet or experience protein deficiencies related to crash dieting. Obesity is not classified as a psychiatric disorder, but it may include features of binge eating disorder and depression.

Society often views morbidly obese individuals as undesirable. They may be abused by strangers and treated with contempt by family members. Even health-care professionals may view them as emotionally disturbed, though there is no increased incidence of psychopathology in morbidly obese people. Others may

Table 18-1 Comparison of Anorexia Nervosa and Bulimia

	Anorexia Nervosa	Bulimia
Epidemiology	• More than 95% female • Younger adolescent onset fairly rare	• 90% female • Young adult onset more likely • 2–3 times more frequent than anorexia
Appearance	• Emaciated • Below normal weight	• Normal or overweight • Weight fluctuations
Family	• Rigid, perfectionistic • Overprotection	• More overt conflict
Behavior	• Introverted • Socially isolated • High achiever • Excessive exercise	• Impulsive • More histrionic, acting out • Depressed
Signs	• Cachexia • Hair loss • Amenorrhea • Dry skin • Pedal edema	• Dehydration • Chronic hoarseness • Chipmunk facies (parotid gland enlargement)
Prognosis	• 5%–18% mortality rate • Frequent lifelong problems with food • Bulimia • Depression	• Death is rarer • Lifelong problems with food

Source: Gorman and Sultan (2008). Psychosocial Nursing for General Patient Care, 3rd ed. Philadelphia: F.A. Davis Company, with permission.

Box 18-3 Example of Body Mass Index Calculation

BMI = Weight (in kilograms) ÷ Height in meters squared

Example:

What is the BMI of a 180-pound woman who is 5 feet tall (60 inches)?

First convert pounds to kilograms and inches to meters:

180 pounds ÷ 2.2= 81.81 kg

60 inches = 1.52 meters

1.52 x 1.52 = 2.31 (meters squared)

81.81 ÷ 2.31 = 35.41 BMI

Tool Box |▶ BMI Calculator:
www.bmi-calculator.net/ (also see Box 18-3)

Cultural Considerations

Morbid obesity affects all ages and races, although it is much more common in lower socioeconomic groups. Obesity is equally distributed between men and women. Childhood obesity is also considered a national health problem that can lead to a lifetime of problems.

view these individuals as lazy, unkempt, and lacking in self-control. Many experts promote viewing these individuals as having a chronic illness rather than a cosmetic problem.

Morbidly obese people face discrimination particularly in the workplace because they are viewed as less healthy, less diligent, and less intelligent than their thinner peers. Certainly, with this kind of reaction, it is no wonder that these people often experience poor self-esteem, feelings of isolation and helplessness, and loss of control. Morbidly obese individuals often have subjected themselves to many weight-loss strategies only to regain the weight, which increases the stress on the body.

Some educators have noted that fewer than 50% of health-care professionals advise obese patients to lose weight (Goldsmith, 2000). Reasons for this low percentage include discomfort about addressing the subject, lack of time to talk with the client, and a belief that this recommendation will not make any difference. Yet it has been found that a client is more likely to try to lose weight if he or she is advised to do so by a health-care professional. However, extremely obese people may avoid regular medical care because of shame about their weight. The U.S. Preventive Services Task Force has recommended that health-care providers identify people with a BMI greater than 30 and refer them for weight loss counseling (2012).

Obesity in children and teens is a serious health concern in the United States and globally. Long-term emotional effects include depression, social isolation, poor self-esteem, and poor academic performance. These can lead to lifelong problems (Cornette, 2008).

All nurses will encounter morbidly obese patients in their practices. Sensitivity to the patient's fears, embarrassment, and coping mechanisms should be incorporated in the treatment plan. Having properly sized equipment like wheelchairs and beds and scales can avoid embarrassment.

Etiology of Morbid Obesity

Causes of morbid obesity are complex. Genetic factors are considered a predisposing factor. Abnormalities in the brain related to satiety, abnormalities of the thyroid gland, and decreased insulin production are some of the many factors that may contribute to morbid obesity. Psychological theories include tendency toward depression and use of food to comfort oneself related to past traumas such as sexual abuse. Overeating as a learned response to stress, tension, and boredom, along with a sedentary lifestyle and poor nutrition, must be incorporated into the complex picture.

Treatment of Morbid Obesity

Obesity is a complex issue, and any weight-loss program needs to include a multidisciplinary approach. The U.S. Preventative Services Task Force (2012) developed federal guidelines for clinicians to help their patients lose weight. It recommends that successful weight-loss programs need to include:

- Behavioral management activities such as setting weight-loss goals

- Improving diet or nutrition and increasing physical activity
- Addressing barriers to change; self-monitoring
- Strategizing how to maintain lifestyle changes.

When these measures have been unsuccessful, some people pursue surgical interventions, called bariatric surgery. The most common surgeries are the lap band and the gastric bypass. The lap band creates restriction of the stomach using a silicone band, which can be adjusted by addition or removal of saline through a port placed just under the skin. This operation can be performed laparoscopically. In gastric bypass, a small stomach pouch is created with a stapler device and connected to the distal small intestine. Generally, bariatric surgery is considered only for people with a BMI greater than 40 or for those with a BMI greater than 35 with serious medical complications related to the excess weight, such as diabetes. After weight loss surgury, patients need support and education to adjust to their new bodies.

Behavioral approaches to address triggers for overeating can be part of counseling. Self-help groups like Overeaters Anonymous or Weight Watchers can be a major source of support. Web-based support programs to manage weight are increasingly popular. These support programs can be helpful even after bariatric surgery.

Clinical Activity

Attend an Overeater's Anonymous meeting in your community.

Cultural Considerations

Some cultures are more accepting of obesity than others. Knowing the patient's cultural group can give some insight into whether obesity is considered a problem to the patient.

Critical Thinking Question

Your 35-year-old patient is in the hospital for complications from a recent abdominal surgery. This man weighs more than 400 pounds. He is withdrawn and appears depressed. When you bring in his dinner tray, he tells you to take it away as he does not want to eat because the doctor told him he has to lose 100 pounds quickly. How should you respond? What options can be given to this patient?

Nursing Care of Patients With Eating Disorders

Common nursing diagnoses in patients with eating disorders include the following:

- Body image, disturbed
- Coping, ineffective
- Nutrition, imbalanced: less than body requirements
- Powerlessness
- Self-esteem, disturbed

Pharmacology Corner: Morbid Obesity

In 2012 the FDA approved two weight loss drugs—the first new drugs in more than 12 years. Qsymia (formerly called Qnexa) combines the appetite suppressant phentermine and the anti-seizure/migraine drug topiramate. Phentermine was once widely prescribed as the "phen" part of the fen-phen weight loss drug that was popular in the 1990s. This combination was withdrawn from the market after its use was linked to high blood pressure in the lungs and heart valve disease. The problems were related to the "fen" or fenfluramine part of the combination, not the phentermine. The other drug approved for weight loss is Belviq (lorcaserin), which promotes a small amount of weight loss with fewer side effects by activating serotonin receptors that affect appetite. Both of these new drugs should not be used in pregnancy. Xenical is the only other FDA-approved weight loss drug and is sold over the counter as Alli.

- Nutrition, imbalanced: more than body requirements

General Nursing Interventions

1. *Promote positive self-concept:* Gaining the patient's trust and giving positive reinforcement for the progress the patient makes will help the patient learn to change his or her lifestyle.
2. *Promote healthy coping skills:* Nurses who understand that developing healthy coping skills is time consuming and difficult for anyone with an eating disorder are able to demonstrate confidence that the patient can change. Empathy for the depth of these disorders will help gain the patient's trust and cooperation. The nurse must be careful not to be manipulated into negative behaviors by the patient with anorexia. Setting limits on behavior is part of the plan of care. Having the patient consistently stay within those limits is part of teaching new lifestyle behaviors.
3. *Promote adequate nutrition:* The physician and dietitian or nutritionist will meet with the patient to discuss calorie and nutrient requirements. Most of these patients will have nutritional deficiencies—even those who are overweight. Nurses are responsible for monitoring the patient's ability and willingness to consume the specified amount of food. Usually, smaller and more frequent meals are tolerated better than the traditional three larger meals. For a person with an aversion to food, presenting a large tray of food can be overwhelming and discouraging. Positive reinforcement for complying with caloric intake can be helpful. *Note:* When implementing this type of behavior modification, the nurse would be better served to praise the caloric intake or the healthy food choices, *not* the weight change. How nurses word the reinforcement can be crucial to the patient's willingness to continue the plan of care (Berkman et al., 2006; Crisafulli, Von Holle, & Bulik, 2008; Silber, Lyster-Mensh, & DuVal, 2011).
4. *Promote self-acceptance:* Anxiety over one's body image is a frequent contributor to distress in these patients. Promoting self-acceptance, feedback, and realistic expectations are all important. Encourage the patient to think about accomplishments unrelated to body weight.

See Table 18-2 for specific interventions for each eating disorder.

> **Critical Thinking Question**
> You are caring for a 21-year-old woman with anorexia nervosa. She is in the hospital receiving enteral feedings due to extreme weight loss. She just started eating small amounts of food as well. When you walk in the room, you see the patient staring at her tray and looking very anxious. She tells you, "Take this away." How should you respond? What factors might have triggered this reaction?

The nursing care plan for patients with eating disorders is provided in Table 18-3.

> **Classroom Activity**
> - If caring for an anorexic patient, review the care plan so consistent behavioral approaches are followed.
> - Review recommendations from the nutritionist.
> - For the morbidly obese patient, identify ahead of time what resources are available to assist in patient care, for example, scale, bed, proper size wheelchair, and proper size patient gown.

Table 18-2 Nursing Interventions for Eating Disorders

Type	Nursing Interventions
Anorexia Nervosa	• Promote positive self-concept and healthy body image. • Promote healthy coping skills. • Promote adequate nutrition. • Support patient being open about fears and concerns. • Report any evidence of patient sabotaging treatment plan. • Encourage patient to talk about his/her body image and promote realistic image. • Allow some control in decision making. • Monitor patient during meal times and right after for support for anxiety as well as to control sabotage. • Monitor for hiding food. • Establish goals with patient and team for weight gain. • Establish appropriate behaviors in terms of exercise and food preparation. • Avoid focusing on food all the time. Encourage other interests.
Bulimia Nervosa	• Approach with positive, realistic expectations of food intake. • Help patient identify feelings when he or she gets the urge to binge or purge. • Encourage eating in public. • Monitor for eating in secret. • Provide support during meals and discourage use of bathroom after eating. • Promote a realistic body image by discussing how patient views self. • Help patient identify feelings associated with eating. • Incorporate ways to promote improved self-concept.
Morbid Obesity	• Work with patient, family, physician, and dietitian to formulate healthy meal plans. • Encourage patient to participate in groups to promote acceptance of self and development of self-esteem. • Make efforts to promote improved self-concept. • Respect privacy. • Work with patient to identify small, achievable goals in weight loss plan. • Encourage keeping a diary of food intake. • Discuss feelings associated with eating. • Work with team to develop a realistic exercise regimen. • Help patient look at weight loss in small increments rather than total weight loss goal. • Promote dignity by being sensitive to patient's appearance in public. • Plan ahead to right-size equipment available, such as wheelchairs. • Promote positive self-image and acceptance of body by emphasizing personal traits other than weight. • Continue to provide support and education after weight loss surgery.

Table 18-3 Nursing Care Plan for Patients With Anorexia

Assessment	Nursing Diagnosis	Goal	Interventions	Evaluation
Emaciated patient describes self as fat; Wears baggy clothes	Body image disturbance	Refers to her body in a more positive way	Avoid overreacting or insincere response to self-deprecating comments. Rather, listen to patient and then comment on how you see her. Encourage discussion of positive traits.	Makes one positive or less negative comment about herself

Key Concepts

1. Eating disorders of one type or another affect large numbers of people in the United States.
2. Though most common in women, anorexia and bulimia are increasingly common in men.
3. Bariatric surgery is becoming far more common than in years past. There are many physical and emotional considerations required when caring for patients undergoing this surgery.
4. Eating disorders are serious and can be fatal as a result of malnutrition and electrolyte disturbances.
5. Eating disorders may be related to emotional or physical causes. Obesity may have genetic and emotional causes.
6. Nursing interventions for eating disorder center on promoting self-esteem and trust.

CASE STUDY

Penny is a 22-year-old woman who has recently graduated from college. She has struggled with her weight all her life. She frequently refers to herself as fat and unattractive though her weight appears normal for her height. Friends frequently encourage her to be more accepting of herself. She is currently job hunting and spends most days at a coffee shop searching for jobs on her computer. She rarely eats during the day, but while alone in her apartment at night she becomes increasing anxious. Penny has kept bags of cookies and potato chips hidden and often eats entire packages of these items. While she is eating these items, she reports feeling relaxed, but shortly after, her stomach aches and she feels anxious and guilty. She often reduces her anxiety by sticking her finger down her throat to induce vomiting. After vomiting, she collapses in bed and often cries herself to sleep.

1. What disorder is Penny most likely suffering from?
2. How could Penny get help for her eating disorder?
3. If Penny came to your mental health clinic, what nursing interventions should be considered?

REFERENCES

American Psychiatric Association. (2006). Treatment of patients with eating disorders. *American Journal of Psychiatry 163*(7 Suppl), 4–54

American Psychiatric Association. (2013). *Diagnostic and Statistical Manual of Mental Disorders 5.* Washington, DC, Author. (Known as DSM-5)

Anderson, A.E., & Yager, J. (2009). Eating disorders. In B.J. Sadock, V.A. Sadock, & P. Ruiz (Eds.), *Kaplan & Sadock's Comprehensive Textbook of Psychiatry.* 9th ed. Philadelphia: Wolters Kluwer/Lippincott Williams & Wilkins.

Berkman, N.D., Bulik, C.M., and Brownley, K.A. (2006). Management of eating disorders. *Evidence Report/Technology Assessment (Full Report) (135),* 1–166.

Cornette, R. (2008). The emotional impact of obesity on children. *Worldviews of Evidence-Based Nursing, 5*(3), 136–141.

Cotton, M.A., Ball, C., and Robinson, P. (2003). Four simple questions to help screen for eating disorders. *Journal of General Internal Medicine 18*(1), 53–56.

Crisafulli, M.A., Von Holle, A., and Bulik, C.M. (2008). Attitudes towards anorexia nervosa: The impact of framing on blame and stigma.

International Journal of Eating Disorders, 41(4), 333–339.
Goldsmith, C. (2000). Obesity: Epidemic of the 21st century. *Newsweek,* May 8, 2000.
Gorman, L., and Sultan, D. (2008). *Psychosocial Nursing for General Patient Care.* 3rd ed. Philadelphia: FA Davis.
Hoek, H.W., and Van Hoeken, D. (2003). Review of the prevelance and incidence of eating disorders. *International Journal of Eating Disorders, 34*(4), 383–396.
Ogden, C., and Carroll, M. (2010). Prevalence of overweight, obesity and extreme obesity among adults through 2007-8. Retrieved from cdc.gov/nchs/fastats/overwt.htm
Silber, T.J., Lyster-Mensh, L.C., and DuVal, J. (2011). Anorexia nervosa: Patient and family-centered care. *Pediatric Nursing, 37*(6), 331–333.
Townsend, M. (2012). *Psychiatric Mental Health Nursing.* 7th ed. Philadelphia: F.A. Davis.
U.S. Preventive Services Task Force. (2012). Screening for and management of obesity in adults. Retrieved from www.uspreventiveservicestaskforce.org/uspstf11/obeseadult/obesesum.htm
Yager J. (2006). *Treatment of Patients With Eating Disorders.* 3rd ed. Retrieved from http://psychiatryonline.org/content.aspx?bookid=28&sectionid=1671334
Yager, J., and Andersen, A.E. (2005). Clinical practice. Anorexia nervosa. *New England Journal of Medicine, 353*(14), 1481–1488.

Test Questions

Multiple Choice Questions

1. The eating disorder that is characterized as an aversion to food is called:
a. Morbid obesity
b. Bulimia nervosa
c. Anorexia nervosa
d. Pica

2. Your patient with anorexia is admitted to your medical surgical unit for malnutrition. She tells you she does not want to eat when her tray is delivered. Which statement is the best response?
a. "The doctor said you will need a feeding tube if you don't eat."
b. "Tell me what happens to you when you see the food tray."
c. "I will ask the doctor to order an appetite stimulant."
d. "You have to eat or you will starve."

3. Your 19-year-old patient has a diagnosis of anorexia nervosa. You notice that she seems to spend more time playing with her food than eating it. You know that patients with anorexia:
a. Will eat normally if ignored
b. Fear being fat
c. Have an accurate body image
d. Will binge and purge

4. An appropriate nursing diagnosis for a patient with anorexia might be:
a. Altered nutrition; less than required amount, as evidenced by distress in eating
b. Altered nutrition; more than required amount, as evidenced by eating meals of 2000 calories or more six to seven times per day
c. Altered body image as evidenced by stating the wish that others look as good as the patient
d. Fluid excess related to increased weight gain

5. A key nursing intervention to help patients with eating disorders is:
a. Let the patient know he or she will be watched closely at mealtimes.
b. Have the patient chart his or her own intake and output.
c. Lock the patient's bathroom door for 2 hours after meals.
d. Encourage the patient to express underlying feelings about food, body image, and self-worth.

6. Bulimia nervosa is characterized by all the following *except:*
a. Binging on food
b. Purging the food after eating it
c. Being able to control eating pattern
d. Obsession with body shape and size

7. Donald has just been admitted to your surgical unit. He has just had stomach stapling surgery. You prepare your list for postoperative care and include therapeutic communication statements such as:
a. "You must be so relieved to be on your way to being thin."
b. "What is the first meal you plan to eat?"
c. "I'm interested to know if the rest of your family is also heavy."
d. "I'm here to help you any way I can."

8. It is Donald's second postoperative day. He is scheduled to have his first oral liquids. As you check on his progress at lunch, you note he has not touched his food. "I'm afraid to eat," he tells you. Your response might be:
a. "It's OK for you to eat now. You won't choke."
b. "Afraid to eat, meaning. . .?"
c. "It's important that you eat, or the doctor may need to order the IV feedings again."
d. "Why are you afraid to eat?"

Test Questions

cont.

9. Your new admission, a 14-year-old female, presents with multiple symptoms including recent extreme dieting, use of laxatives and diuretics, thoughts of suicide, impulsive behavior, and erosion of the enamel on her teeth. The patient's medical diagnosis most likely is:

a. Anorexia nervosa
b. Binge eating
c. Bulimia nervosa
d. Morbid obesity

10. In bulimia, the purging is done to achieve which of the following?

a. Feelings of euphoria at getting rid of the food
b. A need to gain attention
c. A release of tension followed by depression and guilt
d. A way to gain control

UNIT 3

Special Populations

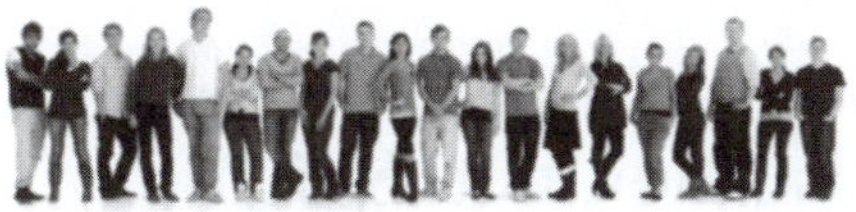

CHAPTER 19

Childhood and Adolescent Mental Health Issues

Learning Objectives

1. Identify child and adolescent populations at risk for mental health disorders.
2. Describe the impact of autism spectrum disorder on the family.
3. Define three mental health conditions of childhood/adolescent age groups.
4. Identify treatment modalities used in childhood/adolescent age groups.
5. Identify two medications used to treat attention-deficit/hyperactivity disorder.
6. Identify age-appropriate nursing care for two selected mental health issues.

Key Terms

- Attention-deficit/hyperactivity disorder (ADHD)
- Autism spectrum disorder
- Bipolar disorder
- Bullying
- Conduct disorder
- Cyberbullying
- Hyperactivity
- Impulsivity

Today, children are displaying behaviors and being diagnosed with mental disorders that two or three generations ago were nonexistent or at least not so readily observed in society. Many factors contribute to this, including greater access to mental health information by parents and teachers. However, stresses on children today are much different than in previous generations and are contributing as well. The fast pace of life, the Internet, social media, continuous exposure to news, instant access to information, and exposure to violence at a young age all lead to children growing up more quickly and having to deal with many issues that previous generations never addressed until they were much older. The growing trend toward **bullying** and especially **cyberbullying**, where the Internet is used to embarrass or shame peers, has added another stressor that young people may encounter. The frequency of divorce, less traditional family roles, and parents working outside of the home has led to a generation that must cope with stresses earlier in life. Many children are dealing with anxieties that were unknown in previous generations, which contributes to a variety of disorders.

Children and adolescents are at risk for developing many of the same mental health disorders as adults. Family history of substance abuse, schizophrenia, and bipolar disorder will impact the development of mental health problems in children and adolescents. Family dynamics will influence the development of many disorders as well.

The Centers for Disease Control and Prevention's National Health and Nutrition Examination Survey (NHANES) data show that approximately 13% of children ages 8 to 15 had a diagnosable mental disorder within the previous year (CDC, 2013). The most common disorder among this age group is **attention-deficit/hyperactivity disorder (ADHD)**, which affects 8.5% of this population. This is followed by mood disorders broadly at 3.7% and major depressive disorder specifically at 2.7%. Other less common disorders include conduct, anxiety, and eating disorders. Mental disorders in children can lead to a lifetime of problems including poor peer relationships, problems in school, substance use and risk-taking behaviors as well as being more likely to develop a chronic psychiatric illness. Forty percent of children with mental disorders will develop a second one (CDC, 2013). Of concern is that many children do not get adequate early treatment, perhaps due to denial on the part of parents and teachers; lack of mental health services, especially in the schools; lack of funding; and stigma. This chapter will discuss depression, bipolar disorder, suicide, ADHD, autism spectrum disorder, and conduct disorder.

Neeb's Tip

- The parents of children with any mental health disorder are under tremendous stress. This stress may be expressed as frustration, irritability, extreme fatigue, depression, and increased use of alcohol/drugs.

Neeb's Tip

- Other siblings in the home are also at high risk for acting out, as they often feel ignored with all the attention on their sibling with the mental health disorder.

Classroom Activity

- Participate/volunteer in a pediatric camp for children and teens with emotional problems.

Clinical Activity

Review the patient's medical chart for family history and social worker's notes on family dynamics and coping when caring for a child with mental health issues.

Depression, Bipolar Disorder, and Suicide in Children and Adolescents

Depression

Children and adolescents do exhibit symptoms of major depressive and dysthymic disorders. The symptoms are the same as in the adult illness (see Chapter 11). In addition to the classic general symptoms of depression, children may exhibit a change in their school routines, such as truancy or dropping sports/clubs, changes in sleep habits, and extreme irritability. They may become inattentive, experience a drop in grades, lose interest, or become anxious about being at school. Adolescents who become depressed may show all of the classic symptoms of depression and those connected with childhood but may also be trying to deal with changes happening in their bodies, hormones adjusting, and social role and peer group changes. Adolescent symptoms of depression may include rebellion, intense ambivalence, anger, rage, pessimism, and low self-esteem (Figs. 19-1 and 19-2). Estimates are that 8.2% of youths between ages 12 and 17 suffer from major depression in the past year, with girls at twice the risk (SAMHSA National Survey on Drug Use and Health, 2008). In children, it is believed that the major factor in development of depression is family influence. If parents are depressed, the children are three times more likely to be depressed than their age-mates. Environment and biochemical imbalances in the brain are also possible causes.

Tool Box | National Institute of Mental Health Information on Childhood and Adolescent Depression:
www.nimh.nih.gov/health/topics/depression/depression-in-children-and-adolescents.shtml

Neeb's Tip

Depression in children and teens may be masked as withdrawn, antisocial behavior; avoiding school; or loss of confidence.

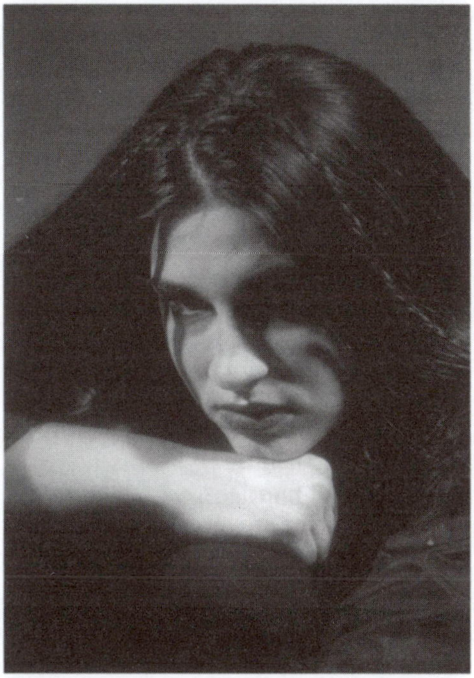

Figure 19-1 Adolescent symptoms of depression may include rebellion, intense ambivalence, anger, rage, pessimism, and low self-esteem.

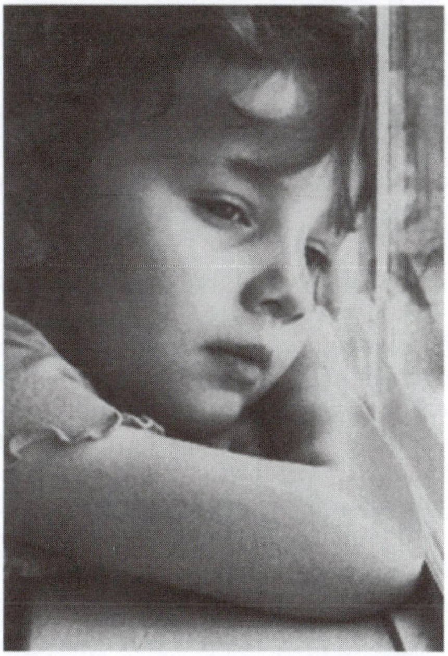

Figure 19-2 Children who are depressed may seem bored and unusually irritable.

Bipolar Disorder

Bipolar disorder is more difficult to diagnose in childhood and may be confused with **conduct disorder** or attention-deficit/hyperactivity disorder (ADHD). Some experts think bipolar disorder has been overdiagnosed in children and teens. DSM-5 requires bipolar disorder to include distinct episodes of mania that differ from baseline personality with or without depression episodes. (See Chapter 12 for more information on bipolar disorder.) Children with bipolar disorder generally do not have the typical cycling of mania to depression as seen in adults. Some behaviors associated with childhood mania include episodes of:

- Hyperactivity
- Grandiose delusions
- Irritability
- Rapid speech/racing thoughts
- Reduced need and desire for sleep

Hopefully, more accurate diagnosis of bipolar disorder in children will lead to improved treatment. Interestingly, in the past, children who were diagnosed with bipolar disorder (perhaps inaccurately) had a greater tendency toward anxiety and depression as adults rather than bipolar symptoms. DSM-5 has a new diagnostic category under Depressive Disorders named Disruptive Mood Dysregulation Disorder. This disorder is characterized by severe temper outbursts with irritable or angry mood in at least two settings in children but no clear manic episodes. This new diagnostic category may include some children that were previously diagnosed as bipolar. Substance use could also contribute to symptoms of this disorder.

Children and teens with any of the following need a thorough evaluation by a child psychiatrist to obtain an accurate diagnosis: extreme mood swings of depression and hyperactivity, delusions of grandeur, pressured speech, euphoria, and decreased need for sleep. Accurate diagnosis is essential so the appropriate medications and other treatments can be started. As with adults, the major contributor to this disorder is family history.

Tool Box |▶ NIH brochure for children and teens and their parents on bipolar disorder: www.nimh.nih.gov/health/publications/bipolar-disorder-in-children-and-teens-easy-to-read/who-develops-bipolar-disorder.shtml

Suicide

Suicide is the second leading cause of death in teenagers (Fig. 19-3). The frequency of suicide attempts in adolescents has taken an alarming increase in recent years. Eleven and a half percent of females and 5.4% of males of high school age have attempted suicide (National Institute of Mental Health Statistics on Suicide, 2012). Peer pressures with the increased use of social media and the presence of bullying have left some vulnerable teens viewing their lives as hopeless. In addition, young people may view suicide in a more romanticized way and be desensitized to death, which may be a contributor in suicide pacts. Depression and bipolar disorders are major contributors to suicide risk, but others, including substance abuse and ADHD, can also be factors. Younger children can also attempt suicide and may think of it as a magical way to get back at parents or others. Lesbian, gay, bisexual, and transgender youths are at especially high risk as they struggle with fitting in with their peers. Gender dysphoria, also known as gender identity disorder, where the child or teen is struggling with his/her sexual identity, can increase the risk for depression and suicide.

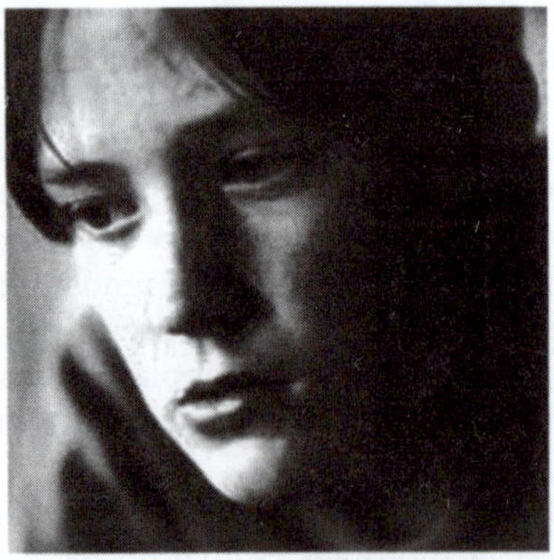

Figure 19-3 Suicides among teenagers are growing alarmingly. Many of the teens who attempt suicide state feelings of anger and frustration about not being listened to or not being taken seriously as the reason for their action. *(Courtesy of Centers for Disease Control and Prevention, National Center for Injury Prevention and Control, Atlanta, GA.)*

Signs of suicide risk can include:

- Talking a lot about death
- Asking questions about death
- Giving away possessions
- Artwork or play with death themes
- Loss of interest in friends/sports
- Evidence of substance abuse
- Poor sleeping habits
- Expression of hopelessness, self-hate
- Previous suicide attempts

Young people's methods of suicide may be similar to those of adults, for example, using firearms or hanging, but also include impulsive acts (especially common in young children) such as jumping out of a window or running in front of cars. As with adults, talking about suicide and previous attempts are common warnings that must be taken seriously.

Neeb's Tip Children can be very sensitive to rejection, which can lead to suicidal thoughts and impulsive acts. Any time a child mentions any thought about suicide, investigate fully. Never minimize his/her concerns.

Clinical Activity
Be aware of your patient's changes in behavior that can signal exacerbation of depression, bipolar disorder, or suicidal intent.

Cultural Considerations

These conditions cross all ethnic groups. In the past, these disorders were less frequently diagnosed in non-Caucasian society, but now parents and the education system are more informed to improve earlier identification across all groups.

Critical Thinking Question

Your new patient is a 10-year-old boy who has just been admitted to the pediatric unit after being hit by a car. His injuries are not life threatening. A neighbor told the paramedics she saw the boy run into the street right at the car. She thought he did it on purpose in a suicide attempt. The boy's parents report he has been bullied by two older boys lately and has been very upset, but they refuse to consider this a suicide attempt. What other information would you want to know about the patient and family? What interventions should the staff consider for this boy?

Treatment of Children and Adolescents With Depression, Bipolar Disorder, and Suicide

Treatment of depression and bipolar disorder in these age groups is challenging. Group therapy, family therapy, individual psychotherapy, and partial or day-hospital programs have been shown to be helpful for many in this age group. Treatment should focus on strengthening coping skills and support. Parental involvement is essential for recovery. Psychoeducation focuses on teaching patients and parents life skills, communication, problem solving, and early signs of relapse to cope with these disorders.

Any sign of suicide risk in a child/teen requires immediate intervention including psychiatric evaluation. See Chapter 13 for specific interventions.

Neeb's Tip Denial of a child's suicide risk can lead to tragedy when the call for help is not recognized out of a belief that a child would not attempt suicide.

Tool Box Compassionate Friends is a national support program for parents whose children have died, including those who have died from suicide. Information on Surviving Your Child's Suicide: www.compassionatefriends.org/Brochures/surviving_your_childs_suicide.aspx

Pharmacology Corner: Depression, Bipolar Disorder, and Suicide

Antidepressants are not always helpful and can be dangerous in the younger age group with depression. In September 2004, the Food and Drug Administration (FDA) of the United States recommended that a strong caution be placed on antidepressant medications for children and teenagers due to increased risk of suicide. The caution that suicide can be a side effect of antidepressants led to the black box warning that is now on all antidepressants. Doctors and parents need to weigh the benefits against potential risks of using these medications. SSRIs including fluoxetine and escitalopram have been approved for treatment in adolescents.

Monoamine oxidase inhibitors (MAOIs) are not often used because of the food contraindications associated with them. Some tricyclic antidepressants can cause cardiac arrest and death in children and adolescents. Still, medications may be needed and should be used cautiously and monitored carefully.

Bipolar disorder is treated with mood stabilizers as in adults as well as with antipsychotics if needed. See Chapter12. Children and adolescents may need to remain on medications for years, so accurate diagnosis and long-term management of side effects is essential.

Suicidal behavior is treated with antidepressants and anti-anxiety medications. See Chapter 13.

When children are diagnosed with a serious psychiatric disorder early in life, the long-term side effects of effective medications are a major concern and must be weighed with the potential benefits. Parents may be faced with difficult choices and will need counseling and support as these decisions are needed.

Tool Box FDA black box warning info on antidepressants: www.fda.gov/Drugs/DrugSafety/InformationbyDrugClass/UCM096273

Neeb's Tip Ensure that parents are familiar with all potential side effects and required monitoring for their child.

Nursing Care of Children and Adolescents With Depression, Bipolar Disorder, and Suicidal Behavior

Common nursing diagnoses for children and adolescents with depression include the following:

- Anxiety
- Coping, ineffective
- Hopelessness
- Injury, risk for
- Self-esteem, low

General Nursing Interventions

1. *Communicate* honestly and effectively and at an age-appropriate level.
2. *Identify limits and boundaries.* Explain what is appropriate behavior and what is not acceptable. Be clear and concise. Place the emphasis in the "positive." For example, to an angry individual a nurse might say, "You may hit the punching bag in the gym, but not another person."
3. *Focus on child/adolescent's strengths.* They should be structured but able to flex frequently with the child/adolescent's needs.
4. *Support the individual*; encourage verbalization of feelings and thoughts. Do not minimize the child's fears and concerns. Young children especially can benefit from art therapy to express their feelings.
5. *Encourage the completion of simple tasks.* Give the child honest feedback on all successes.
6. *Provide a safe environment* where the child feels comfortable to share fears and concerns and has an outlet for pent-up energy and frustration.
7. *Respond to any self-destructive behavior* with concern and action to maintain safety. Encourage the child who has self-destructive thoughts to talk with an adult. Children should be taught to never keep secret another's suicidal plan.

See Chapters 11, 12, and 13 for more interventions for depressive disorders, bipolar disorders, and suicide. See Nursing Care Plan in Table 19-1.

Critical Thinking Question

The mother of your 14-year-old patient who has been admitted after a suicide attempt asks to talk to you. She is understandably quite distressed and asks you to make sure the doctor starts her son on an antidepressant. What teaching needs to be given to the family about antidepressants and teens who have suicidal thoughts?

Attention-Deficit/Hyperactivity Disorder

Attention-deficit/hyperactivity disorder (ADHD) is a pattern of behavior involving inattention and/or **hyperactivity/impulsivity**. For this diagnosis the child must display symptoms in more than one setting for example at home,

Table 19-1 Nursing Care Plan for the Depressed Child

Data Collection	Nursing Diagnosis	Plan/Goal	Intervention	Evaluation
Child is increasingly isolated, refusing to go to school, drops out of sports, is irritable, reports feeling unable to meet teachers' and parents' expectations	Low self-esteem	Child will demonstrate increased feelings of self-worth	Encourage the child to talk about his fears and insecurities in a supportive setting without judgment; Plan activities that provide opportunities for success; Avoid minimizing his fears; Give immediate feedback on any successes	Child returns to one activity he previously enjoyed; Able to verbalize his strengths and successes

in church, at school, or while in the shopping mall. This disorder leads to problems in social, education, and/or work performance. It is grouped under Neurodevelopmental Disorders in DSM-5. The diagnosis is generally made by the age of 12. ADHD can continue into adulthood, and generally adults with ADHD remember having behavior problems by the age of 12. About half of children with ADHD continue to have troublesome symptoms of inattention or impulsivity as adults. However, adults are often more capable of controlling behavior and masking difficulties. ADHD in children younger than age seven is a bit more challenging to diagnose, since the younger child is prone to shorter attention as a result of the child's developmental stage. ADHD is more common in males and does seem to have a pattern of running in families. The troublesome behaviors must be present for at least 6 months to a degree that is maladaptive and inconsistent with developmental level to confirm this diagnosis.

The symptoms of ADHD are divided into inattentive and hyperactivity/impulsivity (Box 19-1). Children can have one or both categories of symptoms to receive this diagnosis.

ADHD can be confused with depression, lack of sleep, learning disabilities, bipolar disorder, tic disorders, and general behavior problems. Every child suspected of having ADHD should be carefully examined by a doctor to rule out other possible conditions or reasons for the behavior before pursuing a diagnosis with other professionals such as teachers, psychologists, and other therapists.

Because children with ADHD put great demands on family life, they may be at higher risk for punitive responses from parents and teachers, which can increase their distress. The presence of ADHD puts the child at risk for a lifetime of maladaptive behaviors and impaired social relationships, so early identification and treatment are important. In addition, children with ADHD are prone to substance abuse, depression, anxiety, conduct disorders, and learning disabilities. Children with this disorder are generally of average or above-average intelligence

Box 19-1 Symptoms of ADHD

Inattentive symptoms:

1. Fails to give close attention to details or makes careless mistakes in schoolwork
2. Has difficulty keeping attention during tasks or play
3. Does not seem to listen when spoken to directly
4. Does not follow through on instructions and fails to finish schoolwork, chores, or duties in the workplace
5. Has difficulty organizing tasks and activities
6. Avoids or dislikes tasks that require sustained mental effort (such as schoolwork)
7. Often loses toys, assignments, pencils, books, or tools needed for tasks or activities
8. Is easily distracted
9. Is forgetful

Hyperactivity/Impulsivity symptoms:

1. Fidgets with hands or feet or squirms in seat
2. Leaves seat when remaining seated is expected
3. Runs about or climbs in inappropriate situations
4. Has difficulty playing quietly
5. Is often "on the go," acts as if "driven by a motor"
6. Talks excessively
7. Blurts out answers before questions have been completed
8. Has difficulty waiting for his/her turn
9. Interrupts others

Source: Adapted from Diagnostic and Statistical Manual of Mental Disorders, Fifth Edition (Copyright 2013). American Psychiatric Association.

Cultural Considerations

In the past, ADHD was diagnosed mainly in Caucasians and under recognized in other ethnic groups. Now with improved diagnostic tools and more awareness, this disorder is recognized in many ethnic groups. Cultural norms also need to be taken into consideration when determining what is considered "normal" behavior for children within a particular group. Children need to be assessed in their native language to avoid confusion about their concerns.

but do not always perform at their level of intelligence.

A definitive cause of ADHD has not been confirmed. See Box 19-2 for list of potential causes. Combinations of organic, genetic, and environmental factors may put a person at higher risk. It is common that parents of the ADHD child showed signs of hyperactivity in their childhoods, indicating a strong genetic component. Abnormal levels of neurotransmitters are associated with many of the symptoms of ADHD, as is abnormal brain function. Chaotic family life is also a factor. Some children have benefitted from diet modifications such as eliminating foods like milk products or sugar.

Clinical Activity
Identify triggers in the environment that lead to your ADHD patient's disruptive behavior.

Treatment of Children and Adolescents With Attention-Deficit/Hyperactivity Disorder

Though medications are commonly used to treat ADHD, they should be used in combination with other therapies. Psychotherapy for the child and family is often helpful, along with cognitive behavior therapy that focuses on learning new coping mechanisms. The child needs to learn the consequences of impulsive behavior and identify alternatives, and learn how to improve social skills. Close involvement of the child's teachers can help with learning and behavior.

Parents need to develop skills to address their child's disruptive behaviors. A structured school and home life can make a difference. This can include a system of rewards and consequences to help guide their child's behavior and handle disruptive behaviors. Support groups can help parents connect with others who have similar problems. Parents need ongoing support programs.

Box 19-2 Possible Causes of ADHD

- Genetics—family history is a strong predictor
- Altered secretion of neurotransmitters like dopamine
- Altered brain anatomy
- Prenatal exposure to alcohol
- Exposure to lead
- Reaction to food dyes, additives, sugar
- Chaotic family life

Source: Adapted from National Institutes of Mental Health (2012) and Townsend (2012).

Tool Box National Institute of Mental Health ADHD publication:
www.nimh.nih.gov/health/publications/attention-deficit-hyperactivity-disorder/how-is-adhd-treated.shtml
Children and Adults with ADHD (CHADD) provides resources to children and parents:
www.Chadd.org

Pharmacology Corner: Attention-Deficit/Hyperactivity Disorder

Medications are the most common treatment approach. As with other illnesses affecting young people, use of medication is controversial. Physicians must consider the physical maturity of a child's brain, liver, and kidneys as well as the child's ability to handle other effects of medication before prescribing.

Psychostimulants (also known as stimulants) are the most commonly used ADHD drugs. Although these drugs are called stimulants, they actually have a calming effect on people with ADHD by increasing the levels of neurotransmitters. These medications can increase the child's ability to concentrate and reduce hyperactivity and impulsiveness. New long-acting formulations, liquids, powders that can be sprinkled on food, and transdermal patches are available for some of these medications to help with compliance. The major side effects of these agents include overstimulation, restlessness, insomnia, anorexia, weight loss, headache, and irritability (Roman, 2011). See Table 19-2 for the common pharmacological treatment of ADHD.

Nursing considerations for children on stimulant medications include:

- Administer after eating or with meals to reduce effect on appetite.

Pharmacology Corner: Attention-Deficit/Hyperactivity Disorder–cont'd

- Generally administer them no later than 6 hours before bedtime to avoid interference with sleep.
- The school nurse and teachers should be informed that the child needs the medications.
- Some schools require the school nurse to administer the medications.
- Monitor adolescents who may share medications with others.
- Monitor the child's weight and blood pressure.
- Prepare parents to monitor for impact on the child's growth.

Neeb's Tip Children may avoid taking their medication out of fear or anger, or to avoid side effects. They may hide it from their parents or school nurse, so close monitoring and promoting open communication are important.

Nursing Care of Children and Adolescents With Attention-Deficit/Hyperactivity Disorder

Common nursing diagnoses for children and adolescents with attention-deficit/hyperactivity disorder include the following:

- Coping, ineffective
- Family coping, compromised
- Injury, risk for
- Self-concept, alteration in
- Self-esteem
- Social interaction, impaired

General Nursing Interventions

1. *Effective communication*: Therapeutic communication with the child/adolescent and the involved family members is always indicated. Teaching/modeling skills to assist with interpersonal family communication is helpful.
2. *Assist with behavior modification tools:* Limit setting, reward systems, and positive reinforcement may be helpful. Facilitate agreement between the parents and child/adolescent regarding what will be used as the reward, what is fair, and what the consequence to inappropriate behavior will be. Consistency among all parties is crucial in this modality.
3. *Promote self-esteem:* Help the child complete a task and reward with praise or other rewards. Give positive feedback for all appropriate behavior. Teach alternative behaviors. It can be helpful to break down tasks into small steps to reduce frustration from poor attention span. Reinforce socially acceptable behavior rather than giving a lot of attention to negative behaviors.
4. *Low stimulation environment*: Identify the signs when behavior is beginning to escalate and intervene to reduce stimulation. Physical activity can be a good outlet for pent-up energy, followed by a quieter environment.

Table 19-2 Common Pharmacological Treatment of ADHD

Drug Category	Drugs
Psychostimulants	Dextroamphetamine/amphetamine (Adderal) Methylphenidate (Ritalin, among other trade names)
Nonstimulant	Atomoxetine (Strattera)
Miscellaneous	Bupropion (Wellbutrin) Clonidine

Source: Adapted from Townsend (2012): Psychiatric Mental Health Nursing: Concepts of Care in Evidence-Based Practice, 7th ed. Philadelphia: F.A. Davis Company, with permission.

5. *Reinforce information about medications:* The physician should discuss the effects and side effects of any medications ordered. Family members may have further questions for nurses. Be prepared to assist with clarification about the medication(s). Stress the importance of compliance with the regimen to the child and parents.
6. *Promote a safe environment* as these children are susceptible to falls and accidents.
7. *Family support and education*: Living with a child with ADHD can be very stressful for a family.

(Pati, 2011; Primich & Iennaco, 2012)

> **Critical Thinking Question**
> Your 6-year-old patient has recently been diagnosed with ADHD. The patient's mother tells you she has been giving him Ritalin at bedtime so he will sleep better. What teaching would you provide to the mother to minimize side effects for the patient?

> **Critical Thinking Question**
> Your neighbor comes to you for advice with her 10-year-old child. He is failing in school, unable to concentrate, and becomes very antsy in class. Your neighbor wants to change his school as she thinks the teacher is at fault. What suggestions would you make?

> **Classroom Activity**
> - Identify local resources for ADHD in your community.
> - Ask a local elementary school teacher or school nurse to discuss management of a child with ADHD in the classroom.

Autism Spectrum Disorder

Autism spectrum disorder (ASD) is a general term that includes classic autism and Asperger's syndrome. These disorders are now classified as ASD rather than treated as separate disorders (DSM-5). ASD is a complex developmental disorder of brain function accompanied by intellectual and behavioral deficits characterized by persistent difficulties in social communication and social interaction with problems in maintaining relationships as well as repetitive patterns of behavior. It is called a spectrum disorder because it can be present in a mild form with some peculiar behaviors and mild social isolation but otherwise normal behavior; or to the other extreme it can be severe, with profound disability in all aspects of life. Asperger's syndrome is a mild form of ASD. Autism spectrum disorder is a neurodevelopmental disorder in DSM-5. It must be present from infancy or early childhood but may not be detected until later because of minimal social demands and support from parents or caregivers in early years.

> **Classroom Activity**
> - View the movie *Rainman* about an adult with autism.

Neeb's Tip

DSM-5 now views autism spectrum disorder to include what was previously known as Asperger's syndrome, though this is a term that is still commonly used. These individuals have less problems with language and cognition than more severe forms of ASD. This syndrome was originally named after an Austrian pediatrician who first described it. Sometimes these people are referred to as having high functioning autism.

> **Tool Box** ▶ **Pediatric screening tools for autism at the CDC Autism Spectrum Disorders Web site:**
> www.cdc.gov/ncbddd/autism/hcp-screening.html

The single most common symptom or manifestation of ASD is impaired social interaction. Learning disabilities, avoiding making eye contact, and inability to make friends or respond to other people's emotions are other symptoms. Children with this disorder may twirl their hair and/or perform self-injuring or self-mutilating behaviors, such as biting themselves or hitting their head on objects. Repetitive patterns can include excessive adherence to routines, ritualistic behavior, and repetitive speech or motor patterns such as rocking or spinning.

Children with ASD commonly exhibit the following symptoms:

- No response to their name by 12 months
- Not pointing at objects to show interest (e.g., not pointing at an airplane flying over) by 14 months
- Not playing "pretend" games (e.g., pretending to "feed" a doll) by 18 months
- Avoiding eye contact and wanting to be alone
- Having trouble understanding other people's feelings or talking about their own feelings
- Delayed speech and language skills
- Repeating words or phrases over and over (echolalia)
- Giving unrelated answers to questions
- Getting upset by minor changes
- Obsessive interests
- Flapping their hands, rocking their body, or spinning in circles
- Unusual reactions to the way things sound, smell, taste, look, or feel
- Appearing to be in their own world

(Adapted from CDC Facts about ASD, 2012)

To make the diagnosis, doctors may also look at failure to meet certain developmental tasks, such as a baby not babbling or performing gestures (pointing, grasping, etc.) by age 12 months, or, at any age, losing any language or social skills that had been acquired. Sometimes the child may appear to have normal development and then stop gaining new skills. There are several inventories that the physician, psychologist, or psychiatrist might administer to help with diagnosing. Parents often notice the signs by age 2 when the child is not developing language skills and/or showing difficulty with social interaction as in not making eye contact or makes repetitive nonpurposeful movements.

The incidence of ASD is on the rise. The CDC reports that 1 in 88 U.S. children have autism spectrum disorder (Centers for Disease Control and Prevention, "Autism Spectrum Disorders," 2012). This is a 78% increase from 2002, reflecting the increased awareness of parents and doctors to the early signs. ASD affects males three to four times more frequently than it affects females. Sadly, at this point in time, it is not curable and most individuals will require lifelong treatment. Children with severe autism are considered disabled for life. Autism should not be confused with or misdiagnosed as schizophrenia, although some behaviors may be similar.

Causes of autism are not confirmed. Genetics, viral infections, and chemicals found in the environment are suspected causes or contributors to development of autism. For parents with one autistic child, there is about a 5% chance of having a second child with autism. Serotonin levels have been shown to be diminished in the left frontal lobe of many with autism. Fragile X syndrome, congenital rubella, exposure to some medications in utero, and tuberous sclerosis have been suggested as possible causes of ASD. The increased incidence of ASD has led to more emphasis on research.

Neeb's Tip Some people continue to believe that autism is caused by childhood vaccines. This has led some parents to refuse vaccines for their infants, which can expose them to normally preventable illnesses and contribute to endangerment of others. If parents are concerned about vaccines, encourage them to discuss their concerns with the physician before making any decisions.

Tool Box | National Institute of Health Fact Sheet on Autism:
www.ninds.nih.gov/disorders/autism/detail_autism.htm
Services for people with autism and Asperger's syndrome provide resources and support:
aspergersyndrome.org
CDC Fact Sheet about ASD
www.cdc.gov/ncbddd/autism/facts.html

Cultural Considerations

ASD has been underdiagnosed in the Latino and black populations due to lack of awareness by parents and health-care professionals. This has led to later diagnosis and treatment in these populations. Previously viewed as a disorder mainly in Caucasian children, more resources are now available to identify and treat this disorder in other races.

Treatment of Children and Adolescents With Autism Spectrum Disorder

Although there is no cure for autism at this time, early identification is important. Early intervention services help children from birth to 3 years old learn important skills and enhance development by taking advantage of the brain's ability to adapt.

Services can include therapy to help the child talk, walk, and interact with others. Many new treatment programs that incorporate intensive speech, occupational, and physical therapies as well as behavioral training and management may be appropriate for some. These are home- and school-based intensive programs that have shown some success. Therapies may incorporate a structured reward system for responding to people. Each child must be evaluated individually for the best treatment. There are also many unproven treatments that parents will pursue in a desperate effort to treat their child.

Neeb's Tip Having a child with ASD creates tremendous physical, emotional, and financial stress on the family. These families need information on all resources available in the community.

Neeb's Tip Parents may be desperate for alternative treatments and may share approaches that you find questionable. It is important to maintain their trust and encourage them to be open to standard medical treatment and investigate thoroughly any alternative approach.

Pharmacology Corner: Autism Spectrum Disorder

Research trials for drugs to treat autism are ongoing, but so far there is no definitive pharmacological treatment. Doctors may prescribe medication for difficult symptoms such as deliberate self-injury, aggression, and uncontrollable temper tantrums. The FDA has approved the use of risperidone (Risperdal) and aripiprazole (Abilify) for children with these symptoms. Patients on these medications require close monitoring. The dosage is based on the weight of the child and clinical response.

Clinical Activity
Review possible side effects of any medications your ASD patient is taking. Reinforce education on medications to parents and the patient.

Nursing Care of Children and Adolescents With Autism Spectrum Disorder

Common nursing diagnoses for children and adolescents with autism include the following:

- Injury, risk for
- Self-care deficit
- Social interaction, impaired
- Verbal communication, impaired

General Nursing Interventions

1. *Maintain safety:* Therapists may prescribe special equipment or even special clothing, such as helmets and arm covers, to help maintain safety. The goal of this intervention is to discourage and prevent self-destructive behavior. Assisting parents to identify situations that may trigger the unwanted behavior is also helpful in preventing or de-escalating the behavior. Monitor the child closely and remove any items in the environment that may cause injury.
2. *Reinforce medical and counselor teaching:* Work with the parents and child on social skills. Provide praise and positive reinforcement for both the parents and

child. Technology is assisting with interventions for some patients. Virtual reality equipment and tablet computers are being used in some settings and with some success to help with teaching and behavioral training. The child may be able to relate more to these images than through interaction with others. Pet therapy, where a child can interact with a dog, cat, or through horseback riding, has shown success.

3. *Maintain effective communication with all parties:* Speak to the child or adolescent in simple, direct, age-appropriate language. Acceptance of behavior is important. Ensure that the family and others involved in the day-to-day care of the patient feel comfortable discussing concerns.
4. *Maintain consistency of caregivers:* The child may do better with familiar people. Try to reduce the amount of stimulation from strangers. Keep expectations realistic, and recognize that progress is slow and regression to previous behaviors may occur, especially under stress. Support independence where possible.
5. *Avoid overstimulating the child:* Determine if the child becomes more stressed with physical contact. The child may be uncomfortable with being touched. Check with the family on what the child will accept.
6. *Establish a routine schedule* with the child that all staff follows as much as possible.
7. *Parental support:* Having an autistic child affects the entire family on a daily basis. They need support and resources.

See Nursing Care Plan in Table 19-3.

Clinical Activity

- If your ASD patient is hospitalized, encourage his or her family to bring in familiar objects and advise staff about usual routines.
- Talk with a social worker about potential support resources for the parents and siblings in the home.

Classroom Activity

- Identify ASD resources in your community and invite some representatives to your class to discuss.
- Arrange an observation in a school for children with special needs such as autism.

Critical Thinking Question

An 8-year-old boy diagnosed with autism is admitted to your pediatric unit for an upcoming surgery. When you walk into his room, he is standing in the corner staring at one spot and does not respond to your greeting. Identify two approaches you would use to make contact with him.

Conduct Disorder

Conduct disorder is a disorder of childhood and adolescence that involves long-term (chronic) behavior problems associated with physical aggression, defiance, rule breaking, and disturbed peer relationships. Sometimes

Table 19-3 Nursing Care Plan for the Autistic Child

Data Collection	Nursing Diagnosis	Plan/Goal	Intervention	Evaluation
8-year-old autistic boy in the hospital is frequently banging his head on the wall and does not speak to any of the staff	Impaired verbal communication	Child will demonstrate one alternative behavior indicating reaction to caregiver, e.g., facial expression, eye contact	• Assign consistent caregivers • Ask parents to bring in familiar objects from home and review usual routine • Give positive feedback for alternative behaviors	Child has reduced frequency of head banging

these children are viewed as "bad" or delinquent rather than having a psychiatric disorder. These children exhibit a repetitive and persistent pattern of behavior in which the basic rights of others or major age-appropriate societal norms or rules are violated. Conduct disorder is now categorized under Disruptive, Impulse Control and Conduct Disorders in DSM-5. The diagnosis of conduct disorder is based on the presence of a pattern of aggressive behavior to people and/or animals, destruction of property, deceitfulness, or theft and/or serious violation of rules. The diagnosis is much more common among boys. The onset can be in childhood or adolescence. For an accurate diagnosis, the behavior must be far more extreme than simple adolescent rebellion or boyish enthusiasm. It is a pattern of behavior; a one-time incident does not diagnose the condition. Some behavior patterns might be bullying, displaying or using a weapon, arson, lying, fighting, animal abuse, truancy from school, chronic rule breaking, and running away from home (Fig. 19-4).

Careful screening and medical testing are important, as much change is happening developmentally in this age group. Conduct disorder has been known to be a precursor of bipolar disorder and/or antisocial personality in adulthood for some. Conduct disorder can occur with or be confused with ADHD, mood disorders, and learning disabilities. DSM-5 has noted several specific patterns that are sometimes seen in conduct disorder including callousness and lack of remorse. When a person with conduct disorder has these traits, he/she is harder to treat. Conduct disorder may be preceded by oppositional defiant disorder (ODD) in some children, which is a pattern of negativistic and hostile behavior toward authority figures.

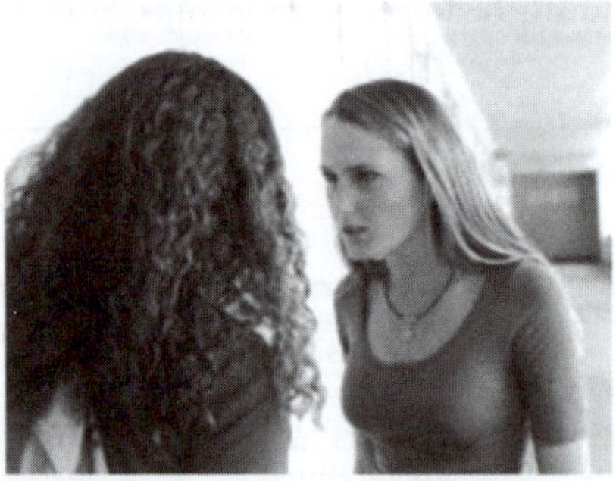

Figure 19-4 Recurrent bullying is a behavior that may indicate a conduct disorder, and it can be found among both boys and girls. *(Courtesy of U.S. Department of Health and Human Services, Office of Women's Health, Fairfax, VA.)*

Causes/contributing factors to conduct disorder include a variety of factors:

- Victim of child abuse/neglect
- Drug addiction or alcoholism in the parents
- Family conflicts
- Genetic defects
- Poverty
- Exposure to toxins
- Head trauma, brain disorder
- Prenatal exposure to cocaine
- History of attention-deficit/hyperactivity disorder
- Substance abuse

Treatment of Children and Adolescents With Conduct Disorder

Medical treatment for conduct disorder first includes a thorough assessment. Sometimes, there is an underlying medical condition in conduct disorder, such as closed head injury or a seizure disorder. The physician will need to assess and treat the underlying disorder as well as the behaviors associated with the conduct disorder.

Once the diagnosis is made, treatment includes counseling for the parents and family as well as the affected child. A child psychiatrist can work with the patient to address past traumas and anger issues. Parenting skills, consistency in limit setting, and progressing maturity of the child may, over time, often lessen or eliminate the behaviors of conduct disorder, especially as the child moves out of adolescence. Parent Management Training is an approach that teaches skills to parents about more effective ways to respond to episodes of aggression. Teachers need to have skills to address these issues. Residential treatment is sometimes prescribed for children with this disorder. Group therapy of some form can help the child relate more appropriately to his/her peer group.

Clinical Activity
When your patient has conduct disorder, recognize possible contributing factors, which can include ADHD, child abuse, substance abuse, and lack of parental guidance.

Neeb's Tip It is important to maintain a calm but firm approach that does not communicate fear or avoidance. The child may have learned to use aggressive behavior to keep people away and maintain power over others.

Tool Box |▶ American Academy of Child and Adolescent Psychiatry has information on Conduct Disorder Resources With Practice Parameters at www.aacap.org/cs/ConductDisorder.ResourceCenter

Neeb's Tip Parents of a child with conduct disorder are faced with many stresses as they must deal with others who are hurt by their child as well as the child's behavior. They need resources to help them, such as legal, emotional, and financial.

Critical Thinking Question
Ben is 11 years old and was brought to your mental health clinic by his single mother after the school has expelled him for repeated "bullying" of younger children. One of the children attempted suicide after being repeatedly humiliated by Ben. Ben's mother is desperate for help and tells you she wants to turn Ben into the juvenile authorities to institutionalize him. What would you say to this mother? What other options might be appropriate?

Pharmacology Corner: Conduct Disorder

Medications such as antipsychotic risperidone can contribute to symptom control for extreme agitation. These work most effectively along with counseling. ADHD medications such as stimulants, along with antidepressants and clonidine, have been used with success for some.

Nursing Care of Children and Adolescents With Conduct Disorder

Common nursing diagnoses for children and adolescents with conduct disorder include the following:

- Coping, defensive
- Injury, risk for
- Other-directed violence, risk for
- Self-esteem, disturbed
- Social interaction, impaired

General Nursing Interventions

1. *Maintain safety:* Maintaining physical safety and psychological and emotional safety is the primary nursing intervention for children and adolescents who have conduct disorder.
2. *Communicate honestly and effectively:* Communicate at an age-appropriate level the behaviors that are acceptable. Communicate the effect that inappropriate behavior has on others around the child. Communicate the consequences of inappropriate behavior and, most importantly, be consistent with enforcing those consequences. Recognize that the child may have poor skills in social situations and may need coaching or positive reinforcement.
3. *Assist with behavior modification tools:* Limit setting, reward systems, and positive reinforcement may be helpful. Set realistic expectations according to the child's age and ability level. Consistency among all parties is crucial.
4. *Model and educate the family with respect to appropriate roles:* In other words, parents need to be parents. The child needs to be the child. The parent should be in "control" of the situation. The child has input; negotiation is healthy, depending on the age of the child, but the child does not always "win." When the child does not "win" and behavior limits are exceeded or violated, the consequences for the inappropriate behavior must be enacted. Parents may find this difficult and exhausting. They will need support

and positive reinforcement from the nurse and medical or counseling staff. When the child is involved in hurting others or in risky behaviors, the adults have to take control to stop these behaviors.

5. *Reinforce information about medications:* The physician should discuss the effects and side effects of any medications ordered. Family members may have further questions for nurses. Be prepared to assist with clarification about medications.

■■■ Key Concepts

1. Children and adolescents do experience threats to their mental health. They have the same illnesses as adults but may manifest them in different ways. Some illnesses continue into adulthood.
2. Medications and therapy are effective for a great many people in these age groups. Recently, black box warnings have been applied to certain antidepressants when used with children and adolescents; some antidepressants may actually increase the chance for suicide.
3. Incidence of autism spectrum disorder has shown a dramatic increase in the last few years. It is a serious disorder that has lifelong effects.
4. Parents, family members, and other primary caregivers need to be involved in the treatment of children and adolescents. Consistency of care is crucial. Parents may need counseling in order to become more effective in their role as parents.
5. ADHD and conduct disorders present challenges to nurses working with children and teens.

CASE STUDY

Sharon, a 15-year-old girl, was brought to your family practice clinic by her mother. Her mother explained that Sharon was suspended from school for assaulting a teacher and needed a "doctor's evaluation" before she could return to class. The history reveals that this is Sharon's tenth school suspension during the past 3 years. She has previously been suspended for fighting, carrying a knife to school, smoking marijuana, and stealing money from other students' lockers. When asked about her behavior at home, Sharon reports that her mother frequently "gets on my nerves" and, at those times, Sharon leaves the house for several days. The family history indicates that Sharon's father was incarcerated for auto theft and assault. Sharon's mother frequently leaves Sharon and her 8-year-old brother unsupervised overnight.

1. Given this information, what suggestions could be made to help this mother cope with the teen's behavior? How would you approach Sharon on first meeting her?
2. What possible diagnoses do you think would be considered?

REFERENCES

American Academy of Child and Adolescent Psychiatry. (2008). The depressed child. Retrieved from http://aacap.org/cs/root/facts_for_families/the_depressed_child

American Psychiatric Association. (2013). *Diagnostic and Statistical Manual of Mental Disorders 5.* Washington, DC, Author. (Known as DSM-5)

Beck-Little, R., and Catton, G. (2011). Child and adolescent suicide in the United States: a population at risk. *Journal of Emergency Nursing, 37*(6), 587–589.

Black, D.W., and Andreasen, N C. (2011). *Introductory Textbook of Psychiatry.* 5th ed. Washington D.C.: American Psychiatric Publishing.

Centers for Disease Control and Prevention. (2012). Autism Spectrum Disorders. Retrieved from http://www.cdc.gov/ncbddd/autism/index.html

Centers for Disease Control and Prevention. (2012). Facts about ASD. http://www.cdc.gov/ncbddd/autism/facts.html

Centers for Disease Control and Prevention. (2013). Mental health surveillance among children—United States, 2005–2011. *Morbidity and mortality reports,* May 17, 2013.

Cooper, G.D., Clements, P.T., and Holt, K. (2011). A review and application of suicide prevention programs in high school settings. *Issues Mental Health Nursing, 32*(11), 696–702.

Goldberg, R.J. (2007). Practical Guide to the Care of the Psychiatric Patient. 3rd ed. St. Louis: Mosby Elsevier.

Kowatch, R.A., et al. (2005). Treatment guidelines for children and adolescents with bipolar disorder: Child Psychiatric Workgroup on Bipolar Disorder. *Journal of the American Academy of Child Adolescent Psychiatry, 44*(3), 213–235.

Lack, C.W., and Green, A.L. (2009). Mood disorders in children and adolescents. *Journal of Pediatric Nursing, 24(*1), 13–25.

Lynch, E. (2010). Making sense of autism. *Nursing Standards, 25*(2), 18–19.

McCann, T.V., Lubman, D.I., and Clark, E. (2012). The experience of young people with depression: A qualitative study. *Jornal of Psychiatry and Mental Health Nursing, 19*(4), 334–340.

McKinney, E.S. (2009). *Maternal-Child Nursing.* 3rd ed. St. Louis: W.B. Saunders.

National Health and Nutrition Examination Survey. (2010). Retrieved from http://www.cdc.gov/nchs/nhanes.htm

National Institute of Mental Health. (2010). Major depressive disorders in children. Retrieved from http://www.nimh.nih.gov/statistics/1MDD_CHILD.shtml

National Institute of Mental Health (2012). Statistics on suicide. Retrieved from http://www.nimh.nih.gov/health/publications/suicide-in-the-us-statistics-and-prevention/index.shtml

National Instititues of Mental Health. (2012). What is attention deficit hyperactivity disorder? Retrieved from http://www.nimh.nih.gov/health/publications/attention-deficit-hyperactivity-disorder/how-is-adhd-treated.shtml

Pati, A. (2011). Early assessment and diagnosis for children with hyperactivity disorder. *Nursing Children and Young People, 23*(7), 5.

Primich, C., and Iennaco, J. (2012). Diagnosing adult attention-deficit hyperactivity disorder: The importance of establishing daily life contexts for symptoms and impairments. *Journal of Psychiatric and Mental Health Nursing, 19*(4), 362–373.

Roman, M.W. (2011). New additions to the psychopharmacopia: Extended release formulations. *Issues in Mental Health Nursing, 32*(11), 717–719.

Shimshock, C.M., Williams, R.A., and Sullivan, B.J. (2011). Suicidal thought in the adolescent: Exploring the relationship between known risk factors and the presence of suicidal thought. *Journal of Child and Adolescent Psychiatric Nursing, 24*(4), 237–244.

Substance Abuse and Mental Health Services Administration (SAMHSA). (2008). SAMHSA's national survey on drug use and health: Youth depression. Retrieved from http://www.samhsa.gov/data/2k8State/Ch6.htm

Substance Abuse and Mental Health Services Administration (SAMHSA). (2012). National Survey on Drug Use and Health at http://www.samhsa.gov

Townsend, M.C. (2012). *Psychiatric Mental Health Nursing.* 7th ed. Philadelphia: F.A. Davis.

Test Questions

Multiple Choice Questions

1. An 8-year-old child is in the waiting room. This child has a diagnosis of conduct disorder. You call another patient to the room but notice this child beginning to act out inappropriately. Your first concern and nursing action would be:
   a. Ask the parent to take the child outside until they are called for their appointment.
   b. Provide an environment of safety for the child and parent.
   c. Change the rooming order and take this parent and child ahead of the patient just called.
   d. Wait a few minutes; the child will probably calm down soon.
2. The child with autism has difficulty with trust. With this in mind, which of the following nursing actions would be most appropriate?
   a. Encourage staff to hold the child as much as possible.
   b. Support different staff caring for child so she gets used to other people.
   c. Encourage the same staff person to care for the child each day.
   d. Avoid talking to the child so she will not be fearful of you.
3. Your 5-year-old patient is not talking to you or the social workers. You suggest giving her some toys and drawing materials. Your rationale for this is:
   a. It gives you one less person to work with at the moment.
   b. You know children can be bribed.
   c. You think she might talk if she were distracted.
   d. Children often communicate feelings through their play.
4. Which of the following activities is most helpful for a child with ADHD?
   a. Checkers
   b. Pool
   c. Video games
   d. Volleyball
5. Which of the following groups of medications are most commonly used with ADHD?
   a. CNS depressants
   b. CNS stimulants
   c. Antidepressants
   d. Antipsychotics
6. Martin is 7 years old and has a diagnosis of ADHD. He has broken his arm and requires surgery to have it set. You are the nurse doing the admission checklist with Martin and his family. You know that people with ADHD:
   a. Have normal or above average intelligence
   b. Are impulsive
   c. Are inattentive or easily distracted
   d. All of the above
7. The single most common symptom of autism is:
   a. Strong ability to make friends
   b. Impaired social functioning
   c. Appropriate emotional responses
   d. Achieving and maintaining age-appropriate developmental tasks
8. The parents of 6-year-old Anna say, "Nurse, why us? The doctors tell us Maria has the most difficult of all childhood developmental disorders to cure. What did we do wrong? What can we do for her?" Your best response might be:
   a. "The doctor is correct."
   b. "Her medications should help calm her somewhat."
   c. "We have specialists here who can help you. I will call someone."
   d. "Maybe she will outgrow the autism."

Test Questions

cont.

9. Which of the following parental traits would be most likely to predispose to conduct disorder in the child?
   a. Overprotective parents
   b. Parents with very high expectations of academic excellence
   c. Chaotic home life with both parents being heavy drinkers
   d. One parent with a physical disability

10. What is the major concern in administering antidepressants to depressed children?
   a. Side effect of dry mouth may affect appetite.
   b. The child may not want to swallow these pills.
   c. The child is at higher risk for suicide.
   d. The child needs to stop drinking milk with these medications.

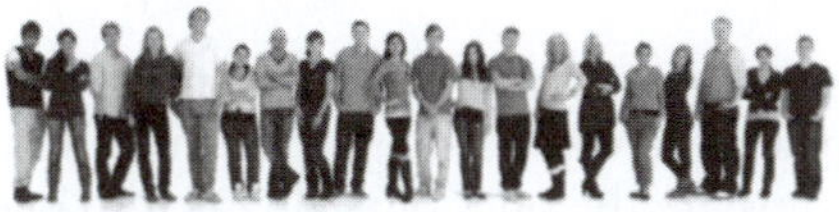

CHAPTER 20

Postpartum Issues in Mental Health

Learning Objectives

1. Differentiate between postpartum blues and postpartum depression.
2. Define postpartum psychosis.
3. Discuss nursing interventions for new mothers who are feeling depressed.
4. Discuss possible side effects of psychotropic medications during pregnancy and breastfeeding.

Key Terms

- Postpartum blues
- Postpartum depression
- Postpartum psychosis

Even though childbirth is exhilarating for most women, **postpartum blues** is a common and normal reaction right after birth. On the other extreme are major psychiatric disorders of **postpartum depression** and **postpartum psychosis** that are much rarer and much more serious. Other issues can include grief response after fetal demise and birth of a sick/imperfect baby. An example is giving birth to an infant that does not meet the mother's expectations, including an infant of the wrong sex or one who is physically challenged. All of these can contribute to poor bonding with the infant that can affect the health of the whole family (Pillitteri, 2007).

Cultural Considerations

Postpartum mental disorders cross all cultures. Each culture has expected behaviors of new mothers, and knowledge of these can make for more accurate screening of possible psychiatric disorders.

■ Postpartum Blues

Postpartum blues (sometimes called transient depressive symptoms) is an extremely common response to the sudden changes immediately after childbirth. It occurs in about 70% of new mothers (Pillitteri, 2007). The major cause is believed to be the plummeting levels of estrogen and progesterone right after birth. The greater the hormone shift, the greater chance of developing postpartum blues (Elder, 2004). Other factors include fatigue and stress of delivery along with the immediate postpartum responsibilities. Symptoms include tears, rapid mood shifts, anxiety, and feeling overwhelmed. The symptoms typically peak at the fourth or fifth day after birth and resolve by day 10 (Ricci, 2007). The disorder is generally self-limiting and does not reflect psychopathology or the care the mother is able to provide to the new baby. The presence of postpartum blues does increase the risk for postpartum major depression.

Treatment of Postpartum Blues

Postpartum blues requires no psychiatric treatment. Families should be educated during the prenatal period of the frequency of this transient condition. Emotional support, compassion, and rest generally help resolve this problem in a matter of days. If the blues go on for a longer period of time (as in more than 2 weeks), there is evidence of intense anxiety about the infant, agitation, feelings of inadequacy, and being overwhelmed most of the time. More intervention is needed. This could signal that postpartum blues has moved into postpartum depression.

Critical Thinking Question

Your postpartum patient is ready to be discharged home. Her family is surrounding her, and they are all thrilled that she had a healthy baby boy. The new mother keeps crying and asks her family to leave her alone. They are shocked and wonder why she is not happy. What would you tell the family? How would you help the patient?

Neeb's Tip

New mothers and their families need to be prepared for postpartum blues and reassured that the mother's response is not abnormal. New mothers may not verbalize their feelings out of fear of appearing to be a bad mother.

Clinical Activity

- Incorporate support, reassurance, and rest in the care of the new mother.
- Provide education and resources, such as a lactation consultant, if needed, to this patient.

Classroom Activity

Promote discussion with classmates who are mothers about their feelings during the postpartum period.

Postpartum Depression

Postpartum depression is a serious disorder that occurs in about 10% of births (Pillitteri, 2007). Some feel this condition is underdiagnosed and undertreated particularly because depression in women in the general population peaks in the 25–44 age group. The symptoms are the ones typically seen in depression (see Chapter 11) with the addition of impaired ability to care for the baby. The majority of sufferers of postpartum depression have had some type of mental health disorder earlier in life, such as a depression. The new mother may hide the symptoms for fear of being viewed as a bad mother. It is not uncommon for the depression to begin during pregnancy so this disorder is sometimes referred to as depression with peripartum onset. The symptoms must occur within 6 months of delivery and be noticeable for at least 2 weeks to be given this diagnosis. This depression can lead to denial of the infant, inability to care for the infant, and even thoughts of hurting the infant, as well as suicidal thoughts or acts in rare, extreme cases.

The strongest risk factor is depression in a previous pregnancy or postpartum depression. See Box 20-1 for symptoms of postpartum depression and Box 20-2 for factors that contribute to postpartum depression.

Tool Box ▶ Edinburgh Postnatal Depression Scale (EPDS) at:
http://www.perinatalweb.org/index.php?option=content&task=view&id=86
This 10-item self-assessment tool can be used by the new mother to monitor her symptoms of depression.

Tool Box ▶ National Alliance on Mental Illness Fact Sheets on Pregnancy and Depression:
http://www.nami.org/Content/NavigationMenu/Inform_Yourself/About_Mental_Illness/By_Illness/Pregnancy_and_Depression.htm

Cultural Considerations

The Edinburgh Postnatal Depression Scale is also available in Spanish:
http://www.perinatalweb.org/index.php?option=content&task=view&id=86

Cultural Considerations

Perinatalweb.org has resources for women from different ethnic groups to address their concerns about postpartum depression.

Box 20-1 Symptoms of Postpartum Depression

- Anxiety
- Irritability
- Loss of interest in new baby
- Views infant as demanding
- Withdrawn
- Irrational guilt
- Sleep disturbances
- Loss of appetite
- Inability to concentrate
- Feels inept at caring for baby
- Does not feel bond or love of new baby
- Excessive anxiety over baby's health
- Feelings of worthlessness
- Poor concentration
- Loss of appetite

Note: For a postpartum depression diagnosis, the symptoms must persist for at least 2 weeks.

Source: Adapted from (Berga, S. L., Parry, B. L., & Moses-Kolka, E. L. (2009). Psychiatry and Reproductive Medicine. In B. J. Sadock, V. A. Sadock, & P. Ruiz (eds.). Kaplan & Sadock's Comprehensive Textbook of Psychiatry (9th ed.), pp. 2539–62. Philadelphia: Lippincott Williams & Wilkins; Pillitteri, A. (2007). Maternal and Child Health Nursing: Care of Childbearing and Childrearing Families (5th ed). Philadelphia: Lippincott Williams & Wilkins;

Box 20-2 Contributing Factors to Postpartum Depression

- Hormone fluctuations
- Personal and/or family history of depression or any mood disorder
- History of premenstrual dysphoric disorder
- Stressful relationship with partner
- Lack of social support
- Major life stressors around the pregnancy
- Ambivalence about the pregnancy
- Sleep disturbance
- Medical problems during the pregnancy or just after birth
- History of a troubled childhood
- Pregnancy under age 20
- Abuse of alcohol, illegal substances

Treatment of Postpartum Depression

Postpartum depression is a serious disorder that requires treatment. Early intervention is associated with a good prognosis. When the diagnosis of postpartum depression is made, the mother is usually placed on antidepressants and begins some form of psychotherapy. If the new mother is breastfeeding, she may be reluctant to take medications. See the Pharmacology Corner for more information on the risks associated with antidepressants. Discussion with the physician and pharmacist can be helpful to determine the risk to the baby. Some women may continue psychotherapy only, pursue alternative treatments such as light therapy, or choose to stop breastfeeding. The woman should be followed closely for at least 6 months after successful treatment. During treatment the family must be involved to provide support and ensure safety of the baby and mother. Treatment will help with establishing a healthy bond between the mother and baby. If left untreated, this depression can continue for months or even years. The mother should be aware that once she is diagnosed with postpartum depression, she is at high risk for recurrence of it with subsequent pregnancies.

A new mother who has any symptoms of or is at risk for postpartum depression should take steps right away to get help. Some helpful tips if a mother is experiencing early signs of postpartum depression include (U.S. National Library of Medicine, 2010; Pearlstein et al., 2009):

- Ask for help in caring for the baby
- Talk about these concerns with the patient's doctor and nurses
- Talk about one's feelings
- Avoid making major life changes during pregnancy or right after delivery
- Encourage realistic expectations of herself
- Take time to get out of the house without the baby, visit with friends, spend time alone with partner, participate in exercise program

- Join a support group with other new mothers
- Ensure adequate rest, e.g., sleep when the baby is sleeping, arrange for child care so mother can sleep
- Comply with any treatment recommendations for depression

Critical Thinking Question

You are working in a postpartum clinic. Your new patient is 4 weeks post-delivery. Her husband approaches you with concerns about why is his wife so tired and irritable. On further questioning, he tells you she is in bed most of the day and family members are caring for the baby. What would you ask the patient when you see her for the initial screening?

Clinical Activity

- Be aware of your postpartum patient's history and family history for psychiatric disorders.
- Review current and past psychiatric medications.

Postpartum Psychosis

Postpartum psychosis is a psychiatric emergency. It is sometimes called puerperal psychosis. It is rare as it occurs in about 0.1–0.2% of pregnancies (Berga, Parry, & Moses-Kolka, 2009). The majority of women with this disorder have had symptoms of mental illness before pregnancy. It is most common in first pregnancies and is generally evident within a few weeks of delivery. This disorder occurs most frequently in women with a history of bipolar disorder pre-pregnancy. Postpartum psychosis can actually be an episode of bipolar illness. See Chapter 12 for detailed information on bipolar disorder. In fact, postpartum recovery time is considered a high-risk period for bipolar disorder recurrence in at-risk women (Sharma & Pope, 2012). Any woman with a history of bipolar disorder should be monitored closely during pregnancy as recurrence of mania symptoms may occur. Women with a history of bipolar disorder are usually advised to discontinue lithium and some other bipolar medications due to possible adverse effects on the fetus. This puts the woman at high risk for recurrence. See the Pharmacology Corner for more information.

The earliest signs of postpartum psychosis are:

- Restlessness
- Irritability
- Insomnia

These can progress quickly to:

- Rapidly shifting moods
- Erratic or disorganized behavior
- Delusions of grandeur or persecution
- Extreme impulsivity
- Disorganized speech and behavior
- Hallucinations
- Disorientation/confusion

Delusional beliefs are common and often center on the infant, as in the infant is evil or the infant can read the mother's mind. Auditory hallucinations that instruct the mother to harm herself or her infant may also occur. The mother may deny the existence of the child, leading to not caring for the infant. Risk for infanticide, as well as suicide, is significant in this population (Massachusetts General Hospital Center for Women's Mental Health, 2010).

In addition to bipolar disorder, postpartum psychosis can also be categorized as Brief Psychotic Disorder with postpartum onset in someone without a psychiatric history (DSM -5, 2013). Postpartum depression can also move to a psychosis with paralyzing depression with hallucinations and delusions in rare cases.

Postpartum psychosis right after delivery needs to be differentiated from delirium. Delirium could be a reaction to many factors during delivery such as anesthesia dehydration.

Tool Box |▶ National Alliance on Mental Illness has information on bipolar disorder and pregnancy at: www.nami.org/Content/NavigationMenu/Mental_Illnesses/Bipolar1/Pregnancy_and_Bipolar_Disorder.htm

Treatment of Postpartum Psychosis

Immediate medical and psychiatric treatment must be instituted when postpartum psychosis is diagnosed (Fig. 20-1). Severe overactivity

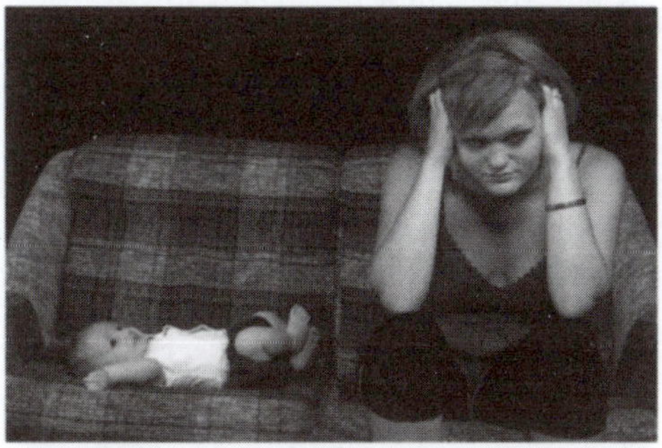

Figure 20-1 New mother with postpartum psychosis is hearing distressing voices.

and delusions may require rapid tranquilization by antipsychotic drugs. Mood stabilizing drugs such as lithium are also useful in treatment and possibly for prevention of episodes in women at high risk (i.e., women who have already experienced manic or psychotic episodes). Immediate safety of the infant must be determined. In some cases electroconvulsive (electroshock) treatment is used. If the woman exhibits signs of psychosis during pregnancy, antipsychotic medications may need to be started. The family needs to consult with experts about the possible risks to the fetus from these medications.

The location of treatment is an issue; hospitalization is disruptive to the family. It is possible to treat moderately severe cases at home, where the sufferer can maintain her role as a mother and build up her relationship with the newborn. This requires the presence, around the clock, of competent adults (such as father or grandparent) and frequent visits by professional staff. If hospital admission is necessary, there are advantages in conjoint mother and baby admission; however, multiple factors must be considered in the subsequent discharge plan to ensure the safety and healthy development of both the baby and mother. This plan often involves a multidisciplinary team structure to follow up on the mother, the baby, their relationship, and the entire family. Family therapy is essential in the treatment process as family members may be traumatized by the patient's bizarre behavior.

Critical Thinking Question

You are doing a home health 6-week follow-up visit for a postpartum patient with a history of bipolar disorder. When you walk in the house, the patient is agitated and tells you the baby is driving her crazy and she wants to get rid of him. What would you do?

Pharmacology Corner

Treatment of postpartum depression and psychosis usually requires psychoactive medications. Concern about the safety of these medications to the infant during pregnancy and during breastfeeding is a major issue in treatment. Informed decisions by the new mother as to the burden and benefit of medications require thorough patient education. In other words, if the medications prevent serious disorders are they worth the risk to the baby. Some concerns include:

- Antidepressants are excreted in breast milk. The infant could be subject to the drug's side effects. The antidepressants that have been identified as safest to the infant include paroxetine, sertraline, and nortriptyline (ACOG Committee Practice Bulletin, 2008). These have been found to have minimal side effects to the infant. The woman should be on the lowest dose possible and time breastfeeding so that it does not occur when concentration of the antidepressants is high. The infant should be monitored closely for side effects and normal growth.
- Some studies report the fetus is at increased risk for complications when exposed to antidepressants during pregnancy. So starting antidepressants during pregnancy or during subsequent pregnancies, must be discussed in detail with the physician.
- Since the risk for postpartum depression and psychosis in women with a history of bipolar disorder is high, considerations about continuing mood

Continued

Pharmacology Corner—cont'd

stabilizers during pregnancy must be discussed and the risks and benefits weighed. Risks to the fetus may include a number of congenital malformations, especially with lithium. In addition, the pregnant woman on lithium is more vulnerable to lithium toxicity due to fluid shifts. The psychiatrist should be consulted for alternative medications if the woman wishes to become pregnant.

- For women with bipolar disorder, breastfeeding may be problematic. First is the concern that on-demand breastfeeding may significantly disrupt the mother's sleep and thus may increase her vulnerability to relapse during the acute postpartum period. Second, there have been reports of toxicity in nursing infants related to exposure to various mood stabilizers, including lithium and carbamazepine, in breast milk. Lithium is excreted at high levels in the mother's milk. Exposure to carbamazepine and valproic acid in the breast milk has been associated with hepatotoxicity in the nursing infant (Massachusetts General Hospital Center for Women's Mental Health, 2010).
- Antipsychotic and anti-anxiety medications are often needed to treat psychosis as well as depression. The psychiatrist will identify those with less risk to the mother and infant. Antipsychotics are generally viewed as having less risk to mother and infant (Berga, Parry, & Moses-Kolka, 2009).

Tool Box |▶ An excellent Web site for monitoring the current knowledge about medications and breastfeeding is http://toxnet.nlm.nih.gov>; click on "LactMed."

Nursing Care of Women With Postpartum Mental Disorders

Nursing diagnoses for women with postpartum mental disorders include the following:

- Anxiety
- Coping, ineffective
- Injury, risk for
- Sleep pattern disturbance
- Thought processes, disturbed
- Violence to self/others, risk for

General Nursing Interventions

1. *Safety:* Maintain safety of the patient and her infant. Any risk factors for this disorder need to be identified early in the pregnancy as a routine part of prenatal care. Anyone at risk should be monitored closely and the patient and family educated on what to look for. If the patient or infant is at any risk, immediate action must be taken to protect them. Safety also involves educating the new mother about risks associated with psychiatric medications.
2. *Compassion and support:* Adequate support for the new family must be in place. Helping the family with options for the mother to get enough rest, resources for infant care, and support groups should be in place.
3. *Ongoing monitoring* for high-risk patients: Be aware that patients with any history of mental disorders, substance abuse, and family conflict are at higher risk for postpartum mental disorders. This information should be identified during pregnancy so adequate support and prevention strategies can be implemented. Listen to family members who may observe the mother's behavior. Home health visits should be arranged for any mother at high risk for postpartum psychiatric disorders. The patient's psychiatrist needs to be involved in the treatment plan.
4. *Education:* The new family needs education about the stresses of pregnancy and

childbirth. Education of the new family about postpartum blues and its transient nature should be included in childbirth classes and doctor visits. Also, education on infant care and breastfeeding can reassure the mother of her skills.

5. *Medication management:* Because the use of psychiatric medications in this population involves some risks, providing support and education is essential.
6. *Further Interventions:* See Chapters 10,11,12, and 15 for specific interventions for anxiety, depression, mania, and psychosis.

Tool Box | PEP (Postpartum Education for Parents) Warmline: (805) 564-3888. Postpartum Distress Support 24/7

Neeb's Tip Monitor coping mechanisms and evidence of family conflict in prenatal visits to give information on how the mother will react after birth.

Neeb's Tip Women often have unrealistic expectations of themselves with a new baby, thinking that other women are better mothers.

Neeb's Tip Lactation consultants can be helpful as a new mother may feel inadequate if having difficulty with breastfeeding.

Clinical Activity

- Obtain information on how psychiatric disorders are addressed in local obstetrics clinics.
- Obtain information on local support groups for new mothers.

The nursing care plan for patients with postpartum issues is provided in Table 20-1.

Table 20-1 Nursing Care Plan for Patients With Postpartum Disorders

Behaviors	Nursing Diagnosis	Goals	Interventions	Evaluation
New mother is avoiding caring for new baby for the first 6 weeks. She has verbalized feelings of inadequacy and lack of attachment to new baby. She cries frequently and expresses feelings that baby would be better off without her.	Ineffective coping	Patient will verbalize her feelings. She will spend more time caring for baby. She will verbalize optimism regarding caring for new baby. Family will maintain safe environment for patient and baby.	Provide support and reassurance. Communicate your observations to MD. Educate patient and family about postpartum depression. Encourage patient to complete small tasks in caring for baby. Reinforce successes in baby care. Assist family in maintaining adequate caregiving for baby. Educate on treatment options for this depression.	Patient verbalizes feelings of competence in caring for baby. Patient and baby remain safe. Patient participates in treatment plan.

Key Concepts

1. Postpartum blues are a very common reaction to plummeting hormones right after delivery. These blues generally do not require any psychiatric treatment.
2. Women with postpartum blues that go on for more than 2 weeks should be evaluated for postpartum depression.
3. Postpartum depression is often associated with a previous history of mood disorders.
4. Postpartum psychosis is a rare disorder and often associated with a history of bipolar disorder.
5. Pharmacological treatment of these disorders may be associated with risks during pregnancy and breastfeeding.
6. Any pregnant woman with a history of psychiatric disorders should have psychiatric follow-up.

CASE STUDY

Janice is a 21-year-old experiencing her first pregnancy. She lives with the father of the baby and has additional support from her mother and grandmother. Janice has a history of substance abuse, including cocaine and opioids, as well as depression, but she denies any drug use during the pregnancy. She is in her 8th month of pregnancy. Upon arrival at the clinic, she appears tearful, unkempt, and sad. Her boyfriend tells you she has been sleeping for days and does not talk to him. He noticed a big change in her behavior 4 weeks ago when she became more withdrawn and tearful. The boyfriend said she told him she does not want to think about the baby and does not want to participate in preparations. She says she is too tired to think about it. The boyfriend works long hours to make ends meet and confides in you that he does not know what they will do when the baby comes, if she remains in this condition. He is considering having Janice's mother take the baby if this continues.

1. Given this information, what would be your primary concern for Janice?
2. What would you ask Janice when you go in to see her?
3. What support options should be recommended for the boyfriend/father?

REFERENCES

ACOG Committee on Practice Bulletins—Obstetrics. ACOG Practice Bulletin: Clinical management guidelines for obstetrician-gynecologists number 92. Use of psychiatric medications during pregnancy and lactation. *Obstet Gynecol. 2008*(111), 1001–1020.

American Psychiatric Association. (2013). *Diagnostic and Statistical Manual of Mental Disorders 5*. Washington, DC, Author. (Known as DSM-5)

Berga, S. L., Parry, B. L., & Moses-Kolka, E. L. (2009). Psychiatry and Reproductive Medicine. In B. J. Sadock, V. A. Sadock, & P. Ruiz (eds.). *Kaplan & Sadock's Comprehensive Textbook of Psychiatry*. 9th ed. pp. 2539–62. Philadelphia: Lippincott Williams & Wilkins.

Elder, C. R. (2004). Beyond baby blues. Nursing Spectrum. Retrieved from nsweb.nuirsingspectrum.com/ce/ce72.htm

Henshaw, C., & Cox, J. (2004). Post natal blues. *J Psychosomatic Obstetrics and Gynecology 25*, 267–72.

Massachusetts General Hospital Center for Women's Mental Health (2010). Postpartum Psychiatric Disorders. Retrieved from http://www.womensmentalhealth.org/specialty-clinics/postpartum-psychiatric-disorders/

McCoy, S, J. (2011). Postpartum depression. *South Med J 104*(2), 128–32.

McKinney, E. S., James, S. R., Murray, S. S., Ashwill, J. W. (2009). *Maternal-Child Nursing.* 3rd ed. St. Louis: Saunders.

Pearlstein, T., Howard, M., Salisbury, A., & Zlotnick, C. Postpartum depression. *Am J Obstet Gynecol. 2009*(200), 357–364.

Pillitteri, A. (2007). *Maternal and Child Health Nursing: Care of Childbearing and Childrearing Families.* 5th ed. Philadelphia: Lippincott Williams & Wilkins.

Ricci, S. S. (2007). *Essentials of Maternity, Newborn and Women's Health Nursing.* Philadelphia: Lippincott Williams & Wilkins.

Sharma, V., & Pope, C. J. (2012). Pregnancy and bipolar disorder. *J Clinical Psychiatry*, 73(11):1447-55.

Townsend MC (2012). Psychiatric *Mental Health Nursing.* 7th ed. Philadelphia: FA Davis.

U.S. National Library of Medicine. (2010). Post Partum Depression. Retrieved from www.ncbi.nlm.nih.gov/pubmedhealth/PMH0004481/

Test Questions

Multiple Choice Questions

1. Which statement reflects postpartum psychosis?
  a. "I wish my baby had more hair."
  b. "My baby has evil eyes."
  c. "I don't think I will be good at breastfeeding."
  d. "I am exhausted and want to sleep rather than see the baby right now."

2. Which of the following statements best reflects postpartum blues?
  a. "I wonder if I will be good at breastfeeding."
  b. "I wish the baby had never been born."
  c. "I am exhausted so I won't feed the baby this morning."
  d. "I can't stop crying every time I look at the baby."

3. Which of the following is true about postpartum blues?
  a. The blues start several months after the baby is born.
  b. The blues occur in the majority of women a few days after childbirth.
  c. The diagnosis of postpartum blues is a psychiatric diagnosis.
  d. The postpartum blues are usually a precursor to poor bonding with the infant.

4. What is the most important risk factor for postpartum depression?
  a. Past history of depression in a previous pregnancy
  b. History of pre-eclampsia in a previous pregnancy
  c. History of conflict within the family during the pregnancy
  d. The baby being born with multiple anomalies

5. Which of the following is a good nursing intervention for a new mother with postpartum blues?
  a. "Let your mother take care of the baby for the first few days."
  b. "Recognize that it is normal to feel very emotional right after the baby is born."
  c. "Let's ask the doctor to order an antidepressant to start today."
  d. "It is important to stop crying around your new baby."

6. You are caring for a woman who has just had a stillbirth. Which of the following statements reflects an understanding of grief after loss of a baby?
  a. "You're young; you can have more children."
  b. "It's best to put this behind you."
  c. "Would you like to have some private time with the baby's body?"
  d. "I will leave you alone so you can have privacy to grieve by yourself."

7. Which of the following is a sign that postpartum blues is progressing to depression?
  a. The new mother is crying for the first 4 days after delivery.
  b. The new mother verbalizes anxiety and fear that she feels nothing for her new baby 2 weeks after delivery.
  c. The new mother tells you that she has heard from her deceased grandmother that the baby is evil.
  d. The new mother wants to sleep for long periods 2 days after delivery.

Test Questions

cont.

8. What is the major risk factor of mood stabilizers during pregnancy?

a. Contributes to pre-eclampsia
b. Increased risk of malformations in neonate
c. Increased risk of postpartum depression
d. Increased cholesterol levels postpartum

9. Which of the following is true about postpartum depression?

a. It is more common than postpartum blues.
b. It is less common in Hispanic women.
c. It can be safely treated with antidepressants.
d. Diet and exercise can usually improve it.

10. What of the following is true about postpartum psychosis?

a. It is a medical emergency.
b. It may be evidence of bipolar disorder.
c. The baby's safety may be compromised.
d. All of the above

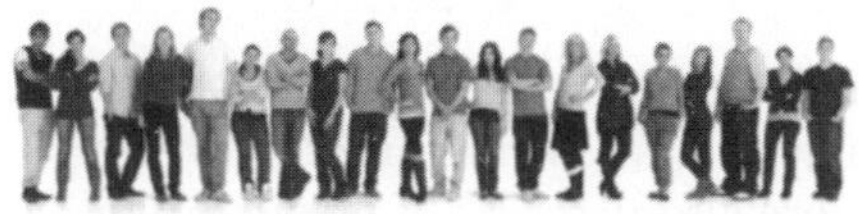

CHAPTER 21

Aging Population

Learning Objectives

1. Discuss concepts of aging.
2. Define ageism.
3. Discuss social trends in the aging population.
4. Identify five mental challenges of the older adult.
5. Identify medical treatment for the older adult.
6. Identify nursing actions for general care of older patients.

Key Terms

- Ageism
- Cerebrovascular disease
- Elder abuse
- Elderly
- Geriatrics
- Gerontology
- Insomnia
- Omnibus Budget Reconciliation Act (OBRA)
- Palliative care
- Restorative nursing

Gerontology means the study of older adults. **Geriatrics** is the branch of medicine caring for older adults. The study of older adults is a specialty in nursing. With more and more North Americans reaching age 65 within the next 10 to 15 years, learning the complications, abilities, and best ways to assist that population is a very timely study. According to the Administration on Aging of the Department of Health and Human Services, "The population of 65+ will increase from 35 million in 2000 to 55 million in 2020."

Neeb's Tip Aging begins at the moment of birth.

Aging happens to everyone, and nobody has control over it. It is a condition of time passing. It is also a condition that researchers are beginning to redefine: What *is* "old age"?

Critical Thinking Question

How do you define your current perception of age-young, young-old, old, or old-old, and what are you using to measure age? What is your view when you meet people in each of these groups?

When children are 10 years old, they cannot wait to be 16 so they can drive a car. Sixteen-year-olds want to be 18 so they can be out on their own. When they turn 30, the idea of time passing begins to take on a different tone for some people. In a society that promotes the image of youth, many people of this age see youth vanishing. They might feel they are not as fast or as thin or as healthy as they were in their 20s. Still, they see healthy, happy people over age 65 working, recreating, and socializing. Life expectancy in the United States is in the 76 for men and the early 81for women (World Health Organization, 2011). So, what *is* this process of aging?

Classroom Activity

- Develop three age range groups in your class and describe what you have in common with the people in your age group.

The majority of people over 65 are intellectually intact and able to care for themselves (Fig. 21-1). Only about 0.4% of people over age 65 live in institutional setting such as

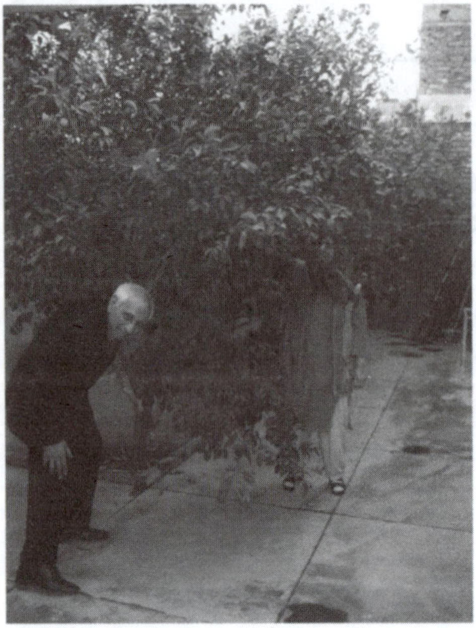

Figure 21-1 Most older adults are independent and fully able to care for themselves. *(Courtesy of Robin Anwar.)*

nursing homes (Administration on Aging, 2011). These numbers are slowly on the rise as children of the 1950s and 1960s (often referred to as "baby boomers") enter advanced age. Older people are usually basically mentally healthy; that is, they are able to accept and deal with the changes and losses they are experiencing.

Of course, many challenges are involved with aging. People aging normally may experience a loss in visual and hearing acuity. Many of these individuals live on fixed incomes that are not adequate to meet their needs for housing, food, and health care. Safety is also an issue. Criminals are finding that older adults are easy targets and are robbing and mugging them in higher numbers than in generations past. For aging adults, the need to face death becomes more of a reality.

Certain illnesses become more prevalent as one ages. Alzheimer's disease (see Chapter 16) may become more prominently manifested in an older person, rendering the individual incapable of caring for himself or herself and possibly requiring a major lifestyle changes. This can include the individual's move to a nursing home or to a family member's home. Coronary disease such as arteriosclerosis and respiratory disorders such as pneumonia occur more frequently in this age group, and patients are less responsive to the treatments than younger people are. Older people are sicker longer. Nutrition is challenged. **Elderly** people may not be able to afford to buy nutritious foods, and the food they do prepare does not taste as it once did because their taste buds are less sensitive. It is essential that this aging group have all of their survival needs met.

A phenomenon called **ageism,** which is occurring in the United States, is discrimination against a group of people on the basis of their age. It assumes that most older people are incapable of functioning in and contributing to society. What thoughts arise as one sees that the car ahead of him is being driven by an older person who can barely see over the steering wheel?

Classroom Activity

- Answer the following questions and share your responses to the questions with your classmates:
  How I will look at 75 years of age?
  Will I be independent?
  What will I be doing at 75?

The retirement age has changed drastically as a result of the economy and Social Security benefits. The expected age for retirement is currently 67 for people currently in the workforce to attain full retirement benefits. Those who have retired from their careers can live a comfortable life provided their retirement funds are adequate (U.S. Social Security Administration, Retirement Planner: Full Retirement Age, 2012).

Whereas people now may conceivably change careers at least five times during their working years, the elderly people of today most likely had one or two jobs over their lifetime and worked 20–30 years at each job. That job probably represented a large part of the person's identity, and retirement may lead to feelings of low self-esteem and depression when the person has to redefine who he or she is. Self-esteem is viewed as a need according to Maslow, and something that was sought after in youth and provides, prestige, and power (Green, 2000).

Retirement also means a decrease in income, which can have a negative impact on a person's lifestyle. Today many elderly people have to make a choice whether to buy groceries or purchase their prescribed medication.

The need for intimacy never leaves us. As human beings, the need to love and be loved is one of the primary needs for survival of the individual and the species (Fig. 21-2). As people age and spouses and friends die, who is there to love older people? Prospects for marriage are slim. Children and grandchildren may live on the opposite side of the country. In addition, older adults may be forced to live with their adult children, which is not always the ideal situation. Older individuals are at risk for **elder abuse** (physical and emotional abuse of older people) by their children or caregivers. Elder abuse is discussed further in Chapter 22.

Aging has many challenges, yet most individuals are able to cope with the changes brought about by aging and progress through this life stage with dignity. They are proud of their families and their personal accomplishments. They can see the contributions that they have passed on to others. People who have learned to adapt to change throughout life have the best chances of progressing through old age with the same kind of resilience.

Older adults with mental illness whether these were diagnosed earlier in life or are a new diagnosis face many challenges on top of the aging process. For example an elderly person with schizophrenia, generalized anxiety disorder, or a personality disorder will need added support as the person declines.

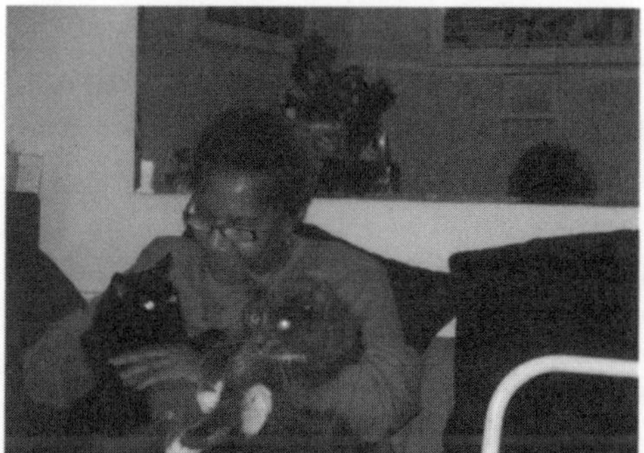

Figure 21-2 Pets can fulfill the need for companionship and intimacy in an older person's life. *(Courtesy of Robin Anwar.)*

The **Omnibus Budget Reconciliation Act (OBRA)** is a federal act that provides standards of care for older adults. One of the provisions of OBRA is ensuring proper assessment of elderly people.

Tool Box |▶ Information About Elders and Mental Health Services
http://www.asaging.org/blog/aca-could-benefit-elders-mental-health-problems-will-it

It is for this reason that only registered nurses (RNs) may conduct or coordinate initial assessments of elderly individuals. The LPN/LVN role is to assist the registered nurse through active listening and competent observation. This responsibility is especially important in long-term care facilities since the role of the LPN/LVN is to administer routine and prn medications. Other health-care team members assist with the registered nurse's assessment by providing input as to the resident's ability and responses to the treatment plan. OBRA also set the standards for providing education for the majority of nurse's aides who are employed by long-term care facilities; the Department of Health and Senior Services regulates the curriculum.

Nurses are caring for the older individual not only in the health-care facility but also increasingly in the privacy of the person's own home (Fig. 21-3). Multidisciplinary teams are

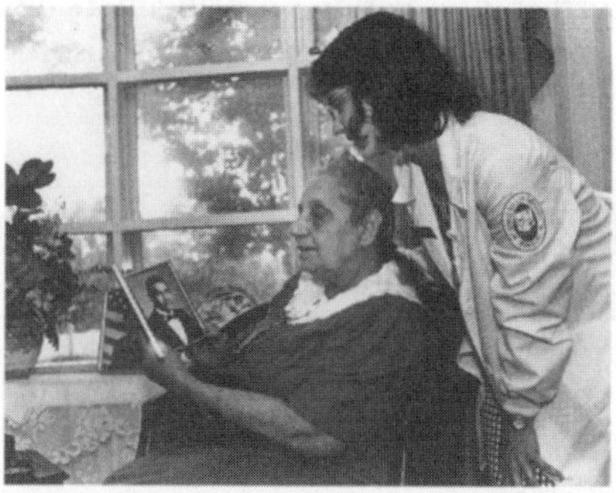

Figure 21-3 Increasingly, nurses are caring for older adults in their own homes. *(From Sorrell and Redmond (2007): Community-Based Nursing Practice: Learning Through Students' Stories. Philadelphia: F.A. Davis Company, with permission.)*

assisting and monitoring the physiological needs of the elderly in the home. Because it is believed that people will stay healthier and maintain more control of their lives if they can stay in their own homes, the home health industry is growing. One of the primary concerns for nurses and others caring for older adults is to help them maintain a good quality of life. Nurses caring for patients in their homes need to be aware of some of the major mental and emotional disturbances they may encounter, as well as the physical diagnoses of the patient. The elderly are prone to a number of major disorders that impact their emotional well-being. These are covered in the next sections (Box 21-1).

Alzheimer's Disease and Other Cognitive Alterations

As stated in Chapter 16, when a person has been diagnosed with **Alzheimer's disease,** it has most likely been taking its toll on the individual for many years. It is in the later stages that the debilitating effects are most observable. This disease may necessitate the person's leaving the home she has lived in all of her adult life. It may mean living apart from a spouse whom she may not appear to remember. Socializing will be curtailed because of the inability to relate to others easily. Alzheimer's disease has an impact not only on the patient but also on all the people in that person's life, which may include the health-care provider.

Further information on Alzheimer's disease and the care of patients with this disorder is included in Chapter 16.

Box 21-1 Some Concerns of Aging Adults

- Alzheimer's disease and other cognitive impairments
- Cerebrovascular (stroke)
- Depression
- Medication concerns
- Paranoid thinking
- Insomnia
- End of Life issues

Cerebrovascular Accident (Stroke)

A **cerebrovascular accident (CVA),** or stroke, is a medical disorder that has implications for mental health workers. A CVA is a devastating and frightening experience for the patient and family. The probability of a CVA in the elderly is higher. Depending on the location and size of the brain and blood vessel involvement, many physical and cognitive functions may be temporarily or permanently affected (Fig. 21-4). Some of the mental health issues associated with CVA are depression and aphasia.

Depression Associated With CVA

Patients realize the losses associated with their stroke. They may not be able to express them verbally or physically, but they do realize that they cannot do things independently. Self-esteem decreases as they realize they may be

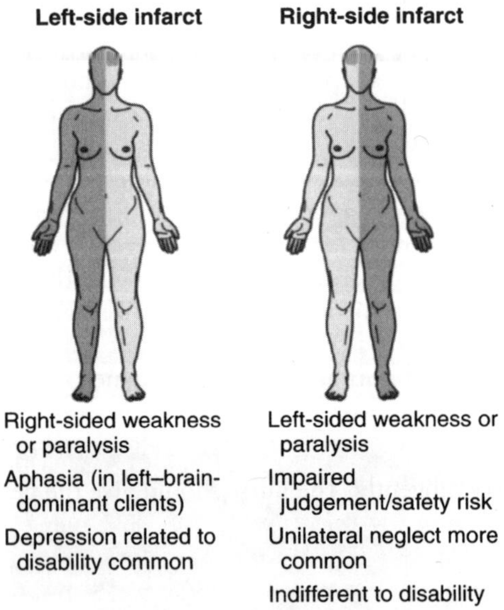

Figure 21-4 The location of a stroke is a key factor in the physical and cognitive functions that may be affected. A stroke on the left side of the brain affects the right side of the body; a stroke on the right side of the brain affects the left side of the body. *(From Williams and Hopper (2011). Understanding Medical-Surgical Nursing, 4th ed. Philadelphia: F.A. Davis Company, with permission.)*

incontinent, unable to eat independently, or unable to communicate with their families. Depression may develop. They worry about the effect of their stroke not only on themselves but also on their spouses and other family members. Will this be permanent or only temporary? Will it happen again? How long will I be this way?

As these worries become more pronounced, the patient may become more depressed. The physicians, nurses, and therapists will try to explain these concerns to the patient and family, but the patient may still feel out of control of his or her destiny. Nurses may see the patient crying and refusing to perform tasks that he or she could do after the stroke. The patient may avoid eye contact with the nurse or refuse to interact with family members. All these behaviors may indicate depression in the patient who has had a CVA. By recognizing and confronting these behaviors, the nurse can help the patient understand that the nurse is really there to help and is concerned with the patient's thoughts and feelings.

Being honest and generous with positive reinforcement for attempts to overcome the feelings of depression will also be helpful in building the patient's confidence and self-esteem.

Aphasia

Aphasia, a speech disorder that may be found in patients who have had a CVA, is classified as expressive, receptive, and/or global (see Chapter 2). A patient with aphasia may need to learn to talk all over again. Communication is such a basic need that the nurse and the patient must work at any threat to this ability very diligently. The nurse should give the person time to speak, write, or show what is needed, and praise him or her for all efforts to communicate. One communication technique that is effective, especially in expressive aphasia, is to associate the object with the word. The more senses a person can engage, the better the reinforcement for the learning.

Neeb's Tip
Patience is mandatory. The goal of communicating with a person who has aphasia is to keep him/her involved in the recovery.

The physician and speech therapist will determine the proper plan of speech therapy. Nurses need to closely follow this plan and document the patient's progress and emotional responses to speech therapy.

Critical Thinking Question
You are celebrating your retirement when the room goes dark. You wake up in a busy room with lights and noise and many people. You think you recognize some of them and you try to call out to them, but they just stand there and look at you. Someone you do not know is trying to say something to you and keeps shining a flashlight in your eye. Your life partner is crying. What happened to you? Why is nobody answering you? What are you feeling now? What do you wish someone would do to help you?

Depression in the Elderly

It is not "normal" to feel depressed all the time despite the fact the person is getting older. Major depression in the elderly population can show itself differently than in other age groups. In addition to the information discussed in Chapter 11, nurses observing and assisting elderly people should collect subjective and objective data for physical symptoms that can mask depression, e.g., confusion, constipation, headaches, and other body aches. Often these patients will discuss these physical symptoms rather than admit to being depressed.

These symptoms are similar to other afflictions common in the elderly population, such as drug side effects (Box 21-2), electrolyte imbalances, and dementia. Nurses must get accurate information, document it, and be certain that appropriate medical care is obtained to rule out other ailments.

Clinical Activity
During clinical preconference at a nursing home, determine how many residents have been diagnosed as depressed. Develop a care plan that will address depression.

Box 21-2 Common Drug Side Effects for Elderly Patients

Dry Mouth
Constipation
Orthostatic hypotension
Urinary complications
Confusion/disorientation/mental sluggishness
fatigue
Mood swings/irritability

Medication Concerns

The process of pharmacokinetics is slower and less complete in older people. Because circulatory, hepatic, and renal function start to decrease normally with age, it is easier for these persons to become toxic. Adverse effects of many medications are more likely to develop in the elderly. Nurses who work in facilities that care for older adults must be very alert to the effects of the medications they give their patients as well as to the possible signs of side effects and toxicity. The nurse needs to report any concerns to his or her charge nurse immediately and document observations accurately. If the state allows a licensed practical nurse/licensed vocational nurse (LPN/LVN) to contact the physician by telephone, the LPN or LVN will also take that responsibility.

Patients who live at home may lose track of their medication routine. They may forget to take medications or forget they have taken them and take another dose. Many pills look alike. When visual acuity is lessened and lighting inadequate, patients may mistake one pill for another—for example, they may take two lanoxin tablets instead of one lanoxin and one furosemide, especially if they put all of their medications in one container. These types of mistakes can be lethal.

To help with this situation, nurses have systems available for teaching patients and families. Containers are available for planning which medications are taken at what time, enabling the nurse and patient to set up the patient's medications for a week or longer and for different times of day. If the patient is reliable, this will serve as a reminder to take a particular dose. If the patient still needs some reassurance, the nurse can instruct the patient to immediately mark on a calendar the appropriate date and time a dose is taken. In this way, the patient can double-check that the medications are taken correctly and will be less anxious about it. Also, new technology is available to create reminder alarms.

Nurses also must be aware of the patient's weight, nutrition, and activity levels. It is very easy for older people to become toxic from their medications, regardless of whether they are at home or in a facility. Patients with drug toxicity or overdose can present with symptoms similar to those of a mental illness or other physical illness. It is not uncommon for a proper dose of a medication for an older adult to be as little as 25% of the "usual" recommended adult dose. It is the nurse's responsibility to ask specific questions of the doctor regarding medication doses.

Similarly, side effects to medications can look like other symptoms. Nurses can teach patients and families about this possibility. Table 21-1 shows some of the common side effects of drugs on older people, disorders that may have similar symptoms, and some nursing actions that can be taken and taught to the patient.

Paranoid Thinking

Paranoid thinking may be a result of fear about the social environment. As stated earlier, certain people see elderly persons as "easy marks." What was once a situation that was not threatening (such as a walk around the block) can become very frightening for the person who has slowed reaction time and diminished physical capacity for self-protection. Paranoid, fearful thinking can be a defense mechanism against these kinds of disabilities, making the fear the reason to avoid leaving the house. This self-imposed isolation can bloom into feelings of loneliness, which can lead to illness that is more serious. Validate what the person is expressing, even when it has taken the form of being paranoid. Investigate the person's fearful thinking. Age-related hearing loss (presbycusis) and vision loss as well as early onset of dementia can all contribute to paranoid thinking. Paranoid thinking can also occur when a patient is entering a long-term care facility and is exposed to new caregivers and a roommate.

Table 21-1 Common Drug Side Effects and Nursing Actions for Elderly Patients*

Side Effect	Other Possibilities	Nursing Actions
Dry Mouth	• Stress response; electrolyte imbalance • Vitamin B deficiency	**1.** Offer sips of water or ice chips. **2.** Offer hard, sugar-free candy (such as lemon drops) if patient is able to suck on them without choking. **3.** Provide oral care with light application of lubricant such as petroleum jelly; saliva substitute. **4.** Review lab work or call physician.
Constipation	• Fluid and nutritional deficiency, hemorrhoids, or rectal pain • Hypothyroidism	**1.** Assess diet for fiber and fluid intake. **2.** Assess area for signs of hemorrhoids or other inflammation. **3.** Assess need for laxatives as ordered by physician. **4.** Discuss need for physical activity as condition warrants.
Orthostatic Hypotension	• Heart disorders • Dehydration	**1.** Assess vital signs. **2.** Teach patient how to get out of bed or chair slowly. **3.** Tell patient to stay sitting for a few minutes until dizziness goes away.
Urinary Complications	• Prostate problems • Bladder problems • Uterus problems • Urinary tract infections • Cancers	**1.** You must: Keep track of frequency, amount, color, and odor of urine, and abdominal girth. **2.** Report signs of urinary tract infection to physician.
Confusion/ Disorientation/ Mental Sluggishness	• Hypoglycemia • Head injury (e.g., fall) • Infection/fever • Depression • Vitamin deficiency • Transient ischemic attack (TIA) • Brain tumor • Dehydration • Alcohol and/or tranquilizer use	**1.** Give sweetened drink. If patient is still confused after 10 minutes, call physician. **2.** Check vital signs and signs of infection. **3.** Attempt to validate whether patient has had recent head trauma.
Fatigue	• Infectious process • Anemia • Hypothyroidism • Stress • Narrowing of coronary arteries	**1.** Assess vital signs. **2.** Assess stress level. **3.** Encourage activity if appropriate. **4.** Assess sleep pattern.
Mood Swings/ Irritability	• Psychological disorders • Electrolyte imbalances	**1.** Use verbal and nonverbal communication skills to assess cause. **2.** Request lab work.

*Always report these side effects to the charge nurse, document carefully, and notify the physician if that is allowed for LPN/LVN practice in your state.

■ Insomnia

Insomnia, or inability to sleep, is seen frequently in the older adult. It can be a result of many conditions, including depression, fear, pain, urinary incontinence, napping during the day, or sometimes a condition nicknamed "sundowner syndrome," in which the person turns around daytime and nighttime hours. These people sleep much of the day and are wide awake and active during the night. This syndrome is sometimes seen in patients who have Alzheimer's disease. Lack of rapid eye movement (REM) sleep from insomnia can have negative effects on anyone, even contributing to psychotic behavior. To someone with Alzheimer's disease or other cognitive problems, the effects of insomnia can intensify the symptoms of the cognitive disorder.

The nurse needs to concentrate on keeping communication open with these patients. Nurses will need to be sure that they and their patients are using words in the same way. For instance, if the patient says, "I do not sleep at night because I am worried," the word *worried* should be explored. What is the patient worried about? What can be done to eliminate the worry? How severe is the worry? Using a 1 to 5 rating scale, the nurse can more objectively document the impact of the "worry" on the patient. In addition, the nurse should ask the patient about his or her definition of not sleeping all night; perhaps the patient had taken naps throughout the night.

End-of-Life Issues

Life can end at any age; however, death is more common among the older population. Nurses who work in areas such as long-term care, home care, or hospice have a great opportunity to learn about and assist people with end-of-life issues. These opportunities also exist when working in acute hospitals and clinics. It may not be feasible for professional counselors to meet the needs of older adults dealing with these profound issues. Many people in this population will prefer the services of their own spiritual leader, but since the duties of many such leaders are overwhelming, the appropriate clergy may not be available at the moment of immediate need. However, nurses are there, and they have all the tools needed to be the helpers.

Neeb's Tip Nurses must take self-inventory of their beliefs surrounding the subjects of death and dying.

It is also very important for nurses to discuss and understand their patients' religious and cultural beliefs about what the end of life means to them. It is the nurse's responsibility and privilege to be able to help someone through this stage of life according to that individual's needs and wants.

One issue a patient may experience is widowhood. The surviving spouse must learn to live independently or face an alternative form of housing. Finances and household chores may have been "gender-specific" in that relationship, and now the surviving person is forced to assume responsibilities formerly done by the deceased. The subjects of dating and working may become delicate issues for the survivor: Families may have strong opinions about what the newly widowed person "should" do. Nurses can play an advocacy role with widowed persons. Active listening skills, validating the person's thoughts and feelings, and offering information about various services available to widowed persons are skills that can be very helpful.

Nurses can be effective in helping people through the dying process. Death of the body as everyone knows it is inevitable. People need to know it is "OK" to die. Elisabeth Kübler-Ross and others who teach about death and dying tell us that helping people to resolve life issues can help them to die with peace and dignity. Again, nurses who choose to work in hospice, home care, and long-term care settings have a special opportunity to be there for people at this very important stage of life. Using humor and laughter appropriately, maintaining the hope patients may still have, and reassuring them that they will not be forgotten after death are some good techniques nurses can learn to use to help people prepare to die. Elisabeth Kübler-Ross's five stages of grieving continue to be taught and used in nursing programs. Not everyone experiences each step nor in the order listed (Kübler-Ross,1969):

1. Denial
2. Anger
3. Bargaining
4. Depression
5. Acceptance

Nurses must not ignore the incidence of suicide among the aging populations. This chapter has alluded to many losses that people are likely to face as they age. Compound the sadness of losing jobs, friends, and other aspects of earlier life with physical illness and altered physical ability, and it may become clearer why some elders feel helpless or hopeless and opt for suicide. According to the National Institute of Mental Health, persons age 65 and older rate of suicide is higher than the national average for all age groups. They account for approximately 13% of the U.S. population, yet they accounted for 14.3% of all suicide deaths in the United States in the year 2007. The highest rates were found in white men age 85 and older. Follow the screening suggestions provided in Chapter 13 when considering the possibility that an older person may be at risk for suicide.

■ Social Concerns

Older adults, like younger adults, in today's world may find themselves in financial trouble. Many are facing financial challenges living on fixed incomes. Many exist only on Social Security benefits. Retirement age has increased over the years, and politicians are discussing raising it yet again, potentially requiring people to continue working longer before they become eligible to receive the Medicare and/or Social Security benefits they have earned. This will impact future generations. Perhaps today's seniors have inadequate personal and supplemental insurance, so they will not seek medical help when they need it. They may find their heat and power cut off due to inability to pay utilities on their fixed income. Most municipalities are enacting laws and emergency funds to help avoid this life-threatening situation. Nurses can help provide the necessary information to help elders who are opting to remain at home or in assisted living.

As baby boomers age, nurses will see a significant increase in this demographic they are caring for. The average age of patients will be older, and the concerns nurses face will relate more frequently to issues pertaining to people in the final stages of life.

It is worth mentioning again at this time that the family unit of the older population may have a different look as well. People are opting to have children later in life. Nurses may see much younger family members than they might anticipate. The upcoming older generation is very diverse. Those of varied ethnic and cultural backgrounds will be seeking assistance in long-term care facilities (Fig. 21-5). Nurses must be prepared to learn about older patients' customs, ask the proper questions upon intake data collecting, and be ready to offer care according to customs that may be different from their own and different from those they were trained in.

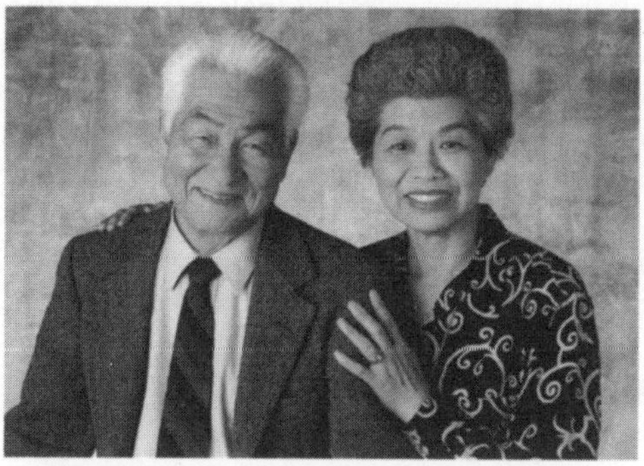

Figure 21-5 The demographic changes in the American population mean that a more ethnically and culturally diverse group will be seeking assistance in long-term care facilities. Nurses must be ready to offer culturally sensitive care.

> ■ ■ ■ Classroom Activity
> - Divide the class into five groups. Each group represents a decade from the past 50 years. Each group should list the music, television shows, and fads popular during their assigned decade and add to a chart.

> ■ ■ ■ Clinical Activity
> Using the chart developed in the classroom activity, ask your patients to provide more information about music, television shows, and fads they believed were popular during those times.

One of the cultural demographics to consider is the group of elders who have lived a gay or bisexual lifestyle. Nurses need to anticipate issues surrounding grooming, roommates, bathroom-sharing, family preferences, and potentially even a different definition of "appropriate behavior" for those with a different lifestyle. Individuals may be reluctant to share this type of information unless nurses communicate acceptance. The nurse's role will need to become even more flexible. Nurses will need to be very open with their communication and with the type of questions they must learn to ask in order to provide the best care to all entrusted to their care.

■ Nursing Skills for Working With Older Adults

The following are some general skills a nurse should learn to use to more effectively work with the elderly population.

1. *Respect:* In the United States, a handshake is a sign of respect and cooperation. It is usually given at the beginning and ending of business meetings, and it is customary to shake hands at more formal social functions or when being introduced to someone new. Shaking the hand of an elderly patient will convey respect and cooperation and is an effective way to begin the nurse-patient partnership. There are citizens and residents of the United States whose culture does not participate in hand shaking, but this does not mean they lack respect for others. If you sense that shaking hands is not acceptable to that patient, then communicate to others that this action should not be used.

Using the proper name of the patient also shows respect for that person. "Mr. Washington" or "Mrs. Jones" is the best way to address the patient. If the patient prefers, the nurse may call him or her by the first name or the name that the person is called socially. Nurses should not do this until invited to do so, however. Also, it is not acceptable to assign nicknames such as granny or honey arbitrarily to patients. In home care and long-term care, there is a danger of becoming too familiar. The facility becomes the residents' home, and they become friendly with each other. This informal atmosphere sometimes spreads among the staff. This is a time when nurses must remember their professional role. They can be pleasant and friendly while still being professional.

Box 21-3 Skills for Working With Older Adults

- Respect
- Goal setting
- Patience and understanding
- Humor
- Safety
- Independence
- Acceptance

■ ■ ■ Critical Thinking Question

You refer to an 87-year-old resident as "grandmom," yet the resident does not have any children as a result of several miscarriages. Describe the emotional effect this title might have on the patient.

Under no circumstances should an older adult be treated as a child. As abilities diminish and the older adult begins to become incontinent and loses the ability to feed and dress himself or herself, some caregivers take on a parental role. It can be easy to deal with an elderly person as one would deal with a child. Elderly patients have had careers and raised families. They are now adults who have special needs in order to help them maintain their adult dignity.

Neeb's Tip It is important to remember that the elderly is a population of people who have been and still are productive members of society.

2. *Goal setting:* When preparing the plan of care with an older patient, nurses must remember to discuss goals that are measurable and attainable. Self-esteem and pride in one's accomplishments are as important when one is 80 as they were when one was 20. Success breeds success, and meeting small goals is an encouragement to the older person to attempt bigger goals. The patient will see that the nurse was there to help reach that goal and, again, the relationship will strengthen.

3. *Patience and understanding:* Older patients who have some challenge to their physical or cognitive functioning may be slower to respond to verbal cues and may not be able to sprint down the halls at the pace that nurses generally travel. Be patient and recognize the care may take longer than expected. Plan for this. Nurses should convey the message that they have plenty of time (even though they may not). The patient who feels burdensome will be less likely to attempt activities or collaborate in the plan of care. He or she will be very sensitive to any nonverbal communication expressed by the nurses. It is important during these times that the nurse's verbal and nonverbal responses are congruent. It is therefore important to focus entirely on that person at that time. Acknowledge any accomplishment, however small. The focus should be on the residents' strengths and not their weaknesses.

Neeb's Tip Not everyone appreciates humor, and not everyone finds humor in the same things.

4. *Humor:* Humor that is appropriate to the age and condition of the patient will help smooth over some of the harder times for the nurse and the patient.

Nurses should take their cues about humor from the patient. If the patient jokes about a situation, it is probably acceptable to go along with the humor. *Never* embarrass or make fun of the patient. Taking a situation in stride at the patient's suggestion, however, can be a very healthy mechanism for dealing with some of the hardships associated with aging.

5. *Safety:* Ensuring safety in the care facility and teaching safety to the patient who remains at home are very important. With vision, hearing, and other senses losing accuracy, it is easier for the older person to misjudge space, sound, and temperature. This could lead to falls, burns, and inability to hear the doorbell or the telephone ringing.
6. *Independence:* The older adult should be allowed to perform without assistance as much as possible. Do not assume that the older person is unable to do things independently. Follow the guidelines on the patient's care plan. If the level of care is complete, then provide complete care. If the level of care indicates the patient needs partial or complete care, then honor those directions. This is one of the fallacies in long-term care: Too much focus is placed on the staff to provide care by a specific time and not on promoting independence. On the other hand, nurses should offer assistance as necessary. Nurses should let the patient know that they would like to help in whatever way they can. Because of the loss in hearing and visual acuity that often accompanies aging, nurses may need to arrange for adaptive equipment that can help the patient to maintain as much independence as possible with daily activities.
7. *Acceptance:* In rapidly increasing numbers, people of diverse backgrounds and lifestyles are approaching the time of life that may require living in long-term care centers or assisted living communities. Those who will be caring for this diverse population must be in touch with their own thoughts and feelings about working with groups of people and must be prepared to flex care to meet their needs.

Neeb's Tip Remember that humans are much more alike than they are different.

Basic human needs as defined by Maslow and others are important for all groups of people. Table 21-2 summarizes some of the concerns of aging adults and techniques nurses can use to more effectively help this population.

Restorative Nursing

Restorative nursing is part of rehabilitation and focuses on maintaining dignity and achieving optimal function for patients and

Table 21-2 Concerns of Aging Adults and Helping Techniques

Concern	Factors Associated With This Concern	Helping Techniques
Alzheimer's Disease and Other Cognitive Impairments	• Debilitating effects are observable. • Patients may need to leave the home they have lived in all of their adult lives; living apart from a spouse. • Socializing will be curtailed.	Respect for the individual Realistic goal setting Maintaining patience and understanding Effective communication; allowing time for the patient to respond Appropriate use of humor Teaching and promoting safety Promoting independence
Cerebrovascular Accident (stroke)	• Physical and cognitive functions may be temporarily or permanently affected. • Depression is evident. • Aphasia may be present.	See "Alzheimer's Disease" Allowing venting of emotions Assisting with communication techniques Allowing patient to verbalize; not automatically answering for patient
Depression	• Symptoms may be different from those in other age groups. • Constipation; headaches, other pains, and fatigue may be indicators. • Difficulty breathing for which there is no diagnosis may occur.	See "Alzheimer's Disease" Allowing venting of thoughts and feelings Teaching about patient's medications Encouraging involvement in group activities as able Focus on positives
Medication Concerns	• Pharmacokinetics is slower and less complete. • Circulatory and renal function is decreased. • It becomes easier for elderly people to experience side effects or become toxic. • Patients who live at home may forget to take medications or forget they have taken them and take another dose. • Visual acuity is lessened; patients may mistake one pill for another. • Nurse should advise patient to maintain weight, nutrition, and activity levels.	Providing patient with information about medication Instructing patient to notify physician immediately if signs of side effects occur
Paranoid Thinking	• Fear about the environment • Slowed reaction time and diminished physical capacity • Feelings of loneliness and isolation	Allowing venting of feelings Not reinforcing the paranoid thoughts Speaking in terms of the "here and now" Provide aids for hearing and vision loss
Insomnia	• Depression, fear, pain, urinary incontinence, napping during the day are common. • Decreased REM sleep can contribute to psychotic behavior; insomnia can intensify the symptoms of cognitive disorders.	Discussing underlying feelings Teaching relaxation methods Encouraging patient to seek medical evaluation Discourage daytime napping Keep sleep diary

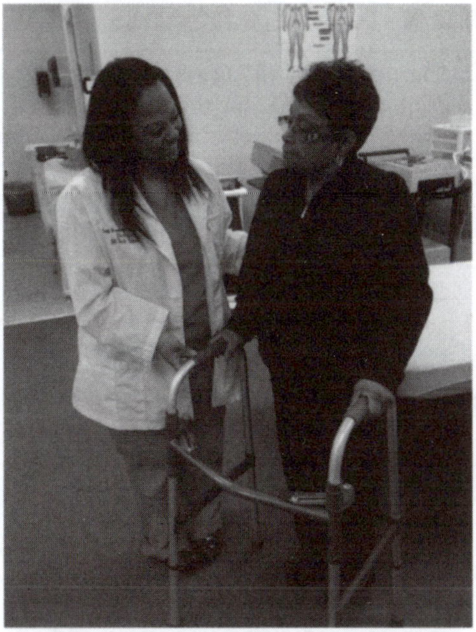

Figure 21-6 Restorative nursing is concerned with providing individualized restorative exercise to help patients achieve maximum function and maintain their dignity.

residents (Fig. 21-6). Some articles refer to restorative nursing as "good, old-fashioned nursing care"—arguably a subjective statement, and likely related to the professional age of the writer. Goals include independence, promoting self-esteem for the patient, and allowing the patient to maintain as much control over his or her life and daily living activities as possible.

Most skilled nursing facilities are required to provide at least one designated nursing assistant and nurse who are specially trained and part of the "restorative" team. They work in conjunction with physical therapy and rehabilitation departments to provide individualized restorative exercise and training to assist residents to achieve their maximum ability.

Restorative nursing is also part of a long-term care facility's documentation and reimbursement requirements. State and federal surveys grade the facility on its restorative program. OBRA long-term care laws require that residents either maintain or improve their condition at the time of admission. Declines in residents' condition that cannot be proven to be medically unavoidable are not allowed. Including restorative nursing care in a patient's care plan can prevent declines in condition that occur gradually, over time, such as loss of mobility, contractures, and loss of self-care ability. Restorative nursing is to be provided to any resident, regardless of his or her cognitive ability: The resident with dementia and the transitional care resident recuperating from knee surgery are equally in need of restorative nursing services.

■ Palliative Care

Palliative care is specialized care for people with serious illness that focuses on addressing management of uncomfortable symptoms and the stress of advanced illness. It is about keeping patients and families comfortable and promoting the best quality of life that one can provide to someone facing an advanced illness. It is often associated with the last phase of life but it can begin earlier in the course of serious illness. Hospice is a specialized aspect of palliative care. Hospice care is specialized services for a patient with a terminal illness with less than 6 months to live. In addition to working with grief and bereavement with the patient and significant persons in that patient's life, nurses choosing to work in a palliative setting will need to be comfortable with issues such as pain, symptom management, sedation and opioid medication, artificial nutrition and hydration, assisted suicide, and coordinating or providing complementary therapies. In addition, nurses will need to sharpen their communication skills and be very cognizant of religious, cultural, ethical, and legal issues, especially surrounding an individual's wishes and advance care planning as the end of life approaches.

It is widely documented that the preferred place of death of a patient is in his or her own home. Sometimes that is not possible. Because of that, many long-term care facilities are designing special units dedicated for palliative care. Organizations such as The Center to Advance Palliative Care are attempting to show the need for hospital-based and out-patient palliative care, as well. Palliative care can be provided in the acute hospital, long-term care facilities, and in the home.

Nurses are receiving special training and certification in this new specialty area. The good news is that LPN/LVN nurses are more than welcome into the fold. To encourage LPN/LVN nurses to participate in palliative nursing, the Hospice and Palliative Nurses Association (HPNA) has developed a set of competencies that can be purchased online (see the Web sites list at end of this chapter). Certification as a hospice and palliative nurse (CHPLN) is also available.

Tool Box |▶ Palliative Training Tools
http://www.capc.org/

Tool Box |▶ Information on certification for LPN/LVNs in hospice and palliative nursing is available at:
www.nbchpn.org
HPNA has a position statement on the value of the LVN/LPN in hospice and palliative nursing, which is available at
http://hpna.org/DisplayPage.aspx?Title=Position Statements

■■■ Key Concepts

1. The concept of old age is changing. People are living longer and better after age 65. Older patients are being cared for in facilities and in their homes. Diversity among aging persons is on the rise. Nurses must be prepared to flex the care required to provide the best care possible to many different groups of elders. Nurses have an active part in helping the patient maintain a good quality of life.
2. Normal conditions of aging include diminished hearing, vision, and other sensory acuity. Alzheimer's disease and other cognitive disorders are not considered a part of normal aging.
3. Afflictions affecting the older adult can be mental or physical, or a combination of these. Medication side effects and drug toxicity can share the same symptoms as disorders that affect the elderly population. Accuracy of observation, documentation, and prompt reporting are crucial to a nurse's responsibility in caring for elderly people. Excellent communication skills are necessary.
4. Palliative care and hospice provide specialized care for people facing advanced and terminal illnesses.

CASE STUDY

Mr. Jacobs is admitted as a new resident in your nursing home. He is 76 years old and has a diagnosis of congestive heart failure (CHF). He has fallen at home several times recently, and his adult children are concerned that he will become seriously injured. They have told him he needs to "go there for a while until you get stronger." They tell the staff, confidentially, that they plan this to be a permanent placement and will be selling Mr. Jacobs's home to pay for his care. Mr. Jacobs will be started on digoxin, furosemide, and potassium for the CHF and has an order for acetaminophen with hydrocodone for pain.

Five days later, Mr. Jacobs has had a change in mood. His family comes to visit and finds that he is combative and forgetful. One of his children is crying. She looks at you and says, "What have you done to him? He's never been like this before." What thoughts cross your mind? How do you respond to the personal attack? How will you attempt to resolve this situation? How would you like to be treated if you were the family member?

REFERENCES

Administration on Aging (2011). A profile of Older Americans 2011. Retrieved at http://www.aoa.gov/Aging_Statistics/Profile/2011/4.aspx

Barry, P. D. (2002). *Mental Health and Mental Illness.* 7th ed. Philadelphia: JB Lippincott.

Ferrell, B. R., and Coyle, N. (2010). *Textbook of Palliative Nursing.* New York: Oxford University Press.

Furman, J. (2005, May 10). *The impact of the president's proposal on social security solvency and the budget.* Retrieved from http://www.cbpp.org/cms/?fa=view&id=261

Green, C. D. (2000, August). *Classics in the history of psychology.* Retrieved from http://psychclassics.yorku.ca/Maslow/motivation.htm

Kaplan, B. J. (November 2002). Gay Elders Face Uncomfortable Realities in LTC. *Caring for the Ages* (American Medical Directors Association), Vol. 3, No. 11.

Kessler, D. (n.d.). *The five stages of grief—Elisabeth Kübler-Ross & David Kessler.* Retrieved from http://grief.com/the-five-stages-of-grief/

Koffman, J., and Higginson, I. J. (2004). Dying to Be Home? Preferred location of death of first-generation Black Caribbean and native-born White patients in the United Kingdom. *Journal of Palliative Medicine,* 7(5):, 628–636.

Kübler-Ross, E. (1969). *On Death and Dying.* New York: Touchstone.

National Institute of Mental Health (2012). *Suicide in the U.S.: Statistics and Prevention* (NIH Publication No. 06-4594). Retrieved from http://www.nimh.nih.gov/health/publications/suicide-in-the-us-statistics-and-prevention/index.shtml

Minnesota Board on Aging. (November 2002). *Spotlight on Aging: A Newsletter for Seniors and Their Families.* St. Paul.

Townsend, M.C. (2012) *Psychiatric and Mental Health Nursing.* Philadelphia: F.A. Davis

U.S. Social Security Administration. (2012). *Retirement planner; full retirement age.* Retrieved from http://www.ssa.gov/retire2/retirechart.htm

World Health Organization. (2011). International Life Expectancy List. Retrieved at http://en.wikipedia.org/wiki/List_of_countries_by_life_expectancy

Test Questions

Multiple Choice Questions

1. One effective communication technique for assisting a patient with aphasia is:
   a. Try to guess the word or finish the sentence.
   b. Associate the word with the object.
   c. Tell the patient to think about it while you make the bed.
   d. None of the above.

2. According to OBRA, who is responsible for completing the assessment of an older adult?
   a. All health staff
   b. Nursing assistants
   c. LPN/LVN
   d. RN

3. Mrs. Brown, who is usually alert and oriented, is showing signs of confusion. Her vital signs are all within normal limits. She has recently been started on furosemide for congestive heart failure. The nurse suspects:
   a. Just normal aging
   b. Stroke
   c. Medication side effect
   d. Depression

4. A 73-year-old patient in your long-term care center has become withdrawn and cranky. You try to find a method to initiate communication and activity with the patient. Which of the following statements is the best choice to try communicating with your patient?
   a. "Why are you staying over here by yourself?"
   b. "Your daughter wants you to make friends here."
   c. "I need a partner for the card game; I'd like to have you be my partner."
   d. "The doctor said the more you do, the better off you'll be."

5. "Losses" that are associated with the process of aging frequently cause:
   a. Presbycusis
   b. Depression
   c. Dementia
   d. CHF

6. When an older patient begins to show signs of dementia, physicians and nurses should assess all of the following *except:*
   a. Medication routines
   b. Nutritional intake
   c. Circulatory function
   d. Behaviors assumed to be part of "normal aging"

7. The speech impairment that affects many people who have had a stroke is called:
   a. Affect
   b. Aphasia
   c. Autism
   d. Ageism

8. Nurses understand that one of the reasons that older people become toxic from their prescription medications is:
   a. Drugs are metabolized faster in older people.
   b. Drugs are metabolized slower in older people.
   c. Drugs are ineffective in older people.
   d. Drugs need to be ordered in stronger doses for older people.

9. Your patient is admitted with bruises on his head and upper arms. His son is with him and jokes about the bruises, stating, "Dad is getting so clumsy. He falls out of his wheelchair a lot." You glance at the patient, who says nothing, is looking down, and is avoiding eye contact. You become alert for the possibility of:
   a. Blood dyscrasias
   b. Vitamin deficiency
   c. Elder abuse
   d. Self-inflicted wounds

Test Questions *cont.*

10. The federal law that mandates special care and assessment skills for the older population is called:
a. OBE
b. OPRAH
c. COBRA
d. OBRA

11. When orienting new nursing assistants and other staff to your long-term care facility, you remind them:
a. Memory loss is a normal part of aging.
b. Memory loss is not a normal part of aging.
c. Stress decreases as people age.
d. All of the above

12. In the orientation class mentioned above, you notice one of the housekeepers crying. She shares with the group that her grandmother has "old timer's or something and she doesn't remember me anymore." You respond to her:
a. "It must be difficult for you to see your grandmother with Alzheimer's disease."
b. "It's called Alzheimer's disease. Many of our residents have that illness."
c. "How old is your grandmother?"
d. "Who else has a relative with Alzheimer's?"

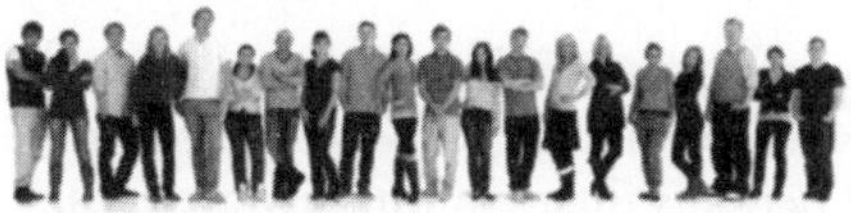

CHAPTER **22**

Victims of Abuse and Violence

Learning Objectives

1. Define abuse.
2. Define victim.
3. Differentiate among different kinds of abuse.
4. Identify characteristics of an abuser.
5. Identify nursing care to help survivors of abuse.

Key Terms

- Abuser
- Child abuse
- Date rape
- Domestic violence
- Economic abuse
- Elder abuse
- Emotional abuse
- Incest
- Neglect
- Physical abuse
- Rape
- Respite care
- Safe house
- Sexual abuse
- Sexual harassment
- Shaken baby syndrome
- Survivor
- Verbal abuse
- Victim

Abuse and violence are unfortunately commonplace in today's society. The news, television dramas, and movies expose people to more violence than they did in the past. Violence in the workplace, road rage, and school violence are commonplace. Violence in the home is on the increase. **Child abuse, domestic violence,** and **elder abuse** are examples of family violence that take a terrible toll on society. All of these have tremendous negative effects. More than 50% of Americans have experienced violence in the family (Carson & Smith DiJulio, 2006). Abuse can take the form of **physical, emotional, sexual,** and **economic abuse,** as well as **neglect**.

Physical abuse includes any action that causes physical harm to another person. Hitting; burning; withholding food, water, and other basic needs; and other activities that go beyond accidental contact are all considered physical abuse. A rule of thumb for defining the line between an accident and physical abuse is when the recipient says, "Stop. You're hurting me," or something similar. If the activity stops and does not repeat itself, that behavior may well have been just an accident. If the behavior persists, if the request to stop is ignored or mocked by the perpetrator, or if the activity is repeated in future situations, there is a strong chance that the perpetrator is guilty of abuse. Neglect can include failure to provide for the basic needs of someone who is dependent on the caregiver, e.g. a child, elderly parent. Emotional abuse can include **verbal abuse**, humiliation, excessive criticism, and lack of emotional support. Sexual abuse can include rape as well as any inappropriate sexual contact without consent.

Victims are often too fearful or ashamed to report abuse, become adept at hiding the signs, and/or use massive denial to convince themselves that the abuse is not that bad. This contributes to the abuse cycle, which can go unnoticed by outsiders. Health-care professionals must be vigilant to recognize the overt and covert signs of abuse. Every state mandates that suspected child abuse be reported, and many states are enacting similar laws for domestic violence and elder abuse. The Joint Commission expects the accredited institutions to provide assessment of potential victims of abuse. Nurses are in a key position to identify and offer help to a potential victim.

■ The Abuser

The **abuser** is usually in a position of dominance or power over a potential victim. The following may cause a person to abuse another:

- History of being a victim: "Violence begets violence. People—especially children—tend to imitate what they see" (Rubin, Peplau, and Salovey, 1993). That statement remains the belief of researchers today. It is accepted that (except in rare situations with a genetic or biological connection) violence, aggression, and abuse are learned behaviors. Children who grow up witnessing violence in the home and perhaps their community are sensitized to believe that this is the right behavior, and they will very likely continue such actions into adulthood. Abusers retreat to these childhood memories and resort to abuse when they are stressed. They may never have developed skills to solve problems or deal with conflict. Rather, they learned that violence is the way to achieve a goal.
- Low self-esteem/need for power: Abusers often have a poor self-image. They feel frustrated and minimized as persons. They have poor interpersonal relationships and may not have had their ideas and accomplishments validated by people important to them. Close relationships are difficult because others become afraid of the abuser. Therefore, they resort to physical, verbal, or emotional abuse of others in an attempt to bring a personal sense of power and importance to themselves. Sexual abuse is almost always not about sex; it is about conquering and winning. It is about demeaning another human being in order to feel a sense of strength. It is a short-term "fix" for the abuser and a lifelong scar for the abused. The abuser may also be isolated and lack a support system in dealing with stress.
- Impairment from alcohol/substance use: Committing abusive acts while under the influence of a substance is a major contributor to violence. When a person's judgment is impaired and his/her ability to control impulses is altered, a person who is prone to these acts may abuse others. Easy access to weapons while impaired adds to the risk associated with substance abuse.
- Biological theories: Brain disorders, alteration in brain function, and genetic influences may also be factors in individuals with a greater tendency toward violence.
- Other factors: The abuser may also be under stress (e.g., poverty) and have limited access to support resources to deal with problems, limited coping

Cultural Considerations

Abuse crosses all cultures, ethnic, and socioeconomic groups. At times some behaviors may appear abusive to us but are culturally appropriate. For example, there can be man's expectation of a wife's subservience in some cultures. This needs to be taken into consideration before assuming she is being abused.

mechanisms to deal with conflict, and difficulty trusting others.

How can an abuser be identified? Abusers may present with some of the following traits in connection with a victim:

- Inconsistent explanation of injuries of the victim
- Failure to show empathy for the victim
- Demand to take victim home and refusal of hospitalization for the injured victim
- Speaks for the victim
- Criticizes the victim
- Abuses family pets

Neeb's Tip Because abuse in a family is often hidden, recognize that it can be difficult to identify an abuser.

The Victim

Though victims of abuse have a broad range of traits, the two most common include:

1. *Low self-esteem:* People who have not learned to be assertive and to say what they think and feel, or to speak out for what they need and want, may not be able to call up the strength they need to ward off an attack. They may be easily manipulated by the abuser into believing either that they deserved the attack or that the abuser is truly repentant and will not abuse again. They will begin to make up reasons to excuse the abuser's behavior and may accept the responsibility for the abuser's actions.
2. *Reliance on the abuser:* People who are reliant on the abuser for financial support as well as emotional and physical support are vulnerable to attacks from the abuser. This holds true for all age groups of people who are abused.

See Table 22-1 for characteristics of victims of child abuse, domestic violence, and elder abuse. Health-care professionals often see victims of abuse without realizing it. Patients who are abused may be fearful of sharing this information but may leave clues. Box 22-1 lists common warning signs of abuse.

Table 22-1 Characteristics of Victims of Abuse

Type of Victim	Characteristics
Child; all ages, with greatest risk under age 4 (including infants) and for fatalities under 2 years of age	• Self-blame for family conflict • Low self-esteem • Fear of parent or caretaker • Cheating, lying, low achievement in school • Signs of depression, helplessness • One child sometimes singled out in family due to being labeled as "difficult," product of unwanted pregnancy, reminds the parents of someone they dislike or even themselves, prematurity (inhibited parent-child bonding), chronic illness
Domestic/spouse/intimate partner	• Low self-esteem • Self-blame for partner's actions • Sense of helplessness to escape abuse • Isolation from family and friends • Views self as subservient to partner • Economic dependence on abuser
Elder	• Older than 75 years of age • Mentally or physically impaired • Isolated from others • Female

Source: From Gorman and Sultan (2008). Psychosocial Nursing for General Patient Care, 3rd ed. Philadelphia: F.A. Davis Company, with permission.

Box 22-1 Common Warning Signs of Abuse

- Delay in seeking treatment for injuries, minimizing injuries
- History of being accident prone
- Pattern of injuries not accidental looking; for example, identical burns on bottom of feet, identical injuries on both sides of head
- Multiple injuries in varying stages of healing
- Conflicting stories from victim and abuser about cause of injury
- Inconsistency between history and injury
- Unusual, even bizarre explanation for injuries
- Repeated visits to emergency rooms or clinics
- Previous report of abuse
- Patient reporting abuse
- Patient fearful of caregiver or partner
- Visits variety of doctors, emergency rooms for treatment to avoid a record of treatment

Source: From Gorman and Sultan (2008). Psychosocial Nursing for General Patient Care, 3rd ed. Philadelphia: F.A. Davis Company, with permission.

Clinical Activity

If your patient has been the victim of abuse, obtain information from the team on the abuser and how to handle this person if he or she is present.

Classroom Activity

- Ask members of local law enforcement to speak to your class about the types of abuse they see in your community and the options for victims of abuse.
- Identify local abuse hotlines and local domestic violence shelters.

Categories of Abuse

The most common categories of abuse include child abuse, sexual abuse, domestic violence (spousal abuse), and elder abuse.

Child Abuse

Child abuse includes physical, emotional, and sexual abuse, as well as neglect. It occurs at all socioeconomic levels. The U.S. Children's Bureau tracks reports of child abuse nationwide and reported that 9.1 per 1000 children were reported as abused or neglected in 2011. Abuse includes neglect (75% reported cases), physical abuse (15% of reported cases), and sexual abuse (10% of reported cases). The youngest children (birth to 1 year) have the highest rates of victimization and those from birth to 2 years have the highest death rate. Reported cases of child abuse have steadily increased over the last few years, but many cases are not reported. Children are a most vulnerable segment of the population because they depend on others for all their needs. Parents are the most common abusers (80% of reported cases). See Box 22-2 for signs of child abuse.

Parents who abuse a child may have unrealistic expectations of a child, such as being able to control crying or following instructions perfectly. **Shaken baby syndrome** is a form of child abuse that occurs when a caregiver shakes a baby in an effort to stop crying, which contributes to infant deaths each year (Center for Disease Control and Prevention, 2010). Sometimes a child with special needs or emotional problems is singled out for abuse as the parents' frustration tolerance is more severely tested.

Box 22-2 Signs of Child Abuse

Child exhibits some of the following:

- Fear of returning home
- Antisocial behavior, such as lying or stealing
- Fear and anxiety when asked about injuries
- Going to lengths to hide injuries
- Lack of reaction to frightening event
- Unexplained, unusual injuries
- Changes in behavior, school performance
- Neglect—malnutrition, lack of medical care

Source: Adapted from Gorman and Sultan (2008). Psychosocial Nursing for General Patient Care, 3rd ed. Philadelphia: F.A. Davis Company, with permission.

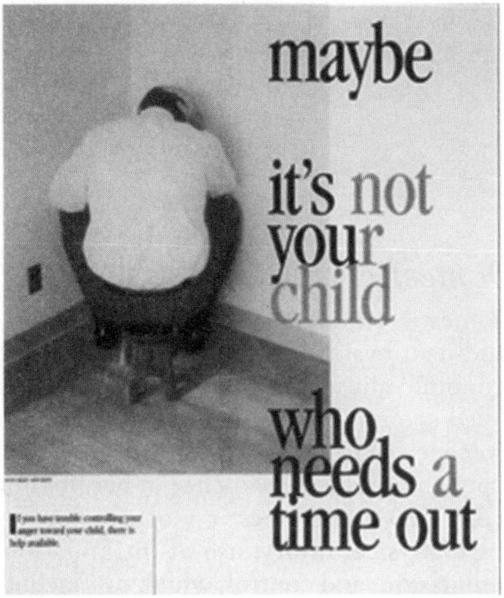

Figure 22-1 Maybe it's not your child who needs a time out.

Each year, newborns are abandoned or even killed when new mothers panic. Many states have passed laws for safe surrender sites of newborns if a mother is unable to keep her child. Rather than abandoning an infant through neglect, mothers can leave the infant at community locations that often include hospitals and fire stations. Many at-risk teenagers who might be pregnant are often not aware of this law, so community education that reaches teens in their communities must be provided to prevent neglect, abandonment, and often death of these infants.

Neeb's Tip It is important to know the law in your state regarding safe surrender sites. This information must be disseminated to pregnant teens and other women.

An early sign of child abuse in the victim can be changes in behavior and school performance. Another sign can be abuse of family pets by the child. Children may try to deal with the situation by controlling another being or seeking an outlet for their anger through a more vulnerable victim.

Victims of child abuse are at an increased risk of becoming abusers as adults. Even though the child may hate the abusive situation, he or she never gets an opportunity to observe healthy parenting or to learn adaptive coping mechanisms to deal with frustration without violence. Other long-term effects of being a victim of child abuse include low self-esteem, high risk for substance abuse, tendency toward depression, difficulty trusting in close relationships, and violent lifestyle including crime. Incarcerated youths frequently have a history of being abused and neglected.

Critical Thinking Question

A 4-year-old child with autism is admitted to your unit from the ER with burns on both hands and bruises on one arm. The child's parents are at the bedside and very concerned. They have told the doctors that the child reached up and put her hands in a pot of hot water on the stove. How would you react to these parents? Describe factors that might indicate this could be child abuse.

Tool Box ▶ National Child Abuse Hotline: 800 4 A Child

Sexual Abuse

Sexual abuse is violent or nonviolent sexual contact or sexual activity that is not wanted by the receiver. It is generally inflicted on someone the abuser considers less powerful physically or emotionally. The abuser is usually a close, significant figure in the abused person's life and knows how to manipulate the potential victim into submission. It can involve unwanted advances, inappropriate sexual contact, **sexual harassment,** and rape.

Girls are the most frequent victims of childhood sexual abuse. Eighty percent of sexually abused children know their abuser, and about 50% of cases involve a parent or caregiver (Mulryan, Cathers, & Fagin, 2000). Long-term effects of sexual abuse include fear of intimacy, sexual problems, eating disorders, and an overwhelming sense of powerlessness. Children may feel threatened, be confused about their feelings, and question if this activity is right. The abuser is usually a trusted person initially to the child, which adds to the confusion. Children do not always have the words to express what is happening to them. They may also be so fearful that they say nothing. They may fear other family members will be hurt if they speak up. Victims may block out the memory of these incidents until later in life, when a major event or trauma triggers memory recall. Exploiting children in pornography has been increasing with access to the Internet and is another facet of sexual abuse. Signs of sexual abuse in children could include frequent urinary tract infections; torn, bloody underclothing; and sudden onset of sexually related behavior in addition to other signs of child abuse as listed above.

Incest is defined as sexual activity between persons so closely related that they are forbidden by law to marry. The most frequent occurrence of incest is in girls under 18, although it can happen to persons of any age group (National Center for Victims of Violent Crimes, 2012).

Rape is forcible, degrading, nonconsensual sexual intercourse accompanied by violence and intimidation. It often goes unreported. When a victim does seek medical care, most hospital emergency rooms and urgent care centers have rape kits to assist in proper collection of evidence such as sperm, hair, and other fibers that may be compared with others to identify a suspect. It is important that the person who was raped not clean up before going to the emergency department. Although evidence must be kept intact, one of the victim's first instincts is to "wash away" the incident both physically and psychologically by showering. Nurses should discourage that activity until evidence and DNA sources can be collected. **Date rape** (also known as acquaintance rape) most frequently occurs among teens and young adults.

An alarming reality in the United States is that rape happens to elderly people. That population is often assaulted in their private residences and in long-term care and assisted living facilities.

> **Clinical Activity**
> Ensure that appropriate tests are completed as part of the workup for victim of sexual abuse (e.g., screening for STIs or sexually transmitted infections, pregnancy test, HIV test).

> **Critical Thinking Question**
> The nurse from the local grammar school calls your clinic asking for help. She tells you a parent of a 6-year-old has accused the teacher of sexually molesting her child. The nurse does not know what to do. What would be your first action?

Domestic Violence

Domestic violence takes many forms, including physical, emotional, sexual, and economic abuse. Domestic violence is also called spousal or intimate partner abuse or violence. One in every four women will experience domestic violence in her lifetime (CDC, 2010). Domestic violence can involve physical injury, use of intimidation, denigration, and control, which can include restricting access to family finances.

Though most often domestic abuse involves women, men can also be victims. They may be less prone to report it out of embarrassment, so the frequency of this is less known.

This type of abuse often incorporates the children. For example, an abusive domestic partner might say, "If you go out with your friends tonight, I'll see to it that your kids are taken away; you're unfit to be their mother (father) if you go out at night and leave them. You do not deserve them!" Or "Leave, and when you get back the kids and I will be gone and you won't see them again!" The children are used as a way to control and intimidate. This type of button pushing is very effective at negatively controlling someone's behavior out of fear of the consequences. Abusers also use the family pet as a means to control; for example, "I will kill the dog if you leave me."

Pediatricians and veterinarians receive training on identifying signs of domestic violence since they may observe clues of a troubled family. In a 2001 study of women visiting a pediatric clinic, researchers found that more than 16%, or 553 mothers, had been physically abused at some point in their lifetime. The researchers strongly encourage screening for domestic violence as part of the office intake protocol (Parkinson, Adams, & Emerling, 2001).

The abuse cycle in domestic violence has been shown to follow a pattern that was originally identified by Walker in 1979.

1. *Tension-building:* The recipient of the abuse is compliant, believing that in some way he or she is at fault and deserves the abuse. These individuals remain accepting and continue to be supportive even though they know the behavior is inappropriate. The victim is probably using denial as a defense mechanism. The perpetrator is using verbal abuse and minor beating, and also is aware that the behavior is not appropriate.
2. *Acute battering incident:* The victim senses that the beating is coming and may even provoke it to get it over with. Some triggering event occurs, which may be something minor like a miscommunication or dropping a dish. The victim may try to hide and will probably not seek help until the next day, if at all. The police may be called, but by the time they arrive, the victim may have already forgiven the perpetrator. This kind of physical abuse usually happens in private.
3. *Honeymoon:* The perpetrator is contrite, loving, and very sad about the incident of abuse that has occurred. He or she may well try to make amends with gifts. The abuser promises to get help but only after discussing how the abuse has taught the other a lesson, such as "Don't make me mad!" The victim wants desperately to believe this, will forgive the perpetrator, and will begin to think that the relationship will return to "normal." The victim is still very much in love with the perpetrator and believes this love will conquer all and the abuse will stop.

This cycle of domestic violence leads to the often-asked question: Why does a victim of domestic violence stay in the relationship? Some of the most common reasons for staying include:

- Fear of retaliation for self or children
- Fear of loss of custody of children
- Dependent financially on the abuser
- Lack of support; does not know where to go if he/she left abuser
- Religious beliefs; will not consider divorce
- Denial; thinks of the good times and hopes that things can improve so there can be good times again

Neeb's Tip Because it is common that a woman may return to a domestic violence situation, staff need to understand they cannot push a patient to leave the abuser. It has to come from the victim. It may take multiple episodes before the patient is able to leave.

In assessing for domestic violence, some signs that a patient might be a victim include: injuries while pregnant when there is resentment of a pregnancy, wearing clothes and makeup to cover up injuries, lack of care for own chronic illnesses, social isolation, use of alcohol or drugs to cover hurt, acting guilty for seeking medical treatment, and history of rape. Sutherland, Fantasia, Fontenot, and Harris (2012) recommend the following questions be incorporated in screening for intimate partner violence.

1. Have you ever been abused or threatened by your partner?
2. In the past year, have you been physically hurt by someone?
3. Have you ever been forced to have sex?

Tool Box ▶ National Domestic Violence Hotline: 1_800_799_SAFE(7233)

Critical Thinking Question

Your pregnant patient has been admitted with a broken ankle from a fall. When you walk into the room, the woman is crying on the phone telling someone she is sorry and it will not happen again. What would be your first action in response to hearing this?

Elder Abuse

Elder abuse includes neglect as well as physical, sexual, and emotional abuse. Exploitation of the person's financial reserves by family, hired help, or strangers is economic abuse (sometimes called fiduciary abuse). Elder abuse can occur in the home or in residential facilities. Elder abuse affects 10% of the geriatric population. (National Center on Elder Abuse, 2013; Gray-Vickrey, 2000). This problem is greatly underreported and will continue to increase as the population grows older.

One problem in reporting it is the inconsistency of laws defining elder abuse. Some states do not include neglect, psychological abuse in their definition, so it is essential for nurses to be aware of how elder abuse is defined in the state where they are working or reside. Because the abuser is often the victim's caregiver, even including the elderly spouse, victims rarely report the abuse. They fear reprisals or abandonment because they are dependent on the caregiver. Society's lack of interest in elderly people may add to the underreporting.

Caring for a loved one with a cognitive impairment increases a caregiver's risk for engaging in abusive behaviors (VandeWeerd, Paveza, & Fulmer, 2005). Caregivers with no history of being an abuser can reach a point of frustration and fatigue that leads to behaviors they would normally find unacceptable, such as slapping or degrading their loved one. Elder abuse can also be difficult to detect by professionals because common signs such as bruising and skin tears may be common in older populations. The patient with dementia is particularly vulnerable because he or she is unable to speak up or will not be believed because of his or her intermittent confusion.

Neeb's Tip Economic or fiduciary abuse can be evidenced when a patient gives hired caregivers liberal access to personal financial information. It is important to determine that the patient is doing this voluntarily and is competent to make reasonable decisions.

Tool Box |▶ Fifteen Questions and Answers About Elder Abuse at: http://www.nlm.nih.gov/medlineplus/elderabuse.html

Caregivers of dementia patients should be counseled about dealing with the stress of this role. They need to be given resources for support and respite care. Local programs such as through the Alzheimer's Association or local senior centers may offer support groups and caregiver resources to help prevent elder abuse.

Specific examples of elder abuse can include:

- Hitting
- Shoving
- Social isolation
- Leaving in soiled linens
- Withholding food/water
- Inappropriate restraints
- Threats
- Being forced to sign over financial affairs, change a will
- Sexual molestation
- Insulting

See Box 22-3 for the characteristics of victims and abusers in elder abuse.

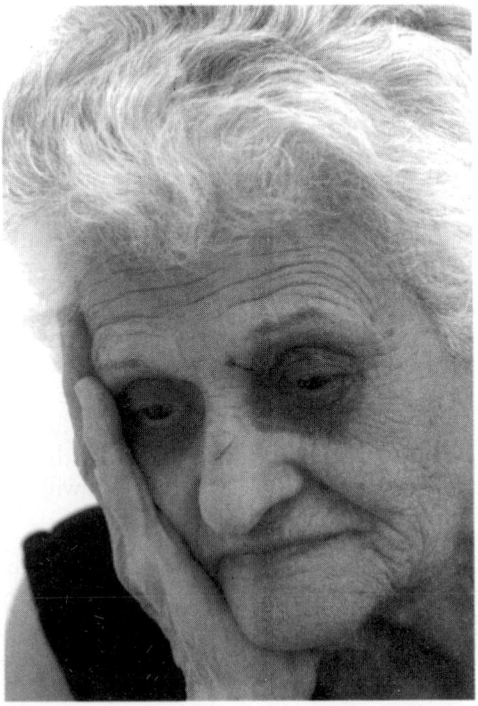

Figure 22-2 Could she be a victim of elder abuse?

Box 22-3 Characteristics of Victims and Abusers in Elder Abuse

Victim

- Evidence of malnutrition, dehydration, poor hygiene, pressure ulcers, not receiving needed medical care
- Unusual injuries such as twisting fractures, cigarette burns on face or back, perforated eardrums from being slapped
- Evidence of sexually transmitted infections, unusual genital injuries
- Deterioration in mental status including confusion and depression
- Sudden lack of funds in person who previously had resources
- Frail, dependent, possible mental impairment requiring care from family member or hired help
- Extreme dependency, attachment to new caregiver
- Evidence of inappropriate use of restraints

Abuser

- Often lives with victim, lacks resources to live elsewhere
- Refusal to allow diagnostic tests, hospitalization
- Often much younger than patient
- Cashes victim's social security or pension checks
- Sudden, intense involvement with patient with little input from other family members
- Discourages patient from contacting others
- Evidence of drug or alcohol abuse or mental illness
- Expects dependent elder to meet his or her needs
- Caregiver overwhelmed with patient's care needs, demonstrates frustration and resentment, isolated with limited assistance
- Elderly spouse with dementia
- Coerces senior to change will to his or her benefit
- Shows no guilt or rationalizes actions

Source: From Gorman and Sultan (2008). Psychosocial Nursing for General Patient Care, 3rd ed. Philadelphia: F.A. Davis Company, with permission.

Critical Thinking Question

You are working in home health care. You visit your 90-year-old patient in her home. The daughter, who is the caregiver, is not home. The door to the house is unlocked and the patient is tied in bed with a restraint. You call your supervisor, and the daughter walks in as you are on the phone. The daughter is frantic and tells you she had to leave for a while to buy groceries. She had no one to watch her mother. What actions should you take? Should this be reported as elder abuse?

Classroom Activity

- Research the elder abuse laws in your state.
- Identify resources for caregivers of dementia patients in your community.
- Talk to staff at local nursing homes and assisted living centers to find out how they address potential elder abuse.

Treatment of Abuse

Victims of abuse often require immediate crisis intervention and then long-term psychological help. The immediate crisis intervention may include getting out of the abusive situation.

Some strategies for crisis intervention that your agency may arrange include: help in providing a domestic violence shelter, arranging **respite care** for an overwhelmed caregiver of a child or elderly parent, immediate social work referral for options if patient cannot return home, and contacting law enforcement. Domestic violence shelters or **safe houses** are available in major cities where women can bring children and even pets and be protected from the abuser. The locations of these shelters are confidential so the victim can feel safe. Victims may need advice on how to seek out help without arousing the suspicion of their abuser. For example, victims may have their computers and cell phones tracked by a suspicious abuser. Anyone who is sexually abused may need testing for sexually transmitted infections, HIV, and pregnancy. Children and teens also need evaluation for substance abuse if they were exposed to drugs as part of the abuse. Children exposed to sexual abuse need access to specialists in the field. Repression of trauma can lead to a lifetime of emotional problems, so therapy is very important. Play and art therapy can be important tools for children to communicate their feelings.

Abusers and victims need specialized counseling programs as well as access to support resources such as local and national hotlines. Ongoing individual and group psychotherapy is often part of the treatment plan for both as well. Mandated therapy for abusers who are convicted of crimes may be part of their rehabilitation. Treatment for abusers can include resources for parenting skills and anger management.

Tool Box |▶ Parents Anonymous is a national organization for parents with issues around child abuse. It is based on the Alcoholics Anonymous model.
http://Parentsanonymous.org

Classroom Activity
- Identify local parenting education programs.

Pharmacology Corner

Victims of abuse may need medications for anxiety and depression. Both victims and abusers may have issues around substance abuse. Abusers may need medications to manage substance abuse, control angry impulses, and manage anxiety.

Neeb's Tip Victims of abuse may seek out drugs or alcohol to self-medicate feelings of fear, anxiety, and shame. Substance use may be the initial symptom that brings the victim to a health-care provider.

Nursing Care of Victims of Abuse

Common nursing diagnoses for the victims of abuse include the following:

- Anxiety
- Caregiver role strain
- Family coping, disabling
- Parenting, impaired
- Post-trauma response
- Powerlessness
- Violence, risk for

General Nursing Interventions

1. *Ensure safety:* The **survivor** of abuse will be confused and fearful. The nurse needs to reassure the patient that everything possible is being done to ensure his/her safety. Social work involvement is essential. The nurse should obtain a list of people who are considered "safe" by the patient, and ask if the patient would like those people to be called. If the patient wishes to press charges, offer assistance with making the appropriate phone calls. Call for assistance from a physician and counselor if none is in the immediate area. Alert security staff members according to agency protocol to prevent the alleged abuser from causing more harm. Maintain a calm milieu. If the abuse victim is a young child or frail elder who cannot speak for himself or herself, immediate involvement of the interdisciplinary team is essential to determine the next steps. Providing a safe, calm, secure environment will reassure the patient.
2. *Know your own thoughts and feelings about abuse:* The nurse is responsible for helping the patient through this initial

horrifying experience. A nurse who has been abused or who has been an abuser may find it difficult to be therapeutic for the patient. Nurses should remember that they may be treating the survivor as well as the abuser. Nurses are responsible to help all patients. Abusers are in need of help as much as the person who is abused. It is worthwhile to mention that nurses face stressful situations daily. Nurses must also be aware of their own safety and avoid putting themselves in a risky situation if a potential abuser threatens violence to someone reporting the abuse.

Neeb's Tip Suspecting someone of abuse can lead to stress for the health-care team. It is important to have a team plan of care when working with a potential abuser. One nurse should not carry all the burden of this difficult situation. Seek out support from coworkers.

3. *Remain nonjudgmental/show empathy:* This is a crisis situation in many ways. Recalling communication skills and helping the patient to verbalize any concerns, thoughts, and feelings are crucial. Remaining technically correct in performing any procedures or sample collections is imperative to avoid contamination. Maintaining professionalism and confidentiality for both the survivor and the abuser is mandatory. Calling for help from counselors, advocates, or people chosen by the patients will help maintain a calm milieu. Nurses are not expected to condone or accept the action but to respect and help the person, regardless of the situation. If a patient who may be a victim wishes to return home with a possible abuser, the nurse can offer support, education, and resources but cannot force a patient into different actions.
4. *Know your agency policy and use your resources:* Every health-care agency has its own policies and procedures for dealing with abuse and violence. Familiarity with these policies and procedures will help save time and convey confidence. The patient may be confused and embarrassed about the situation. It may well have taken every bit of courage the person had just to get to the facility. The nurse's smooth handling of the situation may provide the extra bit of confidence the victim needs to actually go through with the examination. Collection of physical evidence, observations, and screening questions may be part of the nurse's role in potential abuse cases. In most jurisdictions, with the exception of persons legally classified as "vulnerable," notification of police, taking of pictures, etc., may only be done with the patient's consent.

Many hospitals and trauma centers have some sort of abuse-advocacy program. A representative should be contacted immediately to visit the victim. The abuse program representative will be able to offer support and provide information on safe houses and other services that may be available to the victim and his or her children.

Nurses who are caring for a survivor of abuse need to be aware of their state's law regarding children who may have witnessed the abuse. In some states, a child who sees or hears abuse is also considered to have been abused. Nurses and other health-care providers are most likely mandated reporters and, as such, find themselves in an ethical bind: They want to help and support the patient/survivor; however, they must tell that individual that if a child saw or heard the abuse, the nurse must, as a mandated reporter, report this fact to the child protection agency. The patient/survivor may be forced, in a sense, not to divulge the whole situation to the nurse.

The physician or counselor will discuss treatment options with the survivor and the abuser. Legal counsel may be requested as well. A law enforcement agency may be present also. Nurses now can take a more advocacy-oriented role for the patient. Be supportive.

Neeb's Tip Whenever you suspect abuse, get other staff members involved, including your supervisor, social worker, and physician.

See Table 22-2 for a nursing care plan for a child who may be the victim of abuse.

Clinical Activity

Be aware of your emotional reaction when dealing with patients who are victims of abuse or abusers.

Classroom Activity

- Consider an open discussion with classmates about their experiences with any kind of abuse. Each person can use a diary format to write experiences and feelings to keep private or share with others if they wish.

See Table 22-3 for a review of nursing interventions for victims of various types of abuse.

Table 22-2 Nursing Care Plan for a Potentially Abused Child

Data Collection	Nursing Diagnosis	Goal	Interventions	Evaluation
Child admitted with broken bones, burns of unclear etiology. Child abuse by parent is suspected by health-care team.	Family coping, disabling	Keep child safe and provide intervention for parent.	• Ensure the child's safety per agency policy as first priority. • Establish a trusting relationship with child and parent. • Monitor parent interactions with child. • Demonstrate acceptance. • Explain all procedures thoroughly to child and parent. • Encourage parent to talk about stresses. • Ensure that appropriate people are contacted regarding reporting possible abuse.	• Child remains safe. • Parent acknowledges stressors and agrees to help. • Safe, appropriate discharge plan is in place.

Table 22-3 Nursing Interventions for Victims of Abuse

Type of Abuse	Indicators of Abuse	Nursing Interventions
Sexual	• Violent or nonviolent sexual contact or activity that is not wanted by the receiver that could include: foreplay, touching, kissing, and mutual masturbation, as well as oral sex and intercourse • Frequent bladder or vaginal infections • Bloody underwear • Evidence of "incest"—sexual intercourse between persons so closely related that marriage is illegal • Evidence of rape—forcible, degrading, nonconsensual sexual intercourse accompanied by violence and intimidation • "Date rape"—seen frequently in high school and college students (belief surrounding date rape is that the person who pays for the date is entitled to sex from the other person)	• Carefully use rape kit and preserve evidence. • Provide safety and privacy. • Be nonjudgmental. • Show empathy. • Be advocate for patient. • Maintain calm milieu. • Know own thoughts and feelings regarding abuse and abuser. • Know agency policies. • Assist with contacting outside agencies (e.g., lawyer, clergy), as requested by patient.
Physical	• Any actions that cause physical harm to another, such as: • Hitting • Burning • Withholding food, water, and other basic needs • Other activities that go beyond accidental contact • Request to stop ignored or mocked by the perpetrator • Activity repeating itself in future situations • Frequent visits to emergency department (for all forms of abuse) • Excessive bruising or bruising on unusual areas of body • Withdrawal from friends and social groups	• Provide safety. • Be nonjudgmental. • Show empathy and reassurance. • Take the time to develop trusting relationship. • Be advocate for patient. • Maintain calm milieu. • Reinforce self-esteem. • Reinforce that victims should not blame themselves for the abuse. • Know own thoughts and feelings regarding abuse and abuser. • Know agency policies. • Assist with contacting outside agencies (e.g., lawyer, clergy), as requested by patient. • Involve agency social worker.
Emotional	• Willful use of words or actions that undermine self-esteem—includes the "silent treatment" (causes the other person to guess at the problem) and other types of game playing, name calling, frequent degrading and harsh and/or cruel criticism	• Same as for physical abuse • Counter patient's self-depreciating comments. • Reinforce positive traits.

Continued

Table 22-3 Nursing Interventions for Victims of Abuse—cont'd

Type of Abuse	Indicators of Abuse	Nursing Interventions
Child Abuse/ Neglect	• Sexual, physical, and/or emotional abuse—act of commission (doing) or omission (not doing) • Victim may believe that abuse is child's own fault • Child confused about what is happening and why • Abuser often larger, more powerful than the child, which is intimidating • Excessive absences from school • Child may display inappropriate behaviors, e.g., sexual	• Same as for physical abuse • Encourage use of play and art for child to express feelings. • Provide touch and support if the child will accept. • If child uncomfortable being touched, respect that and provide support in other ways. • Accept that child may be mistrustful.
Domestic Violence	• Physical, emotional, sexual, and "button-pushing" kinds of abuse • Most typically reported by women • Kept isolated from friends and family • Withdrawal from friends and social groups • Use of substance abuse to cover distress	• Same as for physical abuse • Recognize that victim may return to abuser initially. • Help identify possible threats that victim is facing, e.g., child custody, loss of financial security.
Elder	• Victim is usually dependent on abuser in some way • May be slapped, burned, tripped, neglected, humiliated • Can include economic abuse where victim's funds are misused or stolen	• Same as for physical abuse • Listen to patient's concerns and report them even if patient is confused. • Provide follow-up in the home.

■■■ Key Concepts

1. Abuse takes many forms and is being reported in higher numbers annually.
2. Victims of abuse are often in a vulnerable position to their abusers, who may have the need to exert power and control.
3. Abuse happens in all age and socioeconomic groups. Men can also be victims, though this is believed to be underreported. The youngest children are the most vulnerable to abuse.
4. Nurses must be sensitive to the needs of the abused person as well as those of the abuser. Careful attention to physical assessment, communication, and emotional support are components of nursing care for people who are suffering the effects of abuse.
5. The nurse has a responsibility to know state laws regarding one's obligation to report evidence of child abuse, domestic violence, and elder abuse.

CASE STUDY

Mrs. Jones leaves your long-term care facility for a weekend with her daughter and son-in-law. She seems apprehensive but tells you, "I just worry that I'm a bother to them." You bathed her and helped her pack, and now you document that she is gone until Sunday afternoon and that you are concerned about her apprehension. You note no other physical or mental abnormalities. Sunday afternoon, she returns with skin tears on both arms and bruises over her right eye and on her right cheek. She is crying. Her daughter says, "Doesn't that look awful? Gram took a tumble from the toilet. "Gram" says nothing until her daughter leaves, then says to you, "I worry about her. Her husband is a nice man, but he gets so mad at us sometimes. I really can't blame him; he has a lot on his mind, and I can't give them any more money."

1. What are your responsibilities according to your facility? According to the state? According to your personal belief system?
2. How would you proceed?

REFERENCES

Carson, V. B., & Smith-Dijulio, K. (2006). Family violence. In E. M. Varcarolis, V. B. Carson, & N. C. Shoemaker (Eds.). *Foundations of Psychiatric Mental Health Nursing.* 5th ed., p. 512. Philadelphia: Saunders.

Centers for Disease Control and Prevention. (2010). Preventing Shaken Baby Syndrome. Retrieved from www.cdc.gov/Concussion/pdf/Preventing_SBS_508-a.pdf

Centers for Disease Control and Prevention. (2010). National Intimate Partner and Sexual Violence Survey. Retrieved from http://www.cdc.gov/violenceprevention/pdf/cdc_nisvs_overview_insert_final-a.pdf

Gray-Vickery, P. (2000). Combating abuse, Part 1: Protecting the older adult. *Nursing 30,* 34–38.

The Joint Commission retrieved at http://www.jointcommission.org/

Mulryan, K., Cathers P., & Fagin, A. (2000). Combating abuse part II: Protecting the child. *Nursing, 30,* 39–45.

National Center on Elder Abuse. (2013). Retrieved from http://www.ncea.aoa.gov/Library?Data/index.aspx

National Center for Victims of Violent Crimes. Retrieved from www.ncvc.org

Parkinson, G.W., Adams, R.C., & Emerling, F.G. (2001). Maternal domestic violence screening in an office-based pediatric practice. *Pediatrics* 108(3):E43.

Rubin, Z., Peplau, H., & Salovey, P. (1993). *Psychology.* Boston: Houghton-Mifflin.

Sutherland, M. A., Fantasia, H. C., Fontenot, H., & Harris, A. L. (2012). Safer sex and partner violence in a sample of women. *Journal for Nurse Practitioners, 8,* 717–24.

Tjaden, P., & Thoennes, N. (2000). National Institute of Justice and the Centers for Disease Control and Prevention. "Extent, Nature and Consequences of Intimate Partner Violence: Findings from the National Violence Against Women Survey."

U.S. Department of Health and Human Services, Administration for Children and Families, Administration on Children, Youth and Families, Children's Bureau. (2012). *Child Maltreatment 2011.* Available from http://www.acf.hhs.gov/programs/cb/research-data-technology/statistics-research/child-maltreatment

Vandeweerd, C., Paveza, G.J., & Gulmer, T. (2005). Abuse and neglect in older adults with Alzheimer's disease. *Nursing Clinics of North America, 41,* 43–56. Vandeweerd

Walker, L. (1979). *The battered woman.* New York: Harper & Row.

Test Questions

Multiple Choice Questions

1. When caring for someone who has been abused, the nurse can be therapeutic by:
   a. Showing empathy
   b. Ensuring safety
   c. Contacting counselors and advocates
   d. All of the above

2. Which of the following is the best approach when caring for a rape victim?
   a. Ask why it happened.
   b. Document the information in the patient's own words.
   c. Offer to take the patient home after your shift.
   d. Ask what the victim was wearing.

3. When a survivor of abuse and the abuser both present at your facility, your responsibility is to care for the:
   a. Survivor only
   b. Abuser only
   c. Both people
   d. Neither one; call the physician

4. Mrs. X has been caring for her mother at home. Mrs. X's mother has stage three Alzheimer's disease and is requiring more of Mrs. X's time. Mrs. X says to you, "I just don't know what to do. I can't stand it anymore. I love my mother, but I don't have any time for myself and I can't afford a nursing home." You say:
   a. "Mrs. X, hang in there. Things have a way of working out."
   b. "Why don't your sisters and brothers help out a little?"
   c. "There are agencies that provide respite care for people in your situation. If you like, I could tell the social worker that you would like some information on this service."
   d. "It's got to be hard to put up with this all day when you aren't trained for it."

5. A 38-year-old female presents to urgent care. She has a 3-year-old and a 4-year-old child with her. She is frightened and badly bruised. "He'll kill us all if he knows we came here," she screams. You:
   a. Ask her to please not scream—she is alarming the other patients.
   b. Ask, "Who will kill you?"
   c. Bring her and her children to a room immediately.
   d. Ask her to sit for a moment while you contact someone who can provide safety for her.

6. Mrs. Smith arrives for her appointment. She has had a positive home pregnancy test and suspects she is pregnant. She has a black eye and a lacerated upper lip, and admits her husband hit her because "I did something stupid. I fell asleep and supper burned. It's my fault. He works hard. He deserves a decent meal. I'm OK." You tell her:
   a. "Nobody deserves to be hit. Here is the name of an organization that can help."
   b. "You need to leave him right away before he hurts your baby too."
   c. "Why do you stay and let him do that?"
   d. "Has he done this before?"

Test Questions

cont.

7. Your 20-year-old female patient in the emergency department has multiple cuts, bruises, and burns. When you ask how she got these, she is vague and says she is just clumsy. She tells you she is anxious to get home to her boyfriend so he will not get angry that she is away from home, but hopes she can get a prescription for a tranquilizer. What does this response indicate to you?

a. She has an anxiety disorder.
b. She is accident prone.
c. She may be caught up in the cycle of abuse.
d. She has a substance abuse problem.

8. A young woman is brought into the ER after a sexual assault. Your primary nursing intervention should be:

a. Help her bathe and clean up to make her feel more relaxed.
b. Discuss the importance of follow-up treatment for possible sexually transmitted disease.
c. Provide her with physical and emotional support during evidence collection.
d. Give her a list of community resources.

9. A woman who was sexually assaulted 6 months ago has been attending a support group for rape victims. She has learned that the most likely reason the man raped her is:

a. He was high and did not know what he was doing.
b. He had a need to control her and dominate her.
c. She met him in a bar and was impaired when they went to her apartment.
d. He had a strong need for sex.

10. Which of the following is not an example of economic abuse in the elderly?

a. Caregiver is using a patient's ATM card for personal use.
b. Patient's son is asking to see patient's will.
c. Caregiver is encouraging patient to no longer see her son and daughter.
d. Hired caregiver is named power of attorney for finances for his elderly patient.

APPENDIX A

Answers and Rationales

CHAPTER 1

History of Mental Health Nursing

1. b. The main goal of deinstitutionalization was to allow as many people as possible to return to the community and lead as normal a life as they could. Not all mentally ill people would be able to do that because of the severity of their illnesses. On the other hand, not all mentally ill people had to be kept in locked units, nor do they today. Community hospitals were to be kept open, but many state hospitals closed because of the decline in census.

2. c. The development of psychotropic (psychoactive) medications in the 1950s was a keystone to allowing people to return to their homes. The Community Mental Health Centers Act came about 10 years later. The Nurse Practice Act dictates the scope of practice for nurses; and electroshock therapy, now called electroconvulsant therapy, took place in hospitals.

3. d. The Nurse Practice Act, which is written specifically for each state, is the set of regulations that dictates the scope of nursing practice. The NLN and the ANA are national nursing associations that set recommendations for the practice, education, and well-being of nurses. The Patient Bill of Rights is a document to protect the patient. Nurses must know the parameters of this document for ethical practice, but it does not dictate the scope of nursing practice.

4. d. Deinstitutionalization and changes in the health-care delivery system encourage people with mental health issues to be treated in a variety of health-care settings. Nurses will care for patients with mental illnesses in all of the settings listed.

5. d. Dorothea Dix is the only one on this list who is not a nurse.

6. b, d, e. AAPINA represents Asian American and Pacific Islander nurses; PNAA represents Philippine nurses; NANAINA represents Alaska Native American Indian nurses.

7. b. Asylums were originally described as places of refuge. The meaning is much different today.

8. d. The National Institute of Mental Health was established in 1946.

9. c. Florence Nightingale recognized the relationship between sanitary conditions and healing.

10. a. Phenothiazines were the first psychotropics drugs introduced in the 1950s.

CHAPTER 2

Basics of Communication

1. b. This option offers assistance in a way that encourages the patient to say what he or she needs. Option A used the word "why," which has negative connotations. C is closed-ended and allows a "yes" or "no" answer. D is also closed-ended. Adding the "please" does not make it a correctly formatted question.

2. c. Nurse-patient communication is purposeful and helpful. Option A would change the focus of the nurse-patient relationship and lower the chances for a successful therapeutic relationship. Sometimes nurses and patients do become friends, but this cannot get in the way of the professional relationship of the nurse to the patient. B suggests that the nurse is somehow "the boss." Patients sometimes have that perception, but the nurse is really a "partner" in collaboration with the patient. D suggests a distance that would place the nurse too far from the patient emotionally. It would be difficult to discuss some of the intimate details the patient needs to discuss if the relationship is too distant and formal.

3. c. This option combines an observation with a closed-ended question. In this instance, it can be effective. Even with the closed-ended question, it is the best of the four choices. Option A implies playing into a hallucination and assumes that the patient intends to be talking to someone else. B is intended to quiet the patient by using guilt. Asking the patient to be quiet will discourage the patient from wanting to confide in you. D uses the word "why" without prefacing it with an observation, thus opening up the possibility of the patient's feeling defensive.

4. d. This option honestly tells the patient that you cannot give that information. The physician must explain the results first. Option A oversteps the boundaries of the nurse. B uses the "why" word. C gives advice, by using the word "should."

5. c. This puts the conversation back to the patient and allows venting of concerns. Options A and B give advice; D gives false reassurance and also belittles the patient's concerns.

6. a. This is correct because it tells the patient the nurse is concerned yet leaves the patient responsible for stating what he or she needs at the moment. B uses the word "why," and C has a very authoritarian tone. D is a command that is very authoritarian and even threatening.

7. a. Here, the nurse tells the patient that he or she understands the special concerns of the religion and culture of Judaism but does not make a promise that the dietitian will come, which would build false hope. Option B is incorrect because it does make that promise. C does not give any indication that compromise is possible or that the nurse is "hearing" the true concern. D is agreeing and is a block to therapeutic communication.

8. d. This is stating an implied thought or feeling. The nurse is checking out the fact that the patient is feeling ignored. Option A makes light of the patient's concern to see the physician. B is not helpful for the patient and shows no sensitivity for the patient's desire to see the physician. C is a block because it shows disapproval for the patient's concern and sides with the physician rather than the patient.

9. a. This option is more correct than B because it offers an observation before using a closed-ended question. B and C are simply closed-ended questions. D is an observation, but it uses "why," which tends to leave people feeling defensive.

10. b. "I feel like" is not a "feeling" statement at all, but rather a thought statement. There is no emotion identified. Option B encourages the nurse and patient to explore what emotional response is being experienced by the patient in a safe environment. Options A and C are nontherapeutic techniques. Option D is nontherapeutic in many ways: changes the subject, does not reflect what the patient has said, and implies the nurse is not interested in pursuing the patient's feelings.

CHAPTER 3

Ethics and Law

1. b. Ethics is a code of professional expectations that does not have legal force behind it. The issues border on legal implications, but ethics comes more out of expectations that patients have of nurses than out of actual legal bounds.

2. c. Each state has a Nurse Practice Act that defines the scope of practice for RNs, LPNs, and LVNs in that state.

3. d. The Patient Bill of Rights is designed to define the rights of all patients in health-care facilities. These will change somewhat from state to state. People who are institutionalized for some reason may be termed "vulnerable" because they may be unable to speak for themselves or provide for their own safety. All who care for people in these facilities must treat them in accordance with the Patient Bill of Rights.

4. b. This is an honest, assertive technique that shows one nurse voicing a concern to another nurse. Options A, C, and D are all forms of blocks to therapeutic communication.

5. d. Most Nurse Practice Acts require that LPNs follow the chain of command. In this situation, speaking with the nurse in charge is the best choice. Option A is a block to therapeutic communication because it is argumentative and voices disagreement with the patient. B is not safe: Even though it is always important to listen to patients, a nurse must never assume the patient is right. C is inappropriate at this time; it must first be determined that an error has occurred. Once this is established, the RN or the LPN, if allowed by state and/or agency policy, should inform the physician.

6. c. The Health Insurance Portability and Accountability Act allows patients to have a greater say in how their records are shared and with whom. It also has regulation relating to other areas of confidentiality and how files are shared among providers. It does not force anyone to treat in a particular facility, but it would raise questions about transporting records in personal vehicles, etc.

7. b. Offer another pain relief technique. Mr. Ouch does have the right to refuse medication. He also has the right to privacy, but the option provided borders on punitive and may be a threat to patient safety. It is also appropriate to discuss acceptable behavior and the effect he is having on the other residents—just not now. Wait for a time when he is reasonably comfortable and willing to negotiate treatment. Bringing in more staff and performing an invasive technique is not only threatening, but it violates many of the Patient Bill of Rights.

8. c. The LPN/LVN works under the direction of the registered nurse or physician and cannot order medication independently. It is not acceptable practice for the LPN/LVN by the Nurse Practice Act.

9. c. It is the LPN/LVN's responsibility to contact his/her supervisor.

10. c. Mr. B should have received a copy of the Bill of Rights. The nurse can review to which right the patient is referring and discuss why he felt his rights have been violated.

CHAPTER 4

Developmental Psychology Throughout the Life Span

1. d. This patient is demonstrating the Electra complex, which is part of the phallic stage of Freud's developmental stages.

2. c. Unsuccessful completion of the anal stage would lead to these behaviors and to more serious disorders, according to psychoanalytic theory. These people would be termed "anal retentive" in some social and professional circles today.

3. d. This option states that Y's behavior is not appropriate and lets Y tell you that the consequences have been discussed. Y is able to make a choice. Options A and B sound harsh and threatening and are not helpful forms of communicating. C is very close to letting the nurse "care-take" for Y. In behavior modification, Y would most likely be responsible for his or her own actions and choices.

4. a. Cell differentiation, the process whereby cells "specialize" into their particular type, is generally complete by the end of the first trimester (third lunar month).

5. d. Women are successfully having children at young ages; however, it is generally believed that a woman's body is not completely mature until the age of 18 years. Because the young woman's body is not completely mature, it is difficult to sustain her health and the life of the fetus. Therefore, infant mortality as well as danger to the mother's health is greatest before this age. Older women are next in line as a risk group for infant mortality because of changing hormones that can jeopardize the woman's ability to support a fetus and carry it to term. Certainly, there are exceptions in both of these age groups regarding pregnancy and successful delivery. These are broad, general beliefs that are held among many in the medical and nursing community.

6. b. Option A describes "animus," the balance to the female, according to Jung.

7. d. According to Erikson, the stage or task for children in the 3- to 6-year-old group is the stage or task of "initiative." The stage or task of "industry" (the stage at which integration of life experiences or the confusion of those experiences develops) covers ages 16–20 years. "Intimacy" (the stage at which the main concern is developing intimate relationships with others) begins at approximately age 18 and continues through approximately age 25.

8. c. It is believed that infants develop in a very similar rate and pattern (physically, behaviorally, and cognitively) until the age of 10 months. Again, this is based on generalizations; there are always exceptions (e.g., a child who is longer than most of his or her particular age group because of the gene pool from parents who are taller than the average).

9. b. Assimilation is the process of taking in and processing information. It is generally learned by experiencing through the senses. "Accommodation" is the process of working with the information that has been assimilated and making that information a working part of the toddler's daily life. "Autonomy" is the stage or task Erikson believes a toddler should be achieving. "Adjustment" is a general term related to change. It is not always a healthy response to change.

10. d. According to Jean Piaget, the 2-year-old child is in the preoperational stage, where the child is demonstrating interest in something other than parents.

CHAPTER 5

Sociocultural Influences on Mental Health

1. b. Proxemics, or spatial distances vary among the cultures. What is comfortable and appropriate for some is not appropriate for others.

2. c. Prejudice means to "pre-judge." It is making a decision about a person, situation, etc., prior to having all necessary information.

3. b. Homelessness is not a mental illness but may be a condition of mental illness. It is difficult for this population of people to access the health-care and community services available.

4. b. Approximately one-third of the homeless in the United States are mentally ill.

5. d. Enlist the assistance of a religious representative to negotiate removal of the item(s) in question. Other safety actions may also be required, but right now, relating to this individual at his or her spiritual level is necessary not only for the patient's religious freedom of expression, but also to get him or her to be able to cooperate with additional nursing actions.

6. d. Actually, all of the responses are correct. Nurses are mandatory reporters for suspected abuse/neglect/endangerment of children. Certainly, the child could ultimately die from uncontrolled diabetes. It is appropriate to call the RN and MD to the exam room, but a stat call would not be necessary. You are there: The best choice is to sit with the family for a time, gain their trust, and collect more information that could be used to modify the care plan or assist the MD in appropriate referrals for the best care of this child and family.

7. b, c, d. Many homeless fall into the "working poor" category and are actually working full-time jobs. Approximately one-third of the homeless also have a mental illness, quite often schizophrenia.

8. a, c, e. Though mental illness is a common cause of homelessness, the economy and loss of assets from health-care expenses has been contributing factors for some.

9. d. Ethnicity is defined by a personal trait or common characteristics relating to a specific group of people.

10. d. Authoritative parenting focuses on the setting of rules and limits setting by the child.

CHAPTER 6

Nursing Process in Mental Health

1. a. Nursing process is a systematic way of collecting data to have consistency in patient care. Options B and C are incorrect, even though nurses do document patient needs and RN and LPN/LVN roles are different in the nursing process. Patient needs are not usually documented as part of the nursing process per se. D is incorrect because the nurse needs to know the difference between medical and nursing care prior to writing the nursing process. Only nursing care is incorporated into the nursing process.

2. c. This is the best choice of those listed. It asks what you need to know, but it asks from the patient's perspective. It is less judgmental than the other choices.

3. b. Return demonstration (redemonstration) is the best method for evaluating the patient's learning. Option A is a method of teaching. C and D are steps in the nursing process and steps in developing a teaching plan.

4. a. Mental status examinations are made as part of the assessment or data collection part of the nursing process.

5. a, b. Planning is the third component in the Nursing Process. In the planning process the nurse plans measurable and realistic goals, both for long and short term.

6. a. The registered nurse initiates the nursing diagnosis from the patient's data collection or assessment. The LPN/LVN can assist in this step.

7. a, b, d. The principle of teaching enhances the patient's understanding of the nurses' rationale for the specific interventions in their care.

8. a, b, d, e. Tone is not part of the mental status exam.

9. d. The North American Nursing Diagnosis Association (NANDA) is a universal and systematic approach in defining a person's needs according to his/her assessment using nursing diagnosis.

10. d. Formal teaching occurs when the patient is ready. The nurse can then prepare a teaching plan. The nurse will also schedule a specific time for teaching and feedback of the learned information.

CHAPTER 7

Coping and Defense Mechanisms

1. c. Rationalization is the defense mechanism that sounds like "excuses."

2. a. Denial is the refusal to accept situations for what they really are. This is a classic example of denial.

3. d. This child is using compensation, which is finding some other strength that will make up for a real or imagined inadequacy.

4. d. He is "blaming" his wife for his actions rather than taking responsibility for his thoughts, feelings, and actions.

5. a. Rationalization. Certainly, eating a meal of burgers and fries does not depict mental illness. Even though the person may be joking, and there is an element of truth, this statement depicts an "excuse" for one's behavior and choice of menu selection.

6. b. Undoing. This is a tricky one. Many may have chosen C, Symbolization. The reason this would be more likely an example of "undoing" is because Tara is trying to make up for a negative behavior that affected her daughter. While words have not been spoken, there is not really an "emotion" that is being represented, as would be the case in symbolization. Rather, Tara seems to be offering the tickets to "undo" the embarrassment she caused her daughter by her drunk and inappropriate public behavior.

7. a, c, d. Shirley is returning to a time when her stress level was minimal. Posing as an adolescent reminded her of being young and innocent. Shirley knew when she pouted at an earlier age that she got her way and was considered cute.

8. c. John blamed the search committee, who are all right handed, for denying him the job instead of the possibility of not being qualified.

9. a. For healthy outcomes, a person has to have effective coping to engage in selecting appropriate choices.

10. a, b, c. The personality is made up of these three components according to Freud's theory.

CHAPTER 8

Mental Health Treatments

1. b. Options A, C, and D are commonly seen in the crisis (or third) phase of crisis; feeling of well-being is observed in the pre-crisis phase of crisis, when the patient thinks and states that everything is "fine."

2. d. The patient needs to know that he or she is away from the stress, even if it is only temporary. The person may not be able to think rationally, and to hear that safety and help are being offered can be the start of stress reduction and intervention. The following explain why the other options are not correct. A: "Why" needs to be avoided when possible to decrease the chance of the statement sounding judgmental and allowing the patient to feel defensive. B: Besides the fact that this is a closed-ended question, the person may not know the answer to this. It may, in fact, be one of the major causes of the stress that led to the crisis. C: This is an open-ended statement and will be valid to ask—later. As one of the first questions a person in crisis hears, it can lead to increased confusion and guilt. He or she might not have a clue as to what led to the attack or may be blaming himself or herself needlessly.

Because nobody deserves to be abused, asking the question of the person experiencing crisis can sound as though the nurse thinks the perpetrator had just cause to abuse.

3. c. Milieu is the therapeutic environment. It should be stress-free, or at least minimally stress-producing, and should make the patients feel comfortable to practice new, healthy behaviors. It might be locked, depending on the patients, but it is not required to be. The patients will not usually be hospitalized "for life" (however, some might be); a 72-hour-hold situation should have a milieu that corresponds to the needs of the patient being held.

4. b. ECT is not used to treat convulsive disorders. That is a mistake people make because of the name "electroconvulsive therapy." The treatment causes a light seizure but does not treat seizure disorders. Options A, C, and D are all true about ECT.

5. d. The use of psychoactive medications can change the person's ability to think and process information and help him or her to feel different about the situation, which may allow other therapies to work in adjunct to the medication, to help the person toward wellness. These medications do not cure mental illness. They are used for more than just violent behavior, and although they may have an effect on pain receptors, that is a side effect rather than a primary use for this group of medications.

6. c. Patients treated with the MAOI group of medications should avoid certain foods and beverages that contain tyramine to avoid hypertensive crisis.

7. b. One of the goals of crisis intervention is to decrease anxiety. The person may feel a temporary increase in anxiety (e.g., at the time of being arrested or taken to the "detox" center), but that should resolve fairly quickly with effective intervention.

8. a. Repression is a defense mechanism and is therefore counterproductive in therapy. All other choices are correct.

9. b. The antianxiety drugs are potentially addictive. Patients with addictive tendencies may become addicted to these medications more easily than they would to drugs from other categories.

10. c. Antidepressants all carry a FDA black box warning that these medications may increase suicide risk in children and adolescents.

CHAPTER 9

Alternative and Complementary Treatment Modalities

1. c. The definition of an alternative therapy is one that is used in place of conventional medicine. Option A suggests that such therapy has no value, which is very dependent upon the patient's beliefs. Option B is the definition of complementary therapies. Option D is incorrect; many cultures and people use alternative modalities as first-line treatment for all types of illness.

2. d. Complementary therapies are used with conventional medicine. Option A is vague; medical treatment is not defined simply by Western standards. Option B is incorrect because a model refers to a picture an idea. Option C infers that conventional medicine is holistic, when in fact it is disease-oriented.

3. a. *Integrative* refers to the use of conventional and less traditional methods in harmony. Option B is incorrect because such combinations are not exclusive to any one belief system. Option C would leave the decision making to a physician without patient input, which is not holistic. Biofeedback, option D, is a complementary therapy.

4. d. The mind-body connection correctly describes why belief and expectation have an effect on health and disease.

Option A is an incorrect definition; complementary therapies are used with conventional medicine. Option B is an opinion based on the notion that the mind and body operate independently of one another. Option C describes a treatment modality rather than a mechanism.

5. b. Regardless of the nurse's own feelings, remaining open and supportive encourages communication and rapport. Option A would have the effect of destroying rapport by making Mrs. Lucas wrong for her beliefs. Option C might be an observation better reported to the physician for his decision. Option D would have the LPN/LVN performing well outside of his or her scope of practice in most states.

6. d. Aromatherapy, biofeedback, and massage are either alternative or complementary. In options A, B, and C, ECT (electroconvulsive therapy), antianxiety medications, and psychotherapy are considered conventional.

7. a. Reiki is a therapy involving energy manipulation and unblocking energy flow. Options B, C, and D are all forms of massage therapy.

8. a. Trance *is* an altered state of consciousness, but it is assuredly *not* sleep. Much of the therapeutic value of the work done in trance is lost if the client falls asleep. Options B, C, and D are all correct statements about trance.

9. c. This statement uses "see" and "clearly" to communicate that the speaker prefers a visual channel. Through the predicates "feels good" and "gut feeling" in option A, the speaker reveals a kinesthetic channel preference. In option B, the speaker demonstrates an auditory preference through the predicates "sounds good" and "paying attention to." Option D reflects the rarely used *olfactory* preference; many practitioners treat these predicates as kinesthetic for therapeutic purposes.

10. b. Presupposing, or assuming, that the patient will not improve will directly and indirectly negatively affect the thoughts, feelings, and actions of the nurse as well as the patient. Often mentally ill patients are more sensitive to unspoken assumption, especially when it is communicated nonverbally. Options A, C, and D will positively impact unspoken communication and improve chances for better rapport.

CHAPTER 10

Anxiety, Anxiety-Related Disorders, and Somatic Symptom Disorders

1. b. The vividness of the description suggests that the person is having a flashback. Auditory hallucinations would most likely involve "voices" or "hearing" the guns. Delusions of grandeur might cause the person to go after the people with guns, while being unarmed himself or herself. Free-floating anxiety would be less descriptive. The person would not know the cause of the anxiety.

2. d. Repetitive behavior that interferes with daily functioning is indicative of OCD.

3. d. This is the best of the four choices because you are simply stating for the patient to relax. You are helping him reoxygenate and refocus and you are calming him by offering to stay with him. It also buys you some time to make a visual assessment. Option A would be appropriate nursing actions, but not as the first priority. Your first action needs to be calming the patient and continuing to assess. B and C are nontherapeutic responses.

4. c, d. Multiple personality disorder (also known as dissociative identity disorder) is considered to be a dissociative disorder rather than an anxiety disorder. Some theorists believe that the dissociative disorders are also anxiety disorders, but most are now differentiating the two types of disorders. Obsessive compulsive disorder has traditionally been classified as an anxiety disorder but that has changed in DSM-5 since it is now known to be neurologically based.

5. d. Rigid and inflexible behaviors are characteristic of OCD. These persons would like to be able to control those behaviors, but without treatment it is very difficult for them. They are not usually hostile, unless they are prevented from performing the obsession or compulsion, because that decreases the anxiety.

6. d. Phobia is an irrational fear that cannot be changed by reason or logic. The patient usually understands it is irrational, but the fear remains.

7. b. A compulsion is a repetitive act; an obsession is a repetitive thought.

8. a, b, c. Luvox (fluvoxemine), Prozac (fluoxetine), and Paxil (paroxetine) are the current drugs of choice for OCD. Venlafaxine is also used in treating many mental disorders. So be careful! All sound similar and are spelled similarly.

9. c. Acrophobia is a form of specific phobia since it is fear of a specific situation (heights).

10. a, e, and **f** are NOT appropriate nursing interventions. Stimuli should be diminished to decrease the stressors present. All changes in behavior and responses to treatment should be documented. Activities should be encouraged, but only those that are enjoyable and do not produce additional stress. People need to acknowledge the stressors and deal with them. Avoiding or creating "diversion" is not the best nursing care. Creating an environment where individuals feel comfortable and want to participate in activities is more therapeutic.

CHAPTER 11

Depressive Disorders

1. a. This is selective reflecting. You have repeated the patient's exact words in a way that encourages her to either explain herself or rephrase her response in some way. Options B, C, and D are all blocks to therapeutic communication. B is challenging her, C uses the word "why," and D is giving advice.

2. b. Selective serotonin reuptake inhibitors like Zoloft typically take anywhere from 2–6 weeks to impact target symptoms like sadness, low energy, loss of appetite, and negative thoughts.

3. c. Communicating in a judgmental manner is always a block to therapeutic, helping relationships.

4. c. Major depression usually manifests itself with symptoms of extreme sadness that is the prevalent mood for a period of at least 2 weeks. Euphoria would be more indicative of bipolar depression.

5. d. This is false reassurance, which is never appropriate in therapeutic relationships. The other choices are all appropriate nursing interventions for a person who is depressed.

6. b. Patients taking monoamine oxidase inhibitors (MAOIs) must avoid processed foods to avoid a hypertensive crisis.

7. d. Rather than pressure the patient to socialize, sitting with the patient shows acceptance and readiness to listen when patient talks.

8. c. Though symptoms of depression are quite normal, using an open-ended sentence demonstrates concern about the changes in behavior.

9. b. You want to know more about the patient's changes in behavior before jumping into a plan of action.

10. a. Though men frequently suffer from depression, it is more common in women.

CHAPTER 12

Bipolar Disorders

1. b. Dehydration can precipitate serious side effects from lithium, including tremors, seizures, and coma.

2. d. One of the main side effects of lithium is dehydration and fluid and electrolyte imbalance. Her dry lips, staggering gait, and feeling confused could all be symptoms dehydration and sodium depletion. We don't have enough information about this situation to know if other factors are involved, such as taking incorrect dose.

3. a. Delusions of grandeur are evidenced by the patient believing that the mayor is seeking out her opinion. This is unlikely and demonstrates an unrealistic sense of self importance.

4. a. 1.0–1.5 mEq/L is the therapeutic serum concentration for acute mania. For maintenance the level is usually lower.

5. b. Olanzapine is an antipsychotic. It may be used in the treatment of psychotic behavior in bipolar disorder but may be used in combination with a mood stabilizer.

6. b. By encouraging the patient to reflect on past disappointments, you are encouraging focus on what the person has been through. At the same time you are not negating the positive feeling he/she has now. Neither are you reinforcing unrealistic thinking.

7. d. The manic patient needs foods that are easy to eat while pacing or moving around. The other foods require the patient to sit down for a meal, and the patient may not be able to do that.

8. c. Given these choices, this patient would benefit from medication to help prevent injury from hyperactivity.

9. d. To be given the diagnosis of Bipolar II the individual must have recurrent depression with bouts of hypomania. The other choices contain incorrect information.

10. a. Stimulants could easily precipitate a manic episode or intensity a current one. All the others may be utilized effectively.

11. a. Cyclothymic disorder is a chronic mood disturbance of at least a 2-year duration involving numerous episodes of hypomania and depressed mood but of less intensity.

CHAPTER 13

Suicide

1. d. Teaching skills to help the patient deal with the problems of day-to-day life will be helpful in the long run. Option B is a mistake made by people who believe the myth that some suicide attempts are not serious. C is a block to therapeutic communication (disagreeing) and may give false hope. The patient does not see that there is much to live for, or the suicide would probably not have been attempted. A is also incorrect because reporting the patient to the police is not required in most communities and could be a threat to the patient.

2. b. People are more likely to carry out the suicide when they appear to feel better. This is when they have the energy to create a plan and carry it out. When they are deeply depressed or confused, they often are not able to think clearly enough to do these things. When people feel loved and appreciated, they are less likely to think about suicide. This may be a temporary feeling on their part, however.

3. c. If a person is talking about suicide, the possibility for carrying it out is very real and must be taken seriously. In very few situations is suicidal ideation a manipulative or attention-seeking behavior. Suicide may be an impulsive act but the person is usually thinking about it for some time.

4. d. This man has definite potential for self-harm. He is not attempting to manipulate his wife's feelings, although she may feel that he is.

5. b. Your first action is to place the patient on one-on-one observation. Some facilities accomplish this by having staff perform rounds at a minimum of every 15 minutes; most facilities assign a staff person to stay with the patient. There is no need to place the patient in a locked unit at this time, nor is it appropriate to publicize the precautions to the whole facility. It would not be appropriate to give him his razor, as this could be an implement he could use to perform the suicide.

6. c. Document the discussion but explain that the precautions remain in effect. It is for his safety and the safety of others that the precautions are policy, generally. You may thank him for sharing his beliefs, and depending on where he is in his treatment, it may become appropriate for him to share his belief system with others.

7. b. Older men who live alone with a history of alcohol abuse are at one of the highest risks for suicide. Though any of the other examples could be suicidal they do not represent the most frequent statistically.

8. d. This response is supportive and empathetic. Responses A and B reflect insensitivity to the patient's distress. Asking the question of response C has nothing to do with the depth of distress this patient must have felt, so it inappropriate.

9. b. By asking the patient directly what she plans to do you are gaining important information and communicating your concern to the patient. Since she told you her plan, you know she is reaching out for help.

10. a. By reaching out to you, she is communicating her mixed feelings about suicide and is indirectly asking for help.

CHAPTER 14

Personality Disorders

1. d. Consequences should always be stated at the time the limits are set, to increase consistency. The problems with options A through C are as follows. A: When the behavior occurs, the patient may be testing, but if the consequences are not known, the patient has not been given enough information to make an appropriate choice. B: Anticipating a behavior is presuming, and you may be presuming incorrectly. This sets up negative expectations from the patient. C: The limits should not be set for the convenience of the staff or family or anyone but the patient. Family should be involved in the care plan if the patient is agreeable.

2. c. David is most likely displaying signs of antisocial personality disorder evidenced by information that he tends to lie, has committed a crime, and his patterns with job and personal relationships. He is not exhibiting signs of suspiciousness or paranoia, nor is he behaving in a dependent manner.

3. a. Manipulation is used frequently by patients with personality disorders. This mechanism can be used with other disorders but it is a primary mechanism in personality disorders.

4. d. Interpersonal relationships are among the most difficult activities for a person with a personality disorder to develop. They can participate in group activities because they can excel and bring attention and gratification to themselves, but developing a close personal relationship is very difficult.

5. c. Antisocial (sociopathic) personality is usually the type of disorder in which a person would be in trouble with the law.

6. b. Schizotypal personality disorder is characterized by bizarre and unusual behaviors—some of which may be also seen in schizophrenia.

7. c. The nurse needs to understand how he/she reacts to the challenging behaviors exhibited by people with personality disorders. Medications, long-term therapy, and in-patient hospitalization are rarely effective.

8. c. Characteristics of narcissistic personality include exaggerated sense of self-importance and lack of concern for the nurse's time.

9. d. Vague communication is not acceptable. Honesty and clarity in communication are always necessary. The patient may feel inferior, which may be part of the manipulation. The nurse needs to confront the feelings of inferiority or any others that the patient might state.

10. b. Borderline personality. This group tends to engage in self-mutilating behaviors.

CHAPTER 15

Schizophrenia Spectrum and Other Psychotic Disorders

1. d. Inviting the patient to the party brings him into the present and allows him to make the choice for himself. This will help increase self-esteem and diminish other symptoms. Option A begins to reinforce the hallucinations, which is never appropriate for nurses. B and C are forms of demands, which may cause the patient to revert to negative and possibly aggressive behaviors.

2. a. Shawna's symptoms are consistent with patients who have catatonic schizophrenia. Option D, schizotypal, is a type of personality disorder but not actually a form of schizophrenia.

3. a. This is an example of a hallucination. The patient is seeing something that is not there. There is nothing actually visible that could be misinterpreted as a snake; if there were, this would be an illusion.

4. c. This is the honest response, and it focuses on returning the patient to reality. The other responses play into the hallucination or border on belittling the patient.

5. c. Patients with schizophrenia do not function well in society without treatment. Even with treatment, some patients have a difficult time. The "reality" of schizophrenic people is their *own* reality and not the reality of the rest of society.

6. b. It is important always to deal with reality and the present when dealing with people with schizophrenia. Never reinforcing hallucinations and directing people away from situations that are stressful or competitive are also important. ECT is not a nursing function.

7. b. This time you are dealing with an illusion. There is something on the ceiling, and the patient is misinterpreting what is there.

8. c. Once again, maintaining honesty and reality is the best response.

9. a. Echolalia is the behavior or symptom of catatonic schizophrenia involving the patient repeating a word or part of a word or phrase over and over. Ecopraxia is repetitive movement or actions.

10. a. Delusions of grandeur include believing one is not subject to the laws of nature.

11. a. Muscle rigidity and protruding tongue are classic symptoms of EPS in addition to restlessness and tremors.

12. c. Decreasing anxiety and promoting trust are both realistic goals. Both of these are a process that can be helped over time.

13. a. We now know that schizophrenia is a brain abnormality.

CHAPTER 16

Neurocognitive Disorders: Delirium and Dementia

1. b. Delirium is probably the best choice, since the patient presented as alert and oriented before surgery. Nothing indicates dementia at this point. She is not delusional; she is having a hallucination. The dilemma may be in what the nurse chooses to do next.

2. a. Your best action is to call your charge nurse and/or physician immediately. Your state Nurse Practice Act will dictate whom you should call first. Turning on the light may be helpful, but asking about the spiders plays into the hallucination, which is not therapeutic. Stopping the patient's pain medications is not an independent nursing function; you need to make that call to the physician first. Checking her medical record should have been done earlier, and it will not be helpful to her right now.

3. c. By reflecting back to Mrs. H your observation, you are promoting good communication and emotional support. The other choices are all blocks to therapeutic or helping communication.

4. b. Aricept can cause insomnia. It can also cause bradycardia not tachycardia.

5. d. Although Alzheimer's type dementia is not a result of aging or arteriosclerosis, these conditions may be present in addition to the dementia.

6. c. You would expect to see memory and other cognitive processes impaired in someone with an organic mental disorder. The person will probably not be oriented to at least one of the three spheres of person, place, or time.

7. b. These symptoms are consistent with a person's having delirium. The admission of alcohol use adds to this conclusion. Time or decompensation of memory and behavior might change this initial diagnosis to a form of dementia. Alcohol-related dementia can develop in someone with a long history of alcoholism.

8. c This is the best option. You are showing concern for the patient, the family, and their situation. You have stated the implied message and offered to get the physician, who must be the one to give the initial information. You have maintained dignity for all, while behaving professionally.

9. d. Vascular or multi-infarct dementia is usually the result of several smaller strokes. The patient has usually had conditions such as high blood pressure for quite some time. The condition displays many of the same behaviors as other types of dementia but is also usually irreversible.

10. d. The patient with delirium receives the greatest benefit from reorientation techniques. In advanced dementia, repeated attempts at orientation can contribute to anxiety.

CHAPTER 17

Substance Use and Addictive Disorders

1. c. Denial is the most common defense mechanism used by people who are chemically dependent. Rationalization is also used by some patients.

2. a. Alcohol is a CNS depressant that can lead to impaired judgment, confusion, lethargy, and coma in large amounts, The "high" that people feel is temporary and very misleading.

3. d. Tremors, confusion, and hallucinations are the classic symptoms of delirium tremens.

4. d. Sally may very well be codependent in her sister's alcohol abuse. Sally is taking responsibility for Susie's behavior instead of having Susie take care of herself.

5. b. This response addresses both sisters and tells them they both need help. It is honest and caring, and puts the responsibility on them to help themselves through this situation.

6. a. Susie should be encouraged to attend weekly AA meetings and Sally to attend weekly Al-Anon meetings. We do not know from the information if they are adult children of alcoholics. There is no need to check into the unit weekly, but they can be told that it is acceptable to call or check in if they choose to do so. The psychologist will tell them the meeting schedule; this would not be a nursing function for discharge planning.

7. c. These behaviors are the classic ones that indicate an addiction.

8. a. Honest communication is necessary for the person and family to heal.

9. b. Codependent. In an effort to be caring, you are inadvertently making excuses and encouraging the drinking behavior.

10. b. Chlordiazepoxide is often used to safely detoxify a person from heavy alcohol use. It is relatively safe and reduces the risk for complications from alcohol such as seizures.

11. d. Alcoholics Anonymous is a lifelong commitment as one admits powerlessness over alcohol and remains in need of this support.

12. a. Methamphetamine abuse often includes appetite suppression and weight loss.

CHAPTER 18

Eating Disorders

1. c. Anorexia nervosa is the fear of food. Bulimia nervosa is termed "binge eating." Pica is an eating disorder seen in young children.

2. b. This response is therapeutic—demonstrating your efforts to help the patient identify the feelings she experiences when trying to eat. Reponses A and D are threats, and appetite stimulants are not useful since the disorder is unrelated to appetite.

3. b. Patients who have anorexia have an intense fear of being fat. They have an inaccurate sense of their size and body image and will not develop normal eating patterns without much help and behavior modification.

4. a. A nutritional deficit, and probably a fluid imbalance, exists in patients who are anorectic. The fluid imbalance is caused by the lack of intake and perhaps vomiting. There is also a body image disturbance, but it is a negative self-perception rather than a positive one.

5. d. Unlocking the feelings surrounding an eating disorder can be very helpful to the patient and treatment team. Focusing on the food and the destructive behaviors associated with the food puts the emphasis on the wrong area.

6. c. Patients with bulimia nervosa cannot control their eating. They binge and purge, and they are overly concerned and preoccupied with body shape and size.

7. d. This statement conveys your desire to help with ANY concern this patient may have postoperatively. The other options do show a concern and interest in this patient, but focusing on food and weight may limit the patient's willingness to offer other needs. The patient may also not be ready to talk about weight yet. This is a hopeful yet traumatic step for many.

8. b. This response is a combination of the therapeutic techniques of parroting and open-ended question. It uses the patient's words and leaves the question open for Donald to elaborate. The other choices are nontherapeutic and do not allow for patient expression.

9. c. These are the classic symptoms of bulimia.

10. c. After binging, the person seeks a release of tension related to shame and guilt by purging.

CHAPTER 19

Childhood and Adolescent Mental Health Issues

1. b. Safety for children with conduct disorder is primary in importance. Chances are that the child will not settle quickly, and asking the parent to leave with the child is not a supportive action for either the parent or child.

2. c. Exposing the child to one new person rather than several will help the child develop a relationship. More than one person and touching the child may increase anxiety. Isolating the child at the same time will reinforce fears.

3. d. Children often act out or draw pictures about what is troubling them. Offering toys or drawing materials and observing the child discreetly can tell you much about what he or she has experienced. It may also serve as a diversion, but offering toys or drawing materials is meant to encourage self-expression rather than serve as a diversion from the situation.

4. d. Physical activity is a good outlet for the ADHD child. Checkers and video games are too sedentary, and pool requires concentration that may be difficult for the child.

5. b. CNS stimulants are effective with ADHD to increase levels of neurotransmitters to elicit a calming effect.

6. d. All of these choices apply to ADHD.

7. b. The most common symptom of autism is impaired social functioning. The patient does not make strong friendships. Emotions may be completely opposite of what would be appropriate, and the patient may achieve an appropriate developmental task and then regress, or may not achieve appropriate developmental tasks at all.

8. c. This is the best choice of the options listed, because it implies the nurse heard the parents' concerns and recognized the need to get them appropriate help right away. The other options are either nontherapeutic or provide false hope to the parents. They may sound polite but are not helpful for the parents, who are concerned they did something wrong and want to know how they can help their child.

9. c. Chaotic home life is a common thread in children with conduct disorder.

10. c. The FDA has issued a black box warning on all antidepressants to monitor children and teens for suicide when taking these medications.

CHAPTER 20

Postpartum Issues in Mental Health

1. b. Projecting evilness onto the infant is a sign of postpartum psychosis. The other responses are all normal reflections of anxiety about the baby or the mother.

2. d. Highly labile emotions related to the baby are a common sign of postpartum blues. Response B and C are signs of more serious disorders that could impact the infant's care. Response A is a normal concern of a new mother.

3. b. Postpartum blues usually start a few days after birth. These blues are common and not a psychiatric diagnosis not reflect problems in bonding.

4. a. Postpartum depression is closely related to depression in a previous pregnancy. The other choices may be factors that could contribute to depression but are not the most important cause. The other responses are not appropriate. Antidepressants are not needed for postpartum blues.

5. b. Giving the new mother information on this being a normal response is an important intervention.

6. c. This response demonstrates sensitivity for the need to grieve this loss. The other responses demonstrate insensitivity to the depth of the loss.

7. b. This statement is concerning that this new mother may be progressing to depression or some other disorder. More follow-up and support is needed. Response C could be an indicator of a postpartum psychosis. A and D are more likely to associated with postpartum blues.

8. b. Mood stabilizers have been linked to malformations in neonates.

9. c. Antidepressants are an effective treatment of postpartum depression. The other responses are inaccurate. Diet and exercise may be helpful in depression but would not be the major treatment for this psychiatric disorder.

10. d. All of these choices must be addressed in postpartum psychosis. This is an emergency for safety of the newborn.

CHAPTER 21

Aging Population

1. b. Reinforce the word by showing or handling the object. Trying to guess the word or finishing the patient's sentence can be frustrating and insulting and can discourage the patient from attempting to communicate. Asking the patient to think about the word while you do something else is distracting.

2. d. Federal regulations require that the assessment be conducted by an RN for purposes of consistency. All other people on the health-care team supply input and documentation to assist with the assessment.

3. c. Medication side effect would be the most obvious possibility, as the medication is a recent change in routine, and normal vital signs should help rule out the possibility of a recent stroke. Depression is a more distant possibility.

4. c. You have been assertive and told the patient what you wanted in a way that encouraged the patient to participate in a specific activity. This also supports the person's self-esteem.

5. b. The losses experienced as people age are frequent causes of depression.

6. d. Dementia is not a part of normal aging. Other possibilities for unusual behavior should be ruled out before diagnosing a person with dementia.

7. b. Aphasia is the speech complication that often results from stroke. Affect can also change after a stroke, but that is not a speech difficulty.

8. b. Drugs are metabolized more slowly in older people, which results in a cumulative effect that leads to toxicity.

9. c. These could be symptoms of elder abuse. The location of the bruises is consistent with shaking or beating. The lack of eye contact or verbal response indicates that the patient may fear. More investigation is needed that the beatings might get worse.

10. d. OBRA stands for Omnibus Budget Reconciliation Act. It establishes standards for the care of the older adult.

11. b. Progressive memory loss is not a normal part of aging. When memory loss is apparent, more evaluation of the causes and nursing interventions to deal with it are important.

12. a. Providing support to a coworker is most important. The other choices are more clinical questions.

CHAPTER 22

Victims of Abuse and Violence

1. d. Showing empathy for the patient, offering to provide further assistance, and reassuring safety will help the patient to trust you and probably to be more comfortable and compliant with examinations.

2. b. Getting a statement in the patient's own words and documenting it in the medical record are required. Option A is information that the patient may not know. The word "why" is counterproductive in therapeutic communication. C is not recommended for reasons of liability for both the nurse and the patient. It is most likely a violation of your agency policy as well as a violation of professional ethics. Option D is inappropriate as it has nothing to do with the rape.

3. c. You need to be helpful to both people. You will need to take care of the physical and emotional health of both patients, and you will do it according to the degree of immediacy called for. A physician must be called if one is not in the area, but until he or she arrives, your nursing care, observation, and documentation will help ensure the best possible care for the patients.

4. c. You let Mrs. X know that you hear her concern and need for help. You are offering the best help you can at the moment, while allowing her to make the decision about speaking to the social worker.

5. c. While some patients may express displeasure at someone going ahead, most will realize something is terribly wrong. Apologize for their inconvenience and have someone assist them as soon as possible. Attending to this woman, her immediate needs, and those of her children is the best nursing choice. You may also let her know that someone will be in who can help her with safety issues, but it is important to get her in a quiet, safe room. After all, the perpetrator may be right behind her. She knows that.

6. a. You are showing empathy, being nonjudgmental, and offering the patient assistance. Offering to her that she needs to leave sounds helpful and may be true, but she has to make that decision on her own. The organization you offered her in option A may assist with that as well. "Why" is a nontherapeutic response. Asking if he's done that before does make an attempt at gathering information and showing concern, but the more immediate need now is to support her and offer her some options for assistance.

7. c. There is evidence to indicate the possibility of the abuse cycle. All the other responses may be accurate, but there is not enough information to determine this. This woman may believe she must return to the home where abuse is probably occurring.

8. c. Physical and emotional support is the most important initial intervention. The other interventions may be needed later in the visit.

9. b. Rape is an act of violence and not related to sexual desire.

10. b. The son may need to see the will to obtain information for financial planning of patient's resources. Responses A and C indicate the caregiver is overstepping his/her boundaries. Would need more information to determine if response D is appropriate.

APPENDIX B

Agencies That Help People Who Have Threats to Their Mental Health

1. **National Institute of Mental Health (NIMH)**
   6001 Executive Boulevard, Room 8184, MSC 9663
   Bethesda, MD 20892-9663
   (301) 443-4513; 1-866-615-6464; 301-443-8431 (TTY)
   Fax: (301) 443-4279
   www.nimh.nih.gov
2. **Depression and Bipolar Support Alliance**
   730 Franklin Street, Suite 501
   Chicago, IL 60610-7224
   (800) 826-3632; Fax: (312) 642-7243
   www.dbsalliance.org
3. **National Alliance on Mental Illness***
   3803 N. Fairfax Drive
   Arlington, VA 22203
   Main: (703) 524-7600;
   Helpline: (800) 950-6264;
   Fax: (703) 524-9094
   www.nami.org

*Most states have a chapter of Alliance for the Mentally Ill (AMI) as well.

4. **Child Welfare Information Gateway**
   www.childwelfare.gov/
5. **Mental Health America (formerly known as National Mental Health Association)**
   2001 N. Beauregard Street, 12th Floor
   Alexandria, VA 22311
   Phone: (800) 969-6642; Fax: (703) 684-5968
   www.mentalhealthamerica.net
6. **American Association of Retired Persons (AARP)**
   Widowed Persons Services
   Social Outreach and Support
   1909 K Street NW
   Washington, DC 20049
   (202) 728-4370
   www.aarp.org
7. **National Hospice & Palliative Care Organization (NHPCO)**
   1731 King Street
   Alexandria, VA 22314
   Phone: (703) 837-1500; Fax: (703) 837-1233
   www.nhpco.org
8. **Child Abuse Prevention Association**
   503 E. 23rd Street
   Independence, MO 64055
   (816) 252-8388; Fax (816) 252-1337
   www.childabuseprevention.org
9. **National Council of Alcohol and Drug Dependence**
   217 Broadway, Suite 712
   New York, NY 10007
   Hope Line: (800) NCACALL; FAX: (212) -269-7510
   www.ncadd.org
10. **Alcoholics Anonymous**
    Mailing Address:
    A.A. World Services, Inc.
    P.O. Box 459, Grand Central Station
    New York, NY 10163
    (212) 870-3400
    http://aa.org

APPENDIX C

Organizations That Support the Licensed Practical/ Vocational Nurse

The following is a partial list of organizations that support and foster the role of the licensed practical/vocational nurse in the United States.

1. National Association for Practical Nurse Education and Service (NAPNES)
   1940 Duke Street, Suite 200
   Alexandria, VA 22314
   (703) 933-1003; Fax: (703) 940-4089
   www.napnes.org

   NAPNES is the oldest association that advocates the practice, education, and regulation of practical and vocational nurses, practical nurse educators, practical nursing schools, practical nursing educators, and students. NAPNES has consistent state members througout the U.S. Publications: *Journal of Practical Nursing.*

2. National Federation of Licensed Practical Nurses (NFLPN)
   111 West Main Street, Suite 100
   Garner, NC 27529
   (919) 779-0046; Fax: (919) 779-5642
   www.nflpn.org

   The Mission of the National Federation of Licensed Practical Nurses, Inc., is to foster high standards of nursing care and promote continued competence through education/certification and lifelong learning, with a focus on public protection.

   NFLPN is committed to quality and professionalism in the delivery of nursing care, working with other organizations and groups in a cooperative progressive spirit to build strong professional and public relationships. Some states have local associations of NFLPN.

3. American Psychiatric Nurses Association (APNA)
   3141 Fairview Park Drive, Suite 625
   Falls Church, VA 22042
   (855) 863-APNA (2762); Fax: (855) 883-APNA (2762)
   www.apna.org/membership

   APNA is a resource for psychiatric mental health nursing. It offers affiliate memberships for LPN/LVNs.

4. American Association for Men in Nursing
   P.O. Box 130330
   Birmingham, AL 35213
   (205) 956-0146; Fax: (205) 956-0149
   www.aamn.org

   Founded in 1973, the purpose of AAMN is to provide a framework for nurses, as a group, to meet, and to discuss and influence factors that affect men as nurses. Check the Web site for local chapter information.

5. NCEMNA, National Coalition of Ethnic Minority Nurse Associations Inc.
   6101 West Centinela Avenue, Suite 378
   Culver City, CA 90230
   (310) 258-9515; Fax: (310) 258-9513
   www.ncemna.org

   NCEMNA is a national collaboration of ethnic minority nurse associations. The site provides announcements about NCEMNA's unique programs and activities, as well as direct links to each member association's Web site.

6. National Association of Hispanic Nurses, Inc. (NAHN)
Mailing Address: 6301 Ranch Drive, Little Rock, AR 72223
DC Office: 750 First Street NE, Suite 700, Washington, DC 20002
501-367-8616 | fax 501-227-5444 | www.nahnnet.org

NAHN promotes the professionalism and dedication of Hispanic nurses by providing equal access to educational, professional, and economic opportunities for Hispanic nurses.

7. National Black Nurses Association, Inc. (NBNA)
8630 Fenton Street, Suite 330
Silver Spring, MD 20910-3803
(301) 589-3200; Fax: (301) 589-3223
www.nbna.org

The National Black Nurses Association's mission is to provide a forum for collective action by black nurses to investigate, define, and advocate for the health-care needs of African Americans and to implement strategies that ensure access to health care that is equal to or above health-care standards of the larger society.

8. Philippine Nurses Association of America, Inc. (PNAA)
8303 Windfern Road
Houston, TX 77040
www.mypnaa.org

PNAA upholds the positive image and welfare of its constituent members, promotes professional excellence, and contributes to significant outcomes to health care and society as well as unifies Filipino-American nurses in the United States and its territories.

APPENDIX *D*

Standards of Nursing Practice for LPN/LVNs

■ National Federation of Licensed Practical Nurses (NFLPN) Code for Licensed Practical/Vocational Nurses

- Know the scope of maximum utilization of the LPN/LVN as specified by the nursing practice act and function within its scope.
- Safeguard the confidential information acquired from any source about the patient.
- Provide health care to all patients regardless of race, creed, cultural background, disease, or lifestyle.
- Refuse to give endorsement to the sale and promotion of commercial products or services.
- Uphold the highest standards in personal appearance, language, dress, and demeanor.
- Stay informed about issues affecting the practice of nursing and delivery of health care and, where appropriate, participate in government and policy decisions.
- Accept the responsibility for safe nursing practice by keeping oneself mentally and physically fit and educationally prepared to practice.
- Accept the responsibility for membership in NFLPN and participate in its efforts to maintain the established standards of nursing practice and employment policies that lead to quality patient care.

■ NFLPN Nursing Practice Standards

Introductory Statement

Definition: Practical/vocational nursing means the performance for compensation of authorized acts of nursing that utilize specialized knowledge and skills and that meet the health needs of people in a variety of settings under the direction of qualified health professionals.

Scope: Practical/vocational nursing comprises the common core of nursing and, therefore, is a valid entry into the nursing profession.

Opportunities exist for practicing in a milieu where different professions unite their particular skills in a team effort for one common objective—to preserve or improve an individual patient's functioning.

Opportunities also exist for upward mobility within the profession through academic education and for lateral expansion of knowledge and expertise through both academic and continuing education.

Standards

Education

The licensed practical/vocational nurse:

1. Shall complete a formal education program in practical nursing approved by the appropriate nursing authority in a state.
2. Shall successfully pass the National Council Licensure Examination for Practical Nurses.
3. Shall participate in initial orientation within the employing institution.

Legal/Ethical Status

The licensed practical/vocational nurse:

1. Shall hold a current license to practice nursing as an LPN/LVN in accordance with the law of the state wherein employed.
2. Shall know the scope of nursing practice authorized by the Nursing Practice Act in the state wherein employed.
3. Shall have a personal commitment to fulfill the legal responsibilities inherent in good nursing practice.
4. Shall take responsible actions in situations wherein there is unprofessional conduct by a peer or other health-care provider.
5. Shall recognize and have a commitment to meet the ethical and moral obligations of the practice of nursing.
6. Shall not accept or perform professional responsibilities which the individual knows (s)he is not competent to perform.

Practice

The licensed practical/vocational nurse:

1. Shall accept assigned responsibilities as an accountable member of the health-care team.
2. Shall function within the limits of educational preparation and experience as related to the assigned duties.
3. Shall function with other members of the health-care team in promoting and maintaining health, preventing disease and disability, caring for and rehabilitating individuals who are experiencing an altered health state, and contributing to the ultimate equality of life until death.
4. Shall know and utilize the nursing process in planning (assessing [data gathering]), implementing, and evaluating health services and nursing care for the individual patient or group.
   - Planning (assessing [data gathering]): The planning of nursing includes:
   - Assessment of health status of the individual patient, the family, and community groups
   - An analysis of the information gained from assessment
   - The identification of health goals
   - Implementation: The plan for nursing care is put into practice to achieve the stated goals and includes:
     - Observing, recording, and reporting significant changes which require intervention or different goals
     - Applying nursing knowledge and skills to promote and maintain health, to prevent disease and disability, and to optimize functional capabilities of an individual patient
     - Assisting the patient and family with activities of daily living and encouraging self-care as appropriate
     - Carrying out therapeutic regimens and protocols prescribed by an RN, physician, or other persons authorized by state law
   - Evaluations: The plan for nursing care and its implementations are evaluated to measure the progress toward the stated goals and will include appropriate persons and/or groups to determine:
     - The relevancy of current goals in relation to the progress of the individual patient
     - The involvement of the recipients of care in the evaluation process
     - The quality of the nursing action in the implementation of the plan
     - A reordering of priorities or new goal setting in the care plan
5. Shall participate in peer review and other evaluation processes.
6. Shall participate in the development of policies concerning the health and nursing needs of society and in the roles and functions of the LPN/LVN.

■ Continuing Education

The licensed practical/vocational nurse:

1. Shall be responsible for maintaining the highest possible level of professional competence at all times.
2. Shall periodically reassess career goals and select continuing education activities which will help to achieve these goals.
3. Shall take advantage of continuing education opportunities which will lead to

personal growth and professional development.

4. Shall seek and participate in continuing education activities which are approved for credit by appropriate organizations, such as the NFLPN.

NFLPN Specialized Nursing Practice Standards

The licensed practical/vocational nurse:

1. Shall have had at least one year's experience in nursing at the staff level.
2. Shall present personal qualifications that are indicative of potential abilities for practice in the chosen specialized nursing area.
3. Shall present evidence of completion of a program or course that is approved by an appropriate agency to provide the knowledge and skills necessary for effective nursing services in the specialized field.
4. Shall meet all of the standards of practice as set forth in this document.

(Reference: NFLPN, Nursing Practice Standards for the Licensed Practical/Vocational Nurse (2003) available at www.nflpn.org/practice-standards4web.pdf.)

APPENDIX E

Assigning Nursing Diagnoses to Client Behaviors

Common behaviors are matched with examples of corresponding nursing diagnoses.

Behavior	Nursing Diagnosis
Aggression, hostility	Risk for injury; Risk for other directed violence
Anorexia or refusal to eat	Impaired nutrition: less than body requirements
Anxious behavior	Anxiety
Body image issues such as negative attitude toward body part	Disturbed body image
Confusion, memory loss	Impaired memory; Confusion; Disturbed thought processes
Delusions	Disturbed thought processes
Denial of problems	Ineffective denial
Depressed mood	Disturbed self-esteem; Disturbed self-concept; Grieving; Hopelessness
Detoxification, withdrawal from substances	Risk for injury
Difficulty sleeping	Disturbed sleep pattern
Difficulty with interpersonal relationships	Impaired social interactions
Expresses anger at God	Spiritual distress
Expresses lack of control over personal situation	Powerlessness
Flashbacks, nightmares, obsession with traumatic experience	Post-trauma response
Hallucinations	Disturbed sensory perceptions; Disturbed thought processes
Highly critical of self	Disturbed self-esteem
Inability to meet basic needs	Self-care deficit
Loose associations or flight of ideas	Disturbed thought processes
Manic hyperactivity	Risk for injury, disturbed thought processes
Manipulative behavior	Ineffective coping; Impaired social interactions
Overeating, compulsive	Risk for imbalanced nutrition: more than body requirements
Phobias	Anxiety; Fear

Continued

Behavior	Nursing Diagnosis
Physical symptoms as coping behavior	Ineffective coping
Potential or anticipated loss of significant entity	Grieving
Projection of blame, rationalization of failures, denial of personal responsibility	Defensive coping
Ritualistic behaviors	Anxiety; Ineffective coping
Inappropriate sexual behaviors	Impaired social interaction
Self-inflicted injuries (non–life-threatening)	Self-mutilation; Risk for self-mutilation
Stress in caring for another person	Caregiver role strain; Compromised family coping
Substance use as a coping behavior	Ineffective coping; Ineffective denial
Suicidal gestures, threats, ideation	Risk for violence to self; Hopelessness
Suspiciousness	Disturbed thought process; Ineffective coping
Violent behavior	Risk for violence; Ineffective coping; Risk for injury
Withdrawn behavior	Social isolation

Source: Adapted from Townsend (2012): *Psychiatric Mental Health Nursing*, 7th ed. Philadelphia: F.A. Davis Company, with permission.

Glossary

Abuse: Physical, verbal, or emotional mistreatment of self or others; misuse of chemicals, food, or other substances.

Abuser: One who mistreats others.

Accommodation: Process of adjusting one's schema to fit changing situations (Piaget).

Accountability: When a health-care worker accepts responsibility for any actions performed while caring for a patient.

Adaptation: The effective coping to changes that are external and internal.

Addiction: A chronic brain disease characterized by compulsive and maladaptive use of a substance or behavior (e.g., gambling).

Advocacy: Act of ensuring that patients, especially those classified as "vulnerable," are being treated in a safe, legal manner.

Affect: The outward display or expression of a feeling or mood.

Ageism: Form of discrimination against people on the basis of age.

Aggressive communication: Form of communication that hurts another and is not self-responsible ("you" statements).

Agnosia: Loss of ability to recognize objects.

Agraphia: Difficulty writing and drawing.

Akathisia: Restlessness; an urgent need for movement.

Alcohol abuse: Compulsive use of alcohol usually lasting 1 month or longer.

Alcohol dependence: Improper use of alcohol with impairment of social or occupational functioning, which leads to signs of tolerance or withdrawal.

Alcoholism: A complex, progressive disease characterized by significant physical, social, and/or mental impairment directly related to alcohol dependence and addiction.

Alternative medicine: Modalities that replace those of conventional medicine.

Alzheimer's disease: A form of progressive dementia.

American Nurses Association (ANA): A national nursing organization established for registered nurses.

American Psychiatric Nurses Association (APNA): A national nursing association dedicated to psychiatric mental health nursing.

Anhedonia: Inability to experience pleasure.

Anorexia nervosa: Serious aversion to food, which can lead to malnutrition and death. Also called *anorexia*.

Antidepressant: Classification of psychoactive medication used to treat depression.

Antimanic agent: Classification of psychoactive medication used to treat manic behavior, such as in bipolar disorder.

Antiparkinson agent: Classification of medication used to treat the symptoms of both drug-induced and non-drug-induced parkinsonism.

Antipsychotics: Classification of psychoactive medications used to treat psychotic behavior found in disorders such as schizophrenia and organic brain disorders.

Antisocial personality disorder: A pattern of irresponsible, exploitive, and guiltless behavior with tendency to fail to conform to the law and exploit and manipulate others for personal gain. Popularly known as *sociopathic personality*.

Anxiety: Feelings of uneasiness or apprehension.

Aphasia: Inability to communicate through speech caused by brain dysfunction.

Apraxia: Inability to carry out motor activities despite intact motor function.

Aromatherapy: Related to herbal therapy; provides treatment by both direct pharmacological effects of the aromatic plant substances and indirect effects of certain smells on mood and affect.

Assertive communication: Self-responsible statements that begin with the word "I" and deal with thoughts, feelings, and honesty.

Assimilation: Taking in, processing, incorporating new information (Piaget).

Asylum: Old term for institution for the care of the needy, especially the mentally ill.

Attention-deficit/hyperactivity disorder (ADHD): The display of a persistent pattern of inattention and/or hyperactivity-impulsivity that is more frequent and severe than is typically observed in individuals at a comparable level of development.

Autism spectrum disorder: A group of disorders that are characterized by impairment in several areas of development, including social interaction, skills, and interpersonal communication.

Autonomy: Development of a sense of self and independence (Erikson).

Avoidant personality: An individual with extreme sensitivity to rejection leading to avoidance of social contacts.

Awareness: Having a realization, perception, or knowledge.

Behavior: Any action or activity that can be observed.

Behavior modification: Form of treatment in which variables are manipulated to encourage and reinforce desired behavioral changes.

Behavioral theorist: Scientists who have developed theories about human thought and behavior including Watson, Pavlov, and Skinner.

Beliefs: Concepts, opinions, and ideas that are accepted as true and are usually not exactly the same for each individual.

Binge drinking: Episodic, excessive drinking. Four or more alcoholic drinks (for women) or five or more alcoholic drinks (for men) on the same occasion on at least one day.

Binge eating disorder: Recurrent episodes of binge eating that leads to feelings of distress. Not associated with purging.

Biofeedback: Method of teaching patients to recognize tension within the body and to respond with relaxation.

Bipolar disorder: A disorder characterized by mood swings from profound depression to extreme euphoria with intervening periods of normalcy.

Body image: Individual's perception of his or her body.

Body mass index (BMI): An approximation of body fat based on a calculation of weight divided by the square of one's height in adults.

Borderline personality: A disorder characterized by a pattern of intense and chaotic relationships with emotional instability and tendency toward self-destructive behavior.

Bulimia: Eating disorder in which a person experiences eating binges along with purging. Also called *bulimia nervosa*.

Bullying: A form of aggressive behavior manifested by the use of force or coercion to affect others, particularly when the behavior is habitual and involves an imbalance of power.

Catatonia: Rigidity and inflexibility of muscles, resulting in immobility or extreme agitation.

Cerebrovascular disease: A disorder of the blood vessels related to the brain.

Chemical restraint: The use of medication as a restriction to manage behavior or restrict patient freedom of movement.

Child abuse: The physical, emotional, or sexual mistreatment of children.

Civil law: Body of laws dealing with rights of private citizens.

Codependency: Maladaptive coping behaviors that reinforce another person's addictive behavior by allowing that person to avoid consequences of his/her actions. Also called *enabling*.

Cognitive: Pertaining to the thought process and the ability to think.

Cognitive Behavior Therapy (CBT): Psychotherapeutic approach that combines behavior therapy with cognitive psychology, It is a problem-focused and action-oriented short-term therapy.

Collaborative: Form of care in which nurses work together and with other disciplines for the betterment of patient care.

Commitment: The act of forced hospitalization, frequently against the patient's will when the patient's safety is compromised.

Communication: Method of transmitting messages between a sender and a receiver. Can be verbal or nonverbal.

Communication block: Method of communication that impedes helpful interactions with patients.

Community Mental Health Centers Act of 1963: A result of President John F. Kennedy's concern for the treatment of the mentally ill.

Complementary medicine: A wide variety of alternative practices such as acupuncture and hypnosis that are recognized and accepted by mainstream medicine; done in conjunction with traditional medicine.

Compulsion: Unwanted, repetitive urge to perform or the actual performance of a behavior.

Conduct disorder: A repetitive and persistent pattern of behavior in which the basic rights of others or major age-appropriate societal norms or rules are violated.

Confidentiality: The act of maintaining privacy of patient information.

Conversion: Transference of anxiety into physical symptoms.

Co-occurring disorder: Existence of both a substance abuse disorder and a serious mental illness. Also called *dual diagnosis*.

Coping: The act of successfully adapting psychologically, physically, and behaviorally to problems or stressors.

Counseling: One of several forms of therapy.

Crisis: A state of psychological disequilibrium.

Culture: Nonphysical traits, rituals, values, and traditions that are handed down to others from generation to generation.

Culture of nurses: Professional values, rituals, and traditions passed down from one generation of nurses to the next.

Cyberbullying: The use of the Internet and social media to harm other people in a deliberate, repeated, and hostile manner.

Cyclothymic: Characterized by chronic mood disturbance involving numerous episodes of hypomania and depressed mood.

DSM-IV: *Diagnostic and Statistical Manual of Mental Disorders,* 4th ed.

DSM-5: *Diagnostic and Statistical Manual of Mental Disorders,* 5th edition. Major psychiatric reference by the American Psychiatric Association.

Data collection: Gathering of information about a patient; part of nursing process.

Date rape: Unwanted sexual intercourse between people who are aqcuainted and in which the party who pays for the date expects sex in return.

Defense mechanisms: Group of behaviors used to reduce or eliminate anxiety. Unconsciously falling into habits that give the illusion of coping but produce ineffective results.

Deinstitutionalization: A policy in which people who had formerly required long hospital stays became able to leave the institutions and return to their communities and homes.

Delirium: Acute brain syndrome; rapid onset of cognitive impairments such as loss of memory and disorientation.

Delirium tremens (DTs): Form of delirium from withdrawal from alcohol in which the person experiences, among other symptoms, tremors, hallucinations, delirium, and diaphoresis.

Delusion: Fixed, false belief relating usually to persecution or grandeur.

Dementia: Gradual progression and deterioration of cognitive functioning that interferes with memory, language, and/or executive functions, such as organizing and abstraction. Also referred to as *major neurocognitive disorder*.

Dependent: Relying on another person or substance.

Dependent personality disorder: Characterized by a pervasive and excessive need to be taken care of.

Depression: An alteration in mood that is expressed by feelings of sadness, despair, and pessimism.

Detoxification: The process of withdrawal of the substance through supervised medical interventions to prevent complications.

Dissociate: To separate a strong emotional response from the consciousness.

Dissociative disorders: Disruption and or discontinuity in the normal integration of consciousness, memory, identity. This category includes dissociative identify disorder (multiple personality).

Doctrine of Privileged Information: A bond between patient and physician. Under this doctrine, the physician has the right to refuse to answer certain questions (e.g., in a court of law) and can cite "privileged physician-patient information."

Domestic violence: Intentionally inflicting or threatening physical injury or cruelty to one's partner. Also known as *intimate partner abuse, spouse abuse.*

Dysfunctional: Having abnormal or ineffective function in mental health pertaining to coping and relationships.

Dysmorphophobia: Preoccupation with an imagined defect in appearance.

Dysphasia: Difficulty in speaking.

Dysthmic disorder: A chronic form of depression with somewhat milder symptoms than major depressive disorder.

Dystonia: A disorder in which the symptoms manifest as bizarre distortions or involuntary movements of any muscle group.

Echolalia: Repetition of phrases, words, or part of a word; often part of catatonia.

Echopraxia: Repeating the movements of others.

Economic abuse: Using another's resources for one's own personal gain without permission or making the victim financially dependent on the abuser. Also called *fiduciary abuse.*

Effective coping: Skills that reduce tension and do not create more problems for an individual.

Ego: Second part of Freud's personality development, balancing the id; the ego meets and interacts with the outside world.

Elder abuse: Physical, emotional, or sexual abuse of older adults.

Elderly: Pertaining to older people, often described as people over 65 years old.

Electroconvulsive therapy (ECT): Electroconvulsive therapy, reserved for types of depression or schizophrenia not responding to other forms of treatment. A current is passed through the patient, resulting in mild seizure and temporary amnesia.

Emotional abuse: Willful use of words or actions that undermine another person's self-esteem.

Empathy: Therapeutic communication technique of understanding another person's emotion without actually experiencing the emotion.

Ethics: The basic concepts and fundamental moral principles that govern conduct.

Ethnicity: The condition of identifying with an ethnic group.

Ethnocentrism: When individuals believe that their particular ethnic or religious group has rights and benefits over those of others.

Eustress: Type of stress that results from positive experiences (experiences such as raises, promotions).

Evaluation: Part of nursing process that summarizes nursing interventions and the outcomes.

Extrapyramidal symptoms (EPS): A variety of responses associated with drugs that antagonize the dopamine receptors outside the pyramidal tract, causing a variety of effects including tremors and rigidity.

Feeling: Emotion.

Feeling statement: Statement that must identify an emotion that one is experiencing or trying to explore (e.g., "I feel proud" or "I feel frightened").

Formal teaching: Teaching that is planned and scheduled.

Free-floating anxiety: Anxiety that has no identifiable cause; feeling of "impending doom."

Free-standing treatment centers: Treatment centers that provide care ranging from crisis care to traditional 21-day stays. They may be called *detoxification* (detox) *centers, crisis centers,* or other similar terms.

Generalized anxiety disorders: An anxiety disorder that has no identifiable cause and that is characterized by excessive worry or severe stress and a feeling of "impending doom;" it typically lasts 6 months or longer.

Geriatrics: Branch of medicine that deals with the illnesses and treatment of elderly people.

Gerontology: The study of aging and old age.

Hallucination: False sensory perception; can affect any of the five senses.

Health-illness continuum: Theory that physical and mental health and illness fluctuate somewhat on a daily basis, while staying within a social norm of behavior.

Health Insurance Portability and Accountability Act (HIPAA): Regulations developed by the Department of Health and Human Services to provide national standards pertaining to the transmission and communication of medical information among patients, providers, employers, and insurers.

Hearing impaired: A loss of hearing function that may be congenital or due to normal aging or other causes. It interferes with communication between the sender and the receiver.

Hill-Burton Act: The first major act or law to address mental illness in the U.S. It provided money to build psychiatric units in hospitals.

Histrionic personality disorder: Associated with extreme dramatic, excessive behaviors in someone who has a pattern of strong emotions.

Holistic view: Viewing a person as a whole.

Homeless: The state of being without a permanent place of residency or home.

Hyperactivity: Excessive psychomotor activity that may be purposeful or aimless.

Hypochondriasis: Condition of unrealistic or exaggerated concern over minor symptoms.

Hypnosis: Form of therapy that is meant to produce a state of increased relaxation and increases openness to suggestions for behavior modification.

Hypnotherapy: The means for entering an altered state of consciousness, and in this state, the use of visualization and suggestion to bring about desired changes in behavior and thinking.

Hypomania: A mild form of mania that is associated with hyperactivity but is not severe enough to cause marked impairment in social or occupational functioning. Also known as *hypomanic episode.*

Id: First part of Freud's personality theory, which is preoccupied with self-gratification.

Illusion: A misperception of a real external stimulus.

Implementation: Part of the nursing process that identifies specific actions a nurse will do to help a patient meet a goal; nursing intervention.

Impulsivity: The trait of acting without reflection and thought to the consequences.

Incest: Sexual activity between people who are so closely related that marriage is illegal.

Ineffective communication: A breakdown either in the sender's process of delivery of a message or how that message is received.

Ineffective coping: The use of coping skills that do not reduce tension and/or that are hazardous to an individual.

Informal teaching: Teaching that is provided at unplanned or unscheduled times.

Insidious: Referring to onset that is so gradual it is hardly noticed.

Insomnia: Difficulty sleeping.

Integrative medicine: The combination of conventional and less traditional treatment methods.

Intentional: An act that may result in injury or property damage, and that is determined to be planned or deliberate.

Judgment: Subjective assessment of a patient's ability to make appropriate decisions.

"La belle indifférence": Inappropriate lack of concern for symptoms.

Laryngectomee: Person who has had a laryngectomy.

Laryngectomy: Partial or total removal of the larynx ("voice box").

Lethality: The level of risk of death in the suicide method.

Lunar month: Twenty-eight–day cycle in prenatal development.

Major depressive disorder: Psychiatric illness characterized by depressed mood or loss of interest or pleasure in usual activities that impacts one's life for at least 2 weeks.

Malingering: Deliberate faking or exaggerating of symptoms.

Mania: Predominant mood that is elevated, expansive, or irritable with frenzied motor activity. Also known as *manic episodes.*

Maslow's Hierarchy of Needs: An orderly progression of development that takes in the physical components of personality development as well as the emotional components.

Memory: Mental function that enables a person to store and recall information.

Menarche: First menstrual period.

Mental health: State of being able to function with successful adaptation to stressors.

Mental illness: Disorders characterized by dysregulation of mood, thought, and/or behavior as recognized by the *Diagnostic and Statistical Manual of Mental Disorders.*

Message: Information that may be verbal or non-verbal and that is transmitted from the sender. It is part of the communication process.

Mild cognitive disorder: Less severe form of cognitive impairment than dementia.

Milieu: Environment for treating patients.

Mind-body connection: An interconnection of the mind and body in which the mind influences the body's responses.

Models: Pictures or ideas that we form in our minds to explain how things work. They help us understand and interact with other people and our environment, and help us to formulate beliefs.

Monoamine oxidase inhibitor (MAOI): Group of antidepressant medications that work by blocking the enzyme monoamine oxidase.

Mood: An individual's sustained emotional tone, which influences behavior, personality, and perception.

Morbid obesity: Condition of being abnormally overweight; weight that is 100 pounds or more above established norms.

Narcissistic personality: A disorder that displays exaggerated self-love and self-importance.

National Association for Practical Nurse Education and Service (NAPNES): The world's oldest nursing organization, it is devoted to promoting quality nursing service through the practice of licensed practical nurses (LPN) and licensed vocational nurses (LVN).

National Federation of Licensed Practical Nurses (NFLPN): An organization in the United States formed for practical/vocational nursing students.

National League for Nursing (NLN): An organization that emphasizes nursing education, development, and leadership.

National Mental Health Act of 1946: Part of the result of the first Congress to be held after World War II, providing money for training and research in nursing care (and other patient care disciplines) to improve care for people with mental illnesses.

Neglect: Deliberate deprivation of necessary and available resources such as medical or dental care.

Neurocognitive disorder: A disorder characterized by deficits in thinking, memory, and/or judgment

Neurolinguistic programming (NLP): The theory that language cues can be used to understand how an individual experiences his or her world, allowing a practitioner to help a patient change her or his experience and respond to problems in a different way; uses visual, auditory and kinesthetic channels.

Nocturnal delirium: Increased confusion and agitation at dusk. Also called *sundowning.*

Nonverbal communication: Actions, the way we use our body, and facial expression that are used in communications.

North American Nursing Diagnosis Association (NANDA): A nursing organization that establishes and oversees standardized language for nurses to improve communication and outcomes.

Nurse Practice Act: An act based on federal guidelines adapted to the needs of individual states that dictates the acceptable scope of practice for the different nursing levels.

Nursing diagnosis: Nonmedical statement of an existing or potential problem.

Nursing Interventions Classification (NIC): A comprehensive standardized language of intervention labels and possible nursing actions.

Nursing Outcomes Classification (NOC): A standardized language that provides outcome statements and a set of indicators that describe the specific patient, caregiver, family, or community states related to outcome.

Nursing process: Established system of data collecting and care planning performed by nurses.

Nurse Practice Act: Act that dictates the acceptable scope of nursing practice for the different levels of nursing.

Obesity: A body mass index greater than 30.

Omnibus Budget Reconciliation Act (OBRA): A federal act that provides standards of care for older adults.

Obsession: Repetitive thought that cannot be ignored by the patient.

Obsessive Compulsive Disorder (OCD): The presence of obsessions and compulsions that the individual feels compelled to think about and perform that interfere with daily functioning.

Obsessive-compulsive personality disorder: Characterized by preoccupation with rules, orderliness, and control.

Operant conditioning: A method of learning that occurs through rewards and punishments for desired or undesired behaviors.

Orientation: Measurement of knowledge of person, place, and time in the mental health assessment.

Palliative care: Specialized care that focuses on patients with advanced illness and their families by providing expert symptom management and the promotion of the best quality of life.

Panic disorder: Condition of having one or more panic attacks, followed by the fear of having others.

Paranoid personality disorder: Consistent pattern of suspiciousness and mistrust that interferes with functioning in society.

Paraphilic disorders: Intense and persistent sexual interest that goes outside the bounds of usual behavior. These include pedophilia, exhibitionism, voyeurism, and sadism.

Parenting: Raising children; referring to styles of raising children.

Parkinsonism: Group of symptoms that mimic Parkinson's Disease including tremors and rigidity.

Patient Bill of Rights: Federal and state guidelines to ensure the civil rights of people who are entrusted to the care of health-care providers in hospitals, nursing homes, and so on.

Patient interview: An interaction between the patient or client and the health-care provider in order to collect patient data.

Patient teaching: Any set of planned education activities designed to improve patients health behaviors and health status.

Person-centered: Humanistic theory of unconditional positive regard for the person, involving treatment of the whole person rather than just the illness.

Personality: Sum of the behaviors and character traits of a person.

Personality disorder: Nonpsychotic, maladaptive behavior that is used to satisfy the self.

Phobia: Irrational fear.

Physical abuse: Any actions by omission or commission that cause physical harm to another.

Physical restraint: Any physical method of restricting an individual's freedom of movement, activity, or normal access to his/her body that cannot be easily removed.

Placebo: A neutral, inactive agent given in place of medication that produces symptom relief or other desired effects based upon the patient's expectations and beliefs.

Plan of care: Nursing process and medical orders that dictate a patient's daily care.

Postpartum blues: A transient, self-limiting period of sadness that occurs in a woman immediately after the birth of her baby.

Postpartum depression: A clinical depression that occurs in a woman shortly after the birth of her baby.

Postpartum psychosis: A sudden onset of psychotic symptoms that occurs in a woman after the birth of her baby.

Post-traumatic stress disorder: Reaction to witnessing or experiencing severe trauma that was not expected (e.g., rape, war).

Prejudice: Prejudging people or situations before knowing all the facts.

Presupposition: Assumptions we make when forming communication.

Primary gain: Relief of anxiety by use of defense mechanisms or the act of remaining physically or mentally unhealthy.

Professional: Referring to performing a skill for pay.

Proxemics: Study of spatial relationships including space, time, and waiting, which are all influenced by one's culture.

Pseudodementia: Depression in the elderly that mimics dementia.

Psychoactive (psychotropic) drugs: Any drug that alters mood, perception, mental functioning, and/or behavior.

Psychoanalysis: Method of psychotherapy based in Freudian theory; uses free association and dream interpretation as part of the treatment. Treatment in this style is usually long-term.

Psychopharmacology: Medications as they are used and prescribed for mental illness.

Psychosexual: Referring to Freud's theory of personality and development in which behavior is related to the sexual gratification or lack of it received in early development.

Psychosis: A mental state in which there is a severe loss of contact with reality.

Puberty: Stage of development at which sexual organs mature and one is capable of reproducing.

Purging: The act of attempting to rid the body of calories by self-induced vomiting or the excessive use of laxatives or diuretics.

Rape: Violent sexual act that is performed against one's will.

Rapport: The matching of speech patterns using auditory, kinesthetic, and visual references, which provide a starting point for meaningful communication.

Rational-emotive therapy (RET): Form of therapy involving a rational balance between thinking and feeling.

Receiver: The recipient of a message (information) sent by a sender.

Reflexology: Massage and manipulation of the feet that acts upon energy pathways in the body, unblocking and renewing the energy flow.

Reiki: A form of energy work incorporating touch that manipulates the client's energy along body meridians or pathways.

Religion: Set of beliefs about one's spirituality, rituals, and worship.

Respite care: Relief supplied to primary caregivers.

Responsibility: Accountability.

Restorative: Pertaining to rehabilitation that focuses on maintaining dignity and achieving optimal function.

Safe house: Specified "secret" place for people who are being abused to go for shelter.

Schizo-affective disorder: A disorder manifested by schizophrenic behaviors with a strong element of mood disorders, including depression or mania.

Schizoid personality disorder: A pattern of extreme detachment from social relationships and a restricted range of emotional responses.

Schizophrenia: Serious mental health disorder characterized by impaired communication, alteration of reality, and deterioration of personal and vocational functioning.

Schizophrenia spectrum disorder: The gradient of psychopathology seen in schizophrenia from least to most severe.

Schizotypal personality disorder: A personality disorder characterized by odd and eccentric behaviors but not to the degree of schizophrenia.

Scope of practice: Terminology used by national and state/provincial licensing boards for various professions that defines the procedures, actions, and processes that are permitted for the licensee.

Secondary gain: Response to illness that results in attention, monetary benefits, and the like.

Self-mutilating behavior: Deliberate, self-injurious behavior such as cutting with the intent of causing nonfatal injury to attain the relief of tension.

Sender: The party who transmits a message (information) to a receiver.

Sexual abuse: Unwanted sexual contact.

Sexual harassment: Unwanted sexual innuendo, often inflicted by a workplace superior on an employee or a subordinate.

Shaken baby syndrome: A condition that results from an infant's being shaken violently by the extremities or shoulders, usually out of frustration and rage over the child's crying.

Signal anxiety: Stress response to a known stressor.

Social communication: The day-to-day interaction with personal acquaintances. Slang or "street language" may be used. Less literal and purposeful in social interactions.

Sociopathic: See *antisocial personality disorder.*

Somatic: Relating to or affecting the body.

Somatic symptom disorders: A persistent pattern of excessive and disproportionate thoughts, feelings, and/or behaviors related to somatic symptoms.

Somatization: Emotional turmoil that is expressed by physical symptoms, often loss of functioning of a body part.

Somatoform disorder: Physical discomfort that resembles a medical condition that has no logical explanation or medical basis.

Somatoform pain disorder: Anxiety that results in severe pain when no physical cause can be found.

Standards of care: Guidelines established by specific health-care organizations with the expectation that care being provided does not fall below the minimum expectations of these organizations.

Stereotype: A general opinion or belief.

Stimulants: Classification of medication that directly stimulates the central nervous system.

Stress: Emotional strain or anxiety.

Stressor: Condition that produces stress in an individual.

Subjective: Based on personal feelings or beliefs; often relates to patients reporting symptoms in their own words.

Substance abuse: The maladaptive and consistent use of a substance accompanied by recurrent and significant negative consequences such as interpersonal, social, occupational, and legal problems.

Substance dependence: A cluster of cognitive, behavioral, and physiological symptoms that indicate that the individual continues use of the substance despite significant substance-related problems.

Suicide: The act of purposefully taking one's own life.

Suicide attempt: Any act with the intention of taking one's own life in which the individual survived.

Suicide contract: Contract between the patient and nurse (or significant other) in which the patient will call the designated person when the patient has thoughts of suicide.

Suicide ideation: Thoughts about harming oneself.

Suicide pact: Agreement made among a group of people (often adolescents) to kill themselves together.

Superego: Third part of Freud's personality theory; the conscience, which deals with morality.

Survivor: One(s) remaining after the death of another.

Survivor guilt: Feeling of guilt at being a survivor; often seen in post-traumatic stress disorder.

Survivor of suicide: Family or friend of an individual who commits suicide.

Sympathy: Nontherapeutic technique of experiencing the emotion along with the patient.

Tardive dyskinesia (TD): Involuntary movements due to side effects of some antipsychotic drugs.

Therapeutic communication: Communication that attempts to determine a patient's needs. Also called *active* or *purposeful communication.*

Thinking/cognition: The mental action or process of acquiring knowledge and understanding through thought, experience, and the senses.

Thought: An opinion, idea, or plan that is formed in one's mind.

Tolerance: The need for increasingly larger or more frequent doses of a substance to obtain the desired effects.

Tort: An action that wrongly causes harm to another but is not a crime and is dealt with in civil court.

Trance: A state of altered awareness of a client's surroundings that brings the individual's focus of attention to an internal experience, such as a memory or an imagined event.

Unconscious: Referring to ideas and behaviors that are concealed from awareness.

Unintentional: An act that may result in injury or property damage and that is determined to be accidental.

Vascular dementia: Dementia caused by disruption in blood flow to brain, as in strokes.

Verbal abuse: Method of harming another by using degrading, harsh, or foul language.

Verbal communication: Process of exchanging information by the spoken or written word; the objective part of the process of communication.

Victim: A person who is harmed by another.

Visually impaired: Describes a person with loss of complete or partial visual functioning.

Withdrawal: Negative physiological and psychological reactions that occur when a substance is reduced or no longer taken.

Index

A

D

E

R

S